Practical Traditional Chinese Medicine & Pharmacology

Medicinal Herbs

By
Geng Junying, Huang Wenquan,
Ren Tianchi and Ma Xiufeng

From Roland; mothers Day March 2001

GW00673794

New World Press, Beiji

First Edition 1991
Second Printing 1997

ISBN 7 – 80005 – 119 – 6

Published by:
New World Press
24 Baiwanzhuang Road, Beijing, 100037, China

Distributed by:
China International Book Trading Corporation
35 Chegongzhuang Xilu, Beijing, 100044, China
P. O. Box 399, Beijing, China

Printed in the People's Republic of China

X ref ç 'A Modern Herbal'
NB although some names x ref, the particular species often seems indigineous to China only

CONTENTS

c) Herbs That Tonify the Blood   *234*

d) Herbs That Tonify *Yin*   *240*

XVIII. Astringent Herbs   *252*

Preface

   This series of "Practical Traditional Chinese Medicine and Pharmacology" consists of five separate books: *Basic Theories and Principles*; *Acupuncture and Moxibustion*; *Medicinal Herbs*; *Herbal Formulas*; and *Clinical Experiences*. These books represent a comprehensive and systematic treatment of the theories and practices of traditional Chinese medicine and pharmacology. This series incorporates a practical approach to the study of Chinese medicine through its use of simple explanations and thorough outlines.

   In the first volume, *Basic Theories and Principles*, the *Yin-Yang* and Five Elements theories are addressed as the basic philosophical elements of traditional Chinese medicine. The theories of physiology, pathology, etiology, diagnostic methodology, and syndrome differentiation in traditional Chinese medicine are explained in a discussion of the *zang-fu* organs (the internal organs) and channels-collaterals. These theories stress the importance of the appropriate holistic treatment according to an accurate diagnosis of the particular complaint. Thus the reader can learn the methods of understanding disease using the vantage point of traditional Chinese medicine and also command a knowledge of its basic theories.

The second volume, *Acupuncture and Moxibustion*, introduces techniques of acupuncture and moxibustion, commonly used acupuncture points, basic laws and methods of selecting points, and details of acupuncture treatment of the common diseases as described in an appendix of typical cases. It enables the reader to learn not only acupuncture techniques for more than forty kinds of diseases and symptoms, but also methods of selecting appropriate points for different symptoms.

The third and fourth volumes, *Medicinal Herbs* and *Herbal Formulas*, provide exhaustive and practicable information on individual traditional Chinese medicinal herbs, and formulas of medicinal herbs. The former presents the theory of the Four Properties and Five Flavors of herbal drugs, the theory of ascending and descending, floating and sinking, and direction of action of medicinal herbs. Also discussed is a description of the origin, property, flavor, and classification of three hundred herbs according to their therapeutic action on diseases of specific channels, general therapeutic action, indications, dispensation of herbal prescription, and contraindications. Readers will learn in the fourth volume the original source and ingredients of one hundred fifty commonly used herbal formulas, and their therapeutic actions, indications, and contraindications. By bringing theories, methods, prescriptions, and individual herbs together, they reflect the philosophy of traditional Chinese medicine which applies treatment on the basis of syndrome differentiation. Readers will not only become acquainted with one hundred fifty commonly used herbal formulas, but also with the laws and methods of differentiating syndromes, the principles of constructing herbal prescriptions, and other aspects of traditional Chinese herbal medicine.

The fifth volume, *Clinical Experiences*, introduces therapeutic methods of treating common internal disease, gynecology, and pediatrics. It associates practical application of theories, methods, herbal formulas, and individual herbs with clinical methods. Moreover, readers can use the fifth volume to learn the basic methods of applying treatment according to syndrome differentiation using the theories of traditional Chinese medicine and pharmacology.

This series on traditional Chinese medicine has been compiled by professionals with many years of experience in teaching, scientific research, and clinical treatment. Each volume has been checked and approved by leading authorities in the field of traditional Chinese medicine and pharmacology. These books present the reader with an easy access to state of the art knowledge on Chinese traditional medicine and pharmacology. The information presented in this series is the product of years of combined research and provides a reference for beginners as well as professionals in the field of traditional medicine. At present it is rare to read English editions which completely and systematically introduce traditional Chinese medical philosophies and methodologies with such conciseness. We hope that this series is able to involve interested readers from all over the world in the development and dissemination of this ancient art for the benefit of the human race.

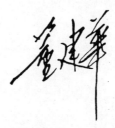

Professor Dong Jianhua

Director of the All-China Association of
Traditional Chinese Medicine
Advisor to the Public Health Ministry of
the People's Republic of China

Chapter One
General Introduction

I. The Properties and Functions of Chinese Herbs

The *Chinese Materia Medica* has properties and functions that can be classed into four basic categories.

a) Four Energies and Five Tastes

The Four Energies indicate the properties of cold, hot, warm and cool. These terms describe the therapeutically significant, energetic characteristics of herbs and their actions. Herbs like Gypsum (Shigao), Anemarrhena rhizome (Zhimu), Coptis root (Huanglian) and Fresh rehmannia root (Shengdihuang), which relieve heat syndromes, are characterized as cool or cold. Herbs such as Prepared aconite root (Fuzi), which relieve cold syndromes, are characterized as warm or hot. Herbs whose properties are neither cold nor hot are termed neutral, such as Poria (Fuling).

The Five Tastes are sour, bitter, sweet, pungent-spicy and salty. When the taste is not obvious, it is known as bland or tasteless. Ancient physicians discovered that a particular property can induce certain therapeutic effects. Pungent-spicy herbs disperse and promote the circulation of *qi* and invigorate the blood. For instance, Ephedra (Mahuang) releases exterior syndromes by causing sweating; Costus root (Muxiang) promotes the circulation of *qi*; and Safflower (Honghua) invigorates the blood.

Sweet herbs tonify, harmonize and moderate. For example, Pilose asiabell root (Dangshen) replenishes *qi*; Prepared rehmannia root (Shudihuang) nourishes blood; and Malted barley (Yitang) and Licorice root (Gancao) moderate and stop pain or harmonize the actions of other herbs. Bland or tasteless herbs transform dampness and promote urination. Sour herbs absorb and control. For instance, Dogwood fruit (Shanzhuyu) and Schisandra fruit (Wuweizi) relieve seminal emissions and spontaneous sweating; and Chinese galla (Wubeizi) controls diarrhea. Also, some herbs are characterized as astringent. They have a function similar to sour herbs. For example, Dragon's bone (Longgu) and Oyster shell (Muli) are used for spontaneous sweating; Red halloysite (Chishizhi) and Pomegranate rind (Shiliupi) stop diarrhea; and Euryale seed (Qianshi) and Raspberry fruit (Fupenzi) treat nocturnal emissions, frequent urination and leukorrhea.

Bitter herbs reduce and dry. For example, Rhubarb (Dahuang) is used to move stool and reduce heat; Lepidium seed (Tinglizi) reduces heat in the lungs and soothes asthma; Atractylodes rhizome (Cangzhu) and Magnolia bark (Houpo) dry and transform turbid dampness; and Phellodendron bark (Huangbai) and Anemarrhena rhizome (Zhimu) dry dampness and tonify *yin*. Salty herbs soften hardness, release hardenings and nodules and purge stool. For example, Glauber's salt (Mangxiao) is used for constipation; and Ark shell (Walengzi) treats subcutaneous nodules and scrofula.

Based on these primary considerations, the ancient physicians generalized the actions of herbs into the theory of Five Tastes. Herbs that have a dispersing function are pungent-spicy; herbs that tonify are sweet; and so on. Consequently, the tastes of herbs described in the classical *Chinese Materia Medica* are approximate. For example, the "pungent" taste of Pueraria root (Gegen), the "sweet" taste of Gypsum (Shigao) and the "salty" taste of Scrophularia (Xuanshen) are not in line with their actual taste in the mouth.

When we speak of the Four Energies and the Five Tastes, we can differentiate degrees of intensity. Herbs may be cold, slightly cold and very cold; bitter, slightly bitter and very bitter; etc. Some herbs, such as Schisandra fruit (Wuweizi), possess several tastes. In any event, every herb is cataloged as having a taste and a property. These two characteristics are used to describe the complicated actions of the herb. Therefore, Ephedra (Mahuang) is pungent-spicy and warm and disperses wind and cold; Lily bulb (Baihe) is sweet and cold and promotes the production of body fluids; and Astragalus root (Huangqi) is sweet and warm and replenishes *qi*.

b) Ascending, Descending, Floating or Sinking

The functional tendencies of ascending, descending, floating and sinking are a clinically useful categorization method. Herbs that ascend and float move upward and outward; they promote sweating, raise *yang*, cause vomiting and open the orifices. Examples include Perilla leaf (Zisuye), Bupleurum root (Chaihu), Cimicifuga rhizome (Shengma) and Black false bellebore (Lilu).

Herbs that descend and sink move downward and inward, conduct *qi* downward, promote urination and defecation, subdue *yang* and calm the mind. Examples include Perilla seed (Suzi), Red ochre (Daizheshi), Rhubarb (Dahuang) and Cinnabar (Zhusha).

In general, the functional tendency of a herb is related to its taste, property, quality and processing. Herbs featured as ascending and floating must be pungent-spicy or sweet in taste as well as warm or hot in property, while herbs characterized as descending and sinking must be bitter, sour or salty in taste as well as cool or cold in property. The well-known doctor Li Shizhen once described the relationships this way: "Sour or salty herbs have no function of ascending, pungent-spicy or sweet herbs have no function of descending, cold herbs have no function of floating and hot herbs no function of sinking."

Herb parts such as flowers and leaves that are light in quality have the functions of ascending and floating; herbs or substances that are heavy in quality such as seeds, fruits and minerals have the functions of descending and sinking. In addition, processing and preparation may change the taste and property of the herb and influence its functional tendencies. For example, frying herbs causes an ascending function; processing with ginger, a dispersing function; baking with vinegar, an astringing function; and preparing with salt, a downward function.

The combination of herbs is also a factor in determining the substance's functional tendency and should be taken into consideration when formulating a herbal prescription. For example, Platycodon root (Jiegeng) has a floating functional tendency, and Cyathula root (Niuxi) has a descending functional tendency. In combination, the functional tendency changes.

c) Herbs Entering Specific Meridians

A herb may selectively act upon a particular part of the body to relieve pathogenic change in specific meridians and organs. The meridians that a herb enters depend on the corresponding symptoms relieved. For example, Ephedra (Mahuang) promotes sweating, soothes asthma and benefits urination. It is indicated for fever, chills and absence of sweating due to invasion by exogenous pathogenic wind and cold, dysuria, edema and so on. Judged by the above indications and analyzed in accordance with the theories of the *zang-fu* organs and meridians, it can be determined that the herbs would enter the lung and urinary bladder meridians. Jujube (Dazao) tonifies *qi* in the spleen and stomach. It is indicated for poor appetite and loose stool due to weakness of the spleen and stomach. So we say that the herb enters the meridians of the spleen and stomach.

The Four Energies, Five Tastes and the meridians are the approaches used to understand the energetic actions of herbs. They are combined so as to relate to and supplement one another. Only by combining these approaches can a comprehensive prescription of herbs be made.

d) Toxicity and Nontoxicity

In the *Chinese Materia Medica*, the words "toxic, nontoxic, very toxic or slightly toxic" often appear. The toxicity of herbs and substances can cause symptomatic reactions as well as have adverse effects on tissues. No overdose of toxic herbs should be given as this may lead to side effects. Nontoxic herbs are moderate in nature and, generally speaking, do not have any side effects. For example, Jujube (Dazao) and Poria (Fuling) are nontoxic herbs, while Prepared aconite root (Fuzi) and Seed of nuxvomica poison nut (Maqianzi) are toxic herbs.

II. The Application of Herbs

a) Combination of Herbs

Two or more herbs are combined to increase or promote their therapeutic effectiveness, to minimize toxicity or side effects, to accommodate complex clinical situations and to alter their actions. Different combinations can cause variations in therapeutic effect. Traditionally, the results for combining herbs are classified as follows.

1. Mutual reinforcement: Two or more herbs with similar properties are used in a combination to reinforce their therapeutic actions. For example, Rhubarb (Dahuang) in combination with Glauber's salt (Mangxiao) reinforces the function of purging downward; Gypsum (Shigao) and Anemarrhena rhizome (Zhimu) used together clear heat and subdue fire.

2. Mutual assistance: Two or more herbs are used in a combination in which one is the principle herb and the others play a subsidiary role to enhance therapeutic action. For example, Astragalus root (Huangqi) combined with Poria (Fuling) replenishes *qi*, strengthens the spleen and promotes urination; Gypsum (Shigao) in combination with Cyathula root (Niuxi) relieves toothache due to excess fire in the stomach.

3. Mutual restraint or mutual counteraction: This refers to the reduction of the toxicity or side effects of one herb by the addition of another. For example, adding Fresh ginger (Shengjiang) to Pinellia tuber (Banxia) counteracts, or restrains, the latter's toxicity.

4. Mutual suppression: In this combination of herbs, the property of one weakens or suppresses the action of the other. For example, Radish seed (Laifuzi), combined with Ginseng (Renshen), weakens the function of the latter in replenishing *qi*.

5. Mutual antagonism: This refers to the ability of two herbs or substances to minimize or neutralize each other's positive effects. Severe side effects may result when two incompatible herbs or substances are used in combination. Traditionally, there existed "eighteen incompatible medicinal herbs" and "nineteen mutual restraining medicinal herbs." Among the eighteen incompatible medicinal herbs, or substances, Tendrilled fritillary bulb (Chuanbeimu), Pinellia tuber (Banxia), Bletilla tuber (Baiji), Trichosanthes fruit (Gualou) and Ampelopsis root (Bailian) are incompatible with Sichuan aconite root (Wutou); Asarum

herb (Xixin), Peony (Shaoyao), White peony root (Baishao), Ginseng (Renshen), Glehnia root (Shashen), Salvia root (Danshen) and Scrophularia (Xuanshen) are incompatible with Black false bellebore (Lilu); Peking spurge root (Daji), Genkwa flower (Yuanhua), Kansui root (Gansui) and Seaweed (Haizao) are incompatible with Licorice root (Gancao).

The nineteen mutual restraining medicaments include Croton seed (Badou), which restrains Pharbitis seed (Qianniuzi); Cloves (Dingxiang), which restrains Curcuma root (Yujin); Ginseng bark (Renshen), which restrains Trogopterus dung (Wulingzhi); Cinnamon bark (Rougui), which restrains Red halloysite (Chishizhi); Sulphur (Liuhuang), which restrains Mirabilite (Poxiao); Mercury (Suiyin), which restrains Arsenic Trioxide (Pishuang); Langdu root (Langdu), which restrains Litharge (Mituoseng), Monkshood root (Chuanwu) and Wild aconite root (Caowu), which restrain Rhinoceros horn (Xijiao); and Mirabilite (Yaxiao, or Poxiao), which restrains Burreed tuber (Sanleng).

b) Precautions and Contraindications

1. The precautions and contraindications in combination: The historical medical literature contraindicates certain herbs and substances. These include the eighteen incompatible medicinal herbs and the nineteen mutual-restraining medicinal herbs.

2. The precautions and contraindications during pregnancy: It is contraindicated to prescribe herbs with strong actions or toxicity, especially Croton seed (Badou), Pharbitis seed (Qianniuzi), Peking spurge root (Daji) and Burreed tuber (Sanleng), for pregnant women. Pungent-spicy and hot herbs that promote circulation of *qi* and remove stagnation of *qi* and blood should be used with caution during pregnancy. These include Peach seed (Taoren), Safflower (Honghua), Rhubarb (Dahuang) and Prepared aconite root (Fuzi).

3. The precautions and contraindications in food intake: Certain foods may influence the action of herbs or bring about some abnormalities. It is advisable, in general, not to eat raw, cold, greasy, strong smelling or spicy food while taking medicine. The historical medical literature records that Dichroa root (Changshan) is contraindicated with onion; Rehmannia root (Dihuang) and Fleeceflower root (Heshouwu) are contraindicated with onion, garlic and turnip; Mentha (Bohe) is contraindicated with turtle meat; Poria (Fuling) is contraindicated with

vinegar; and Turtle shell (Biejia) is contraindicated with three-colored amaranth.

Each herb has its own indications; the clinician should not select herbs at random. He or she must know the properties, tastes and actions of the herbs. For example, Ephedra (Mahuang) is pungent-spicy and warm in taste and property and promotes sweating. It is used to treat fever, chills and absence of sweating due to an invasion of exogenous wind and cold. It is contraindicated in deficiency exterior syndrome with the symptoms metioned above.

Chapter Two
Herbs

I. Herbs That Release Exterior Syndrome

Exterior-releasing herbs are those that dispel pathogenic factors while in the superficial portion of the body. These herbs have a pungent-spicy taste, cause sweating and release the exterior. They are further divided into warm-pungent and cool-pungent classes. The warm-pungent herbs release wind-cold exterior syndromes, while the cool-pungent herbs release wind-heat exterior syndromes. Some of the herbs have additional functions including treating edema, stopping cough and asthma, bringing measles to the body surface, promoting the lungs' dispersing function and strengthening water-metabolism. Some herbs also dispel wind and damp and stop pain. The herbs that release the exterior should be used with caution: overdosage may cause heavy sweating and consumption of *yang-qi* and body fluids, thus weakening the body. These herbs are also contraindicated in the advanced stage of febrile diseases accompanied by exhaustion of body fluids, chronic boils and carbuncles, urinary dysfunction and loss of blood.

a) Warm-pungent Herbs That Release Exterior Syndrome

The main function of warm-pungent herbs is to dispel wind and cold. They are indicated in wind-cold excess exterior syndrome and are accompanied by chills, fever, absence of sweating, headache, thin and white tongue coating and superficial and tense pulse. In addition, these herbs can be used to treat cough, asthma, edema and pain caused by invasion of wind-damp. As warm-pungent herbs may cause heavy sweating, proper dosages should be used.

1. Ephedra (Mahuang)

Pharmaceutical Name: Herba Ephedrae

Botanical Name: 1. Ephedra sinica Stapf; 2. Ephedra equisetina Bunge; 3. Ephedra intermedia Schrenk et Mey.

Common Name: Ephedra, Ephedra Mormon tea

Source of Earliest Record: Shennong Bencao Jing

Part Used & Method for Pharmaceutical Preparations: Herbaceous twigs or stems are collected from the Beginning of Autumn (thirteenth solar term) to Frost's Descent (eighteenth solar term), dried in a shady place and then cut into pieces and used either raw or baked with honey.

Properties & Taste: Pungent-spicy, bitter and warm

Meridians: Lung and urinary bladder

Functions: 1. To promote diaphoresis; 2. To pacify asthma; 3. To benefit urination

Indications & Combinations:

1. Wind-cold type of exterior syndrome manifested as chills, fever, headache, general pain, nasal obstruction, absence of sweating, thin and white tongue coating and superficial and tense pulse. In such cases, Ephedra (Mahuang) is used with Cinnamon twigs (Guizhi) in the formula Mahuang Tang.

2. Cough and asthma due to invasion by exogenous wind and cold. Ephedra (Mahuang) is used with Apricot seed (Xingren) in the formula Sanniu Tang.

3. Edema with exterior syndrome. This disease in traditional Chinese medicine is similar to acute nephritic edema in Western medicine. Ephedra (Mahuang) is used with Gypsum (Shigao) in the formula Yuepi Tang.

13

Dosage: 1.5-10 g

Cautions & Contraindications: This herb causes heavy sweating. It should be used cautiously in deficiency conditions with sweating or asthma and cough due to failure of the kidneys in receiving *qi*.

2. Cinnamon twigs (Guizhi)

Pharmaceutical Name: Ramulus Cinnamomi
Botanical Name: Cinnamomum cassia Presl
Common Name: Cinnamon twigs, Cassia twigs
Source of Earliest Record: Shennong Bencao Jing
Part Used & Method for Pharmaceutical Preparations: The twigs are picked in the spring, dried in a shady place or in the sunshine and then cut into slices or pieces.
Properties & Taste: Pungent-spicy, sweat and warm
Meridians: Heart, lung and urinary bladder
Functions: 1. To promote diaphoresis and relieve exterior syndrome; 2. To promote blood circulation; 3. To warm the meridians and disperse cold

Indications & Combinations:

1. Wind-cold type of exterior syndrome. Cinnamon twigs (Guizhi) used with Ephedra (Mahuang) increases the diaphoretic action of the herb.

2. Wind-cold type of exterior deficiency syndrome manifested as sweating, aversion to wind, fever and superficial and tardy pulse. Cinnamon twigs (Guizhi) is used with White peony root (Baishao) in the formula Guizhi Tang.

3. Arthritic pain caused by invasion of exogenous wind, cold and damp manifested as soreness and pain in the joints, limbs, shoulders and back. Cinnamon twigs (Guizhi) is used with Prepared aconite root (Fuzi).

4. Deficiency of *yang* in the heart and spleen manifested as palpitations, edema and shortness of breath. Cinnamon twigs (Guizhi) is used with Poria (Fuling) and White atractylodes (Baizhu).

5. Weakness of *yang* in the chest (including what is known as Angina pectoria in Western medicine) manifested as pain in the chest, palpitations, or intermittent pulse. Cinnamon twigs (Guizhi) is used with Macrostem onion (Xiebai) and Trichosanthes fruit (Gualou).

6. Amenorrhea abdominal pain due to cold invasion and blood

stasis. Cinnamon twigs (Guizhi) is used with Peach seed (Taoren), Moutan bark (Mudanpi) and Poria (Fuling) in the formula Guizhi Fuling Wan.

Dosage: 3-10 g

Cautions & Contraindications: The herb is contraindicated in warm-febrile disease as well as cases of deficient *yin* with heat signs. It should be used with caution in pregnant women.

3a. Perilla leaf (Zisuye)

Pharmaceutical Name: Folium Perillae

Botanical Name: Perilla frutescens (L.) Britt.

Common Name: Perilla leaf, Purple perilla leaf

Source of Earliest Record: Benjing Jizhu

Part Used & Method for Pharmaceutical Preparations: The leaf is picked in July and August and dried in the shade.

Properties & Taste: Pungent-spicy and warm

Meridians: Lung and spleen

Functions: 1. To release the exterior symptoms and disperse cold; 2. To promote the flow of *qi* in the spleen and stomach; 3. To alleviate fish and crab poisoning

Indications & Combinations:

1. Wind-cold type of common cold manifested as fever, chills, headache, nasal obstruction and cough. Perilla leaf (Zisuye) is used with Fresh ginger (Shengjiang), Tangerine peel (Chenpi), Cyperus tuber (Xiangfu) and Apricot seed (Xingren) in the formula Xing Su San.

2. *Qi* stagnation in the spleen and stomach manifested as nausea, vomiting and fullness sensation in the chest or abdomen. Perilla leaf (Zisuye) is used with Agastache (Huoxiang) for cold manifestations. If there are more heat signs, Perilla leaf (Zisuye) can be prescribed with Coptis root (Huanglian). For cases with *qi* stagnation and accumulation of phlegm, Perilla leaf (Zisuye) is used with Pinellia tuber (Banxia) and Magnolia bark (Houpo). For vomiting during pregnancy, Perilla leaf (Zisuye) is used with Tangerine peel (Chenpi) and Amomum fruit (Sharen).

3. Fish and crab poisoning manifested as vomiting, diarrhea and abdominal pain. Perilla leaf (Zisuye) is used with Fresh ginger (Shengjiang) and Dahurian angelica root (Baizhi).

Dosage: 3-10 g

Cautions & Contraindications: This herb should not be boiled for a long time.

3b. Perilla stem (Sugeng)

Perilla stem (Sugeng) refers to the stem of Perilla frutescens, which is pungent-spicy, sweet and warm. It enters through the lung, spleen and stomach meridians. The herb promotes *qi* in the chest and dia-phram (relieving distention and pain in the chest, abdomen and costal region) and calms restless fetuses. Perilla stem (Sugeng) is usually combined with Cyperus tuber (Xiangfu) and Tangerine peel (Chenpi).

Dosage is 5-10 g. The herb should not be boiled for a long time.

4a. Fresh ginger (Shengjiang)

Pharmaceutical Name: Rhizoma Zingiberis Recens
Botanical Name: Zingiber officinale Willd. Rosc
Common Name: Fresh ginger
Source of Earliest Record: Mingyi Bielu
Part Used & Method for Pharmaceutical Preparations: The rhizomes are dug from September to November. After the fibrous roots have been removed, the rhizomes are washed, cut into slices and pounded to extract the juice, or the skin is peeled off for usage.
Properties & Taste: Pungent and warm
Meridians: Lung, spleen and stomach
Functions: 1. To promote diaphoresis and release the exterior; 2. To warm the spleen and stomach and alleviate vomiting; 3. To warm the lungs and alleviate cough
Indications & Combinations:

1. Wind-cold exterior syndrome manifested as chills, fever, head-ache and nasal obstruction. The herb is used to strengthen the diaphor-etic function.

2. Vomiting due to cold in the stomach. Fresh ginger (Shengjiang) is often used with Pinellia tuber (Banxia). In vomiting due to heat in the stomach, Fresh ginger (Shengjiang) should be used with Bamboo shavings (Zhuru) and Coptis root (Huanglian).

Dosage: 3-10 g

Cautions & Contraindications: This herb is contraindicated in *yin* deficiency with excessive heat in the interior.

4b. Fresh ginger skin (Shengjiangpi)

Fresh ginger skin refers to the skin of the Zingiberis rhizome, which is pungent and cool in property. The herb harmonizes the spleen and promotes water-metabolism. It is mainly indicated in edema. Fresh ginger skin (Shengjiangpi) is often combined with Poria peel (Fulingpi) and Mulberry bark (Sangbaipi) to treat edema. The dosage is 3-10 g.

5. Elsholtzia (Xiangru)

Pharmaceutical Name: Herba Elsholtziae
Botanical Name: 1. Elsholtzia splendens Nakai ex F. Maekawa
Common Name: Elshotzia, Aromatic madder
Source of Earliest Record: Mingyi Bielu
Part Used & Method for Pharmaceutical Preparations: The entire plant, when it is ripe, is gathered, dried in the sunshine and cut into pieces.
Properties & Taste: Pungent and slightly warm
Meridians: Lung and stomach
Functions: 1. To promote diaphoresis and release the exterior; 2. To resolve dampness and harmonize the spleen and stomach; 3. To promote water metabolism and release edema
Indications & Combinations:
1. Wind-cold exterior syndrome occurring in the summer season manifested as chills, fever, headache, absence of sweating, abdominal pain, vomiting and diarrhea. Elsholtzia (Xiangru) is used with Hyacinth bean (Biandou).
2. Edema and dysuria. Elsholtzia (Xiangru) is used with White atractylodes (Baizhu).
Dosage: 3-10 g
Cautions & Contraindications: This herb is contraindicated in deficiency exterior syndrome with sweating.

6. Schizonepeta (Jingjie)

Pharmaceutical Name: Herba seu Flos Schizonepetae
Botanical Name: Schizonepeta tenuifolia Briq.
Common Name: Schizonepeta
Source of Earliest Record: Shennong Bencao Jing
Part Used & Method for Pharmaceutical Preparations: The aerial part of the plant is gathered in autumn and winter, dried in the shade and

cut into pieces. It can be used raw or baked until yellow and black in color.

Properties & Taste: Pungent and warm

Meridians: Lung and liver

Functions: 1. To release the exterior and expel wind; 2. To stop bleeding

Indications & Combinations:

1. Wind-cold exterior syndrome manifested as headache, chills, fever and absence of sweating. Schizonepeta (Jingjie) is used with Ledebouriella root (Fangfeng) and Notopterygium root (Qianghuo).

2. Wind-heat exterior syndrome manifested as fever, headache, sore throat and slight sweating or no sweating. Schizonepeta (Jingjie) is used with Forsythia fruit (Lianqiao), Mentha (Bohe) and Platycodon root (Jiegeng) in the formula Yin Qiao San.

3. Measles and skin eruption with itching. Schizonepeta (Jingjie) is used with Mentha (Bohe), Cicada slough (Chantui) and Arctium fruit (Niubangzi) to bring the rash to the surface and alleviate itching.

4. Hemorrhagic diseases, such as epistaxis, bloody stool and uterine bleeding. Carbonized Schizonepeta (Jingjie) is used with the ohter herbs that stop bleeding.

Dosage: 3-10 g

Cautions & Contraindications: To stop bleeding, this herb should be carbonized (or baked until yellow and black in color).

7. Ledebouriella root (Fangfeng)

Pharmaceutical Name: Radix Ledebouriellae

Botanical Name: Ledebouriella divaricata (Turcz.) Hiroe

Common Name: Ledebouriella root

Source of Earliest Record: Shennong Bencao Jing

Part Used & Method for Pharmaceutical Preparations: The root is dug in spring and autumn, dried in the sun, soaked in water and cut into pieces.

Properties & Taste: Pungent, sweet and warm

Meridians: Lung, liver, spleen and urinary bladder

Functions: 1. To release the exterior and expel wind; 2. To expel wind-dampness and alleviate pain; 3. To alleviate spasms

Indications & Combinations:

1. Wind-cold exterior syndrome manifested as fever, chills, head-

18

ache and general pain. Ledebouriella root (Fangfeng) is used with Schizonepeta (Jingjie) and Notopterygium root (Qianghuo).

2. Wind-heat exterior syndrome manifested as fever, sore throat, red eyes and headache. Ledebouriella root (Fangfeng) is used with Schizonepeta (Jingjie), Scutellaria root (Huangqin), Mentha (Bohe) and Forsythia fruit (Lianqiao).

3. Wind-cold-damp *bi* syndrome manifested as joint pain (arthritis) and spasms of the limbs. Ledebouriella root (Fangfeng) is used with Notopterygium root (Qianghuo) and Chinese angelica root (Danggui).

4. Urticaria and itching of the skin. Ledebouriella root (Fangfeng) is used with Flavescent sophora root (Kushen) and Cicada slough (Chantui) in the formula Xiaofeng San.

Dosage: 3-10 g

Cautions & Contraindications: This herb should be used with caution for spasms due to blood deficiency, and is contraindicated for cases of deficient *yin* with heat signs.

8. Notopterygium root (Qianghuo)

Pharmaceutical Name: Rhizoma seu Radix Notopterygii
Botanical Name: 1. Notopterygium incisium Ting ex H. T. Chang; 2. Notopterygium forbesii Boiss.
Common Name: Notopterygium root
Source of Earliest Record: Yaoxing Lun
Part Used & Method for Pharmaceutical Preparations: The root, or rhizome, is dug in the early spring or autumn, dried and cut into slices.
Properties & Taste: Pungent, bitter and warm
Meridians: Kidney and urinary bladder
Functions: 1. To release the exterior and disperse cold; 2. To dispel wind and eliminate dampness; 3. To stop pain
Indications & Combinations:

1. Wind-cold exterior syndrome manifested by chills, fever, headache and severe general pain. Notopterygium root (Qianghuo) is used with Ledebouriella root (Fangfeng), Dahurian angelica root (Baizhi) and Atractylodes rhizome (Cangzhu).

2. Wind-cold-damp *bi* syndrome manifested as joint pain and soreness and pain in the shoulders and upper back. Notopterygium root (Qianghuo) is used with Ledebouriella root (Fangfeng) and Turmeric (Jianghuang).

Dosage: 3-10 g

Cautions & Contraindications: The herb is contraindicated in joint pain due to deficient blood and headache due to deficient *yin.*

9. Dahurian angelica root (Baizhi)

Pharmaceutical Name: Radix Angelicae Dahuricae

Botanical Name: 1. Angelica dahurica (Fisch. ex Hoffm.) Benth. et Hook. f.; 2. Angelica dauburica (Fisch. ex Hoffm.) Benth. et Hook. f. var. formosana (Boiss.) Shan et Yuan

Common Name: Dahurian angelica root

Source of Earliest Record: Shennong Bencao Jing

Part Used & Method for Pharmaceutical Preparations: The root is dug in the period between summer and autumn, when the leaves turn yellow. The fibrous roots are removed, dried, soaked in water and cut into slices.

Properties & Taste: Pungent and warm

Meridians: Lung and stomach

Functions: 1. To expel wind and release the exterior; 2. To reduce swelling and discharge pus and dampness; 3. To stop pain

Indications & Combinations:

1. Wind-cold exterior syndrome manifested by headache, supraobital pain and nasal obstruction. Dahurian angelica root (Baizhi) is used with Chinese green onion (Congbai), Prepared soybean (Douchi) and Fresh ginger (Shengjiang).

2. Thick and sticky nasal discharge (as in thinitis, nasosinusitis). Dahurian angelica root (Baizhi) is used with Xanthium fruit (Cang'erzi) and Magnolia flower (Xinyi) in the formula Cang'er San.

3. Boils, carbuncles, ulceration and skin diseases. Dahurian angelica root (Baizhi) is used with Trichosanthes fruit (Gualou), Tendrilled fritillary bulb (Chuanbeimu) and Dandelion herb (Pugongying).

4. Damp-cold type of leukorrhea manifested as watery, whitish and profuse leukorrhea with no offensive smell. Dahurian angelica root (Baizhi) is used with White atractylodes (Baizhu), Cuttlefish bone (Wuzeigu) and Poria (Fuling).

5. Damp-heat type of leukorrhea manifested by thick, yellow and profuse leukorrhea with offensive smell. Dahurian angelica root (Baizhi) is used with Phellodendron bark (Huangbai), Plantain seed (Cheqianzi) and Flavescent sophora root (Kushen).

Dosage: 3-10 g

Cautions & Contraindications: This herb is contraindicated in *yin* deficiency.

10. Ligusticum root (Gaoben)   — Louage

Pharmaceutical Name: Rhizoma Ligustici

Botanical Name: 1. Ligusticum sinense oliver; 2. Ligusticum jeholense Nakai et Kitag.

Source of Earliest Record: Shennong Bencao Jing

Common Name: Ligusticum root

Part Used & Method for Pharmaceutical Preparations: The roots are dug in spring. After the fibrous roots have been removed, they are dried in the sun. Then, after soaking them in water, the roots are cut into slices.

Properties & Taste: Pungent and warm

Meridians: Urinary bladder

Functions: 1. To expel cold and release the exterior; 2. To expel wind and dampness; 3. To stop pain

Indications & Combinations:

1. Headache due to invasion by wind and cold manifested by pain at the vertex and migraine headache. Ligusticum root (Gaoben) is used with Dahurian angelica root (Baizhi) and Chuanxiong rhizome (Chuanxiong).

2. Wind-cold-damp *bi* syndrome manifested as joint pain and pain in the limbs. Ligusticum root (Gaoben) is used with Ledebouriella root (Fangfeng), Notopterygium root (Qianghuo), Clematis root (Weilingxian) and Atractylodes rhizome (Cangzhu).

Dosage: 2-10 g

Cautions & Contraindications: This herb is contraindicated during heat syndromes, as well as in headache due to blood deficiency.

11. Xanthium fruit (Cang'erzi)

Pharmaceutical Name: Fructus Xanthii

Botanical Name: Xanthium sibiricum Patr.

Common Name: Xanthium fruit, Cocklebur fruit

Source of Earliest Record: Shennong Bencao Jing

Part Used & Method for Pharmaceutical Preparations: The fruit is gathered in autumn, dried in the sun and then baked till the thorns fall off.

Properties & Taste: Pungent, bitter, warm and slightly toxic

Meridian: Lung

Functions: 1. To open the nasal cavities; 2. To dispel wind and dampness; 3. To stop pain

Indications & Combinations:

1. Rhinorrhea manifested as headache, nasal obstruction, runny nose and loss of smell. Xanthium fruit (Cang'erzi) is used with Magnolia flower (Xinyi) and Dahurian angelica root (Baizhi) in the formula Cang'er San.

2. Wind-damp *bi* syndrome manifested as joint pain and spasms of the limbs. Xanthium fruit (Cang'erzi) is used with Clematis root (Weilingxian), Cinnamon bark (Rougui), Atractylodes rhizome (Cangzhu) and Chuanxiong rhizome (Chuanxiong).

Dosage: 3-10 g

Cautions & Contraindications: This herb is contraindicated in headache due to blood deficiency. Overdosing will produce toxins and give rise to vomiting, abdominal pain and diarrhea.

12. Magnolia flower (Xinyi)

Pharmaceutical Name: Flos Magnoliae

Botanical Name: 1. Magnolia biondii Pamp. 2. Magnolia denudata Desr. 3. Magnolia Sprengeri Pamp.

Common Name: Magnolia flower

Source of Earliest Records: Shennong Bencao Jing

Part Used & Method for Pharmaceutical Preparation: The flowerbuds are gathered in the early spring and dried in the sun.

Properties & Taste: Pungent and warm

Meridians: Lung and stomach

Functions: 1. To expel wind and cold; 2. To open the nasal cavity

Indications & Combinations: Rhinorrhea manifested as nasal obstruction, headache, runny nose and loss of smell. For the cold-type of rhinorrhea followed by white, dilute and profuse nasal discharge, Magnolia flower (Xinyi) is used with Asarum herb (Xixin), Dahurian angelica root (Baizhi) and Xanthium fruit (Cang'erzi). For the heat-type of rhinorrhea with yellow, thick and scanty nasal discharge, Magnolia flower (Xinyi) is used with Mentha (Bohe) and Scutellaria root (Huangqin).

Dosage: 3-10 g

Cautions & Contraindications: Overdosing causes redness of eyes and dizziness.

13. Chinese green onion (Congbai)

Pharmaceutical Name: Bulbus Allii Fistulosi
Botanical Name: Allium fistulosum L.
Common Name: Allium bulb, Wild scallion, Chinese green onion
Source of Earliest Record: Shennong Bencao Jing
Part Used & Method for Pharmaceutical Preparations: The fresh, white bulb is gathered in any season.
Properties & Taste: Pungent and warm
Meridians: Lung and stomach
Functions: 1. To release the exterior and cause sweating; 2. To disperse cold by invigorating *yang-qi*; 3. To alleviate toxins
Indications & Combinations:

1. Initial stage of wind-cold exterior syndrome (the very early stage of common cold). Chinese green onion (Congbai) is used with Fresh ginger (Shengjiang) and Prepared soybean (Douchi).

2. Abdominal pain due to stagnation of *qi* by cold, or retention of urine due to dysfunction of *qi* of the urinary bladder. The heated Chinese green onion (Congbai) is used for external application on the umbilicus.

3. Boils, carbuncles, ulceration and skin disease. The mashed Chinese green onion (Congbai) can be mixed with honey and applied to the affected area.

Dosage: 3-10 g

Cautions & Contraindications: This herb should not be taken with honey.

14. Coriander (Husui)

Pharmaceutical Name: Herba Coriandri
Botanical Name: Coriandrom saticum L.
Common Name: Coriander
Source of Earliest Record: Jiayou Bencao
Part Used & Method for Pharmaceutical Preparations: The entire plant is gathered in August, dried in the sun and cut into pieces.
Properties & Taste: Pungent and warm

Meridians: Lung and stomach

Functions: To promote sweating and bring the rash to the surface

Indications & Combinations: Early stage of measles due to attack of wind and cold manifested as fever, no sweating and measles without a rash. Coriander (Husui) is used with Spirodela (Fuping) and Cimicifuga rhizome (Shengma). The heated herbal tea is applied to the skin to bring the rash to the surface.

Dosage: 3-6 g

Cautions & Contraindications: The herb is contraindicated in measles without a rash on the surface due to excessive toxic heat in the interior.

15. Tamarisk tops (Chengliu)

Pharmaceutical Name: Cacumen Tamaricis

Botanical Name: Tamarix chinensis Lour.

Source of Earliest Record: Kaibao Bencao

Common Name: Tamarisk tops

Part Used & Method for Pharmaceutical Preparations: The leaves are gathered in May and June when the plant flowers, dried in the sun and cut into pieces.

Properties & Taste: Pungent and neutral

Meridians: Lung, stomach and heart

Functions: To promote sweating and bring the rash to the surface

Indications & Combinations: Early stage of measles due to attack of wind and cold manifested as measles without a rash. Tamarisk tops (Chengliu) is used with Arctium fruit (Niubangzi) and Cicada slough (Chantui) in the formula Zhuye Liu Bang Tang.

Dosage: 3-10 g

Cautions & Contraindications: This herb is contraindicated in measles with a rash. A large dosage can cause restlessness.

b) Cool-Pungent Herbs That Release Exterior Syndrome

These herbs are cool and pungent in property. They are not strong enough to promote sweating. They are indicated in wind-heat exterior syndrome manifested as high fever, mild chills, thirst, sore throat, scanty or no sweating, thin and yellow tongue coating and superficial and rapid pulse. Some of these herbs are also effective in promoting the full expression of rashes in measles, and for use on boils and carbuncles on the exterior.

16. Mentha (Bohe)

Pharmaceutical Name: Herba Menthae
Botanical Name: Mentha haplocalyx Briq.
Common Name: Mentha, Peppermint
Source of Earliest Record: Xinxiu Bencao
Part Used & Method of Pharmaceutical Preparations: The entire plant, including leaves, is gathered in any season. The leaves can be picked two or three times each year, dried in a shady place and then cut into pieces.
Properties & Taste: Pungent and cool
Meridians: Lung and liver
Functions: 1. To disperse wind-heat and clear the head and eyes; 2. To promote liver *qi*, allowing it to flow freely; 3. To bring rashes to the surface
Indications & Combinations:

1. Wind-heat exterior syndrome manifested as fever, headache, mild aversion to wind and cold, sore throat and red eyes. Mentha (Bohe) is used with Platycodon root (Jiegeng), Arctium fruit (Niubangzi) and Chrysanthemum flower (Juhua).

2. Early stage of measles with slight rash. Mentha (Bohe) is used with Arctium fruit (Niubangzi) and Pueraria root (Gegen).

3. Stagnation of *qi* in the liver manifested as a full sensation and pain in the chest and costal region. Mentha (Bohe) is used with White peony root (Baishao) and Bupleurum root (Chaihu) in the formula Xiaoyao San.

Dosage: 2-10 g
Cautions & Contraindications: This herb should not be boiled for a long time.

17. Arctium fruit (Niubangzi)

Pharmaceutical Name: Fructus Arctii
Botanical Name: Arctium lappa L.
Common Name: Arctium fruit, Burdock fruit
Source of Earliest Record: Mingyi Bielu

Part Used & Method for Pharmaceutical Preparations: The fruit is gathered in autumn and dried in the sun. The raw fruit can be used, or it can be baked and smashed and then used.

Properties & Taste: Pungent, bitter and cold

Meridians: Lung and stomach

Functions: 1. To disperse wind-heat and benefit the throat; 2. To release toxins and bring rashes to the surface

Indications & Combinations:

1. Sore throat caused by invasion of wind and heat. Arctium fruit (Niubangzi) is used with Platycodon root (Jiegeng), Mentha (Bohe) and Schizonepeta (Jingjie) in the formula Niubang Tang.

2. Incomplete expression of measles rash. To encourage rashes to the surface, Arctium fruit (Niubangzi) is used with Cimicifuga rhizome (Shengma), Pueraria root (Gegen) and Mentha (Bohe).

3. Toxic heat manifested as swelling, carbuncles and mumps. Arctium fruit (Niubangzi) is used with Viola (Zihuadiding) and Wild chrysanthemum flower (Yejuhua).

Dosage: 3-10 g

Cautions & Contraindications: This herb should be used with caution. It is contraindicated in patients with diarrhea.

18. Cicada slough (Chantui)

Pharmaceutical Name: Periostracum Cicadae

Zoological Name: Cryptotympana pustulata Fabricius

Common Name: Cicada slough

Source of Earliest Record: Mingyi Bielu

Part Used & Method for Pharmaceutical Preparations: The slough shed by the cicada is found on the ground or on the branches of trees, then dried in the sun.

Properties & Taste: Sweet and cold

Meridians: Lung and liver

Functions: 1. To disperse wind and clear heat; 2. To bring the rash to the surface and relieve itching; 3. To clear eyes; 4. To stop spasms

Indications & Combinations:

1. Wind-heat exterior syndrome manifested as fever, headache, sore throat and hoarse voice. Cicada slough (Chantui) is used with Boat sterculia seed (Pangdahai), Arctium fruit (Niubangzi) and Platycodon root (Jiegeng).

26

2. Early stage of measles without rash. Cicada slough (Chantui) is used with Pueraria root (Gegen) and Arctium fruit (Niubangzi).

3. Itching due to the surface being attacked by exogenous wind. Cicada slough (Chantui) is used with Tribulus fruit (Baijili) and Schizo-nepeta (Jingjie).

4. Wind-heat of liver meridian manifested as red eyes, watery eyes and blurred vision. Cicada slough (Chantui) is used with Chrysanthemum flower (Juhua) and Shave grass (Muzei) in the formula Chan Hua San.

5. Convulsions and spasms due to tetanus or high fever. Cicada slough (Chantui) is used with Scorpion (Quanxie), White-stiff silkworm (Baijiangcan), Uncaria stem (Gouteng) and Chrysanthemum flower (Juhua).

Dosage: 3-10 g

Cautions & Contraindications: This herb should be used with caution during pregnancy.

19. Prepared soybean (Douchi)

Pharmaceutical Name: Semen Sojae Preparatum
Botanical Name: Glycine max (L.) Merr.
Common Name: Prepared Soja, or Prepared soybean
Source of Earliest Record: Mingyi Bielu
Part Used & Method for Pharmaceutical Preparations: The seeds are gathered and subjected to a process of fermentation.
Properties & Taste: Pungent, sweet, slightly bitter and cold
Meridians: Lung and stomach
Functions: 1. To release the exterior; 2. To relieve restlessness
Indications & Combinations:

1. Wind-cold exterior syndrome. Prepared soybean (Douchi) is used with Chinese green onion (Congbai) in the formula Cong Chi Tang.

2. Wind-heat exterior syndrome. Prepared soybean (Douchi) is used with Arctium fruit (Niubangzi) and Forsythia fruit (Lianqiao).

3. Irritability, restlessness and insomnia following febrile disease. Prepared soybean (Douchi) is used with Capejasmine (Zhizi) in the formula Zhizi Chi Tang.

Dosage: 10-15 g

20. Mulberry leaf (Sangye)

Pharmaceutical Name: Folium Mori

Botanical Name: Morus alba L.

Common Name: Morus leaf, Mulberry leaf

Source of Earliest Record: Shennong Bencao Jing

Part Used & Method for Pharmaceutical Preparations: The leaves are gathered in autumn, during the period of Frost's Descent (eighteenth solar term), then dried in the sun.

Properties & Taste: Sweet, bitter and cold

Meridians: Lung and liver

Functions: 1. To expel wind and clear heat; 2. To clear heat in the liver and benefit the eyes

Indications & Combinations:

1. Wind-heat exterior syndrome manifested as fever, headache, sore throat and cough. Mulberry leaf (Sangye) is used with Chrysanthemum flower (Juhua), Platycodon root (Jiegeng), Mentha (Bohe) and Forsythia fruit (Lianqiao) in the formula Sang Ju Yin.

2. Lung attacked by dryness and heat manifested as cough with sputum and dry nose and mouth. Mulberry leaf (Sangye) is used with Apricot seed (Xingren), Tendrilled fritillary bulb (Chuanbeimu) and Ophiopogon root (Maidong) in the formula Sang Xing Tang.

3. Flaring up of fire in the liver manifested as red, painful and watering eyes. Mulberry leaf (Sangye) is used with Chrysanthemum flower (Juhua), Cassia seed (Juemingzi) and Plantain seed (Cheqianzi).

4. Deficient *yin* of the liver manifested as dizziness and blurred vision. Mulberry leaf (Sangye) is used with Ligustrum (Nüzhenzi), Wolfberry fruit (Gouqizi) and Black sesame seed (Heizhima).

Dosage: 5-10 g

21a. Chrysanthemum flower (Juhua)

Pharmaceutical Name: Flos chrysanthemi

Botanical Name: Chrysanthemum morifolium Ramat.

Common Name: Chrysanthemum flower

Source of Earliest Record: Shennong Bencao Jing

Part Used & Method for Pharmaceutical Preparations: The chrysanthemum flower is gathered and then dried in the shade.

Properties & Taste: Pungent, sweet, bitter and slightly cold

Meridians: Lung and liver

Functions: 1. To dispel wind and clear heat; 2. To release toxins and brighten the eyes; 3. To pacify the liver

Indications & Combinations:

1. Wind-heat exterior syndrome manifested as fever, headache, chills and sore throat. Chrysanthemum flower (Juhua) is used with Mulberry leaf (Sangye), Mentha (Bohe) and Platycodon root (Jiegeng) in the formula Sang Ju Yin.

2. Wind-heat in the liver meridian or an upward attack of liver fire manifested as red, swelling and painful eyes. Chrysanthemum flower (Juhua) is used with Mulberry leaf (Sangye), Cicada slough (Chantui) and Prunella spike (Xiakucao).

3. *Yin* deficiency in the liver and kidneys manifested as blurred vision and dizziness. Chrysanthemum flower (Juhua) is used with Wolfberry fruit (Gouqizi) and Grossy privet fruit (Nüzhenzi) in the formula Qi Ju Dihuang Wan.

4. Hyperactivity of liver *yang* manifested as dizziness, vertigo and blurred vision. Chrysanthemum flower (Juhua) is used with Cassia seed (Juemingzi), Uncaria stem (Gouteng) and White peony root (Baishao).

Dosage: 10-15 g

Cautions & Contraindications: The yellow chrysanthemum flower is mainly indicated in wind-heat exterior syndrome, while the white chrysanthemum flower is used to pacify the liver, expel wind and brighten the eyes.

21b. Wild chrysanthemum flower (Yejuhua)

The entire wild chrysanthemum flower is used. It is pungent, bitter and slightly cold in property. The herb enters the lung and liver meridians. It is used to clear heat and release toxins in furuncles, carbuncles and sore throat. The combination of Wild chrysanthemum flower (Yejuhua), Dandelion herb (Pugongying), Viola (Zihuadiding) and Honeysuckle flower (Jinyinhua) are mainly used. The dosage can be 10-18 g. For external application, the proper dosage should be taken into consideration.

22. Chastetree fruit (Manjingzi)

Pharmaceutical Name: Fructus Viticis

Botanical Name: 1. Vitex trifolia L. var. simplicifolia cham.; 2. Vitex trifolia L.

Common Name: Vitex fruit, Chastetree fruit

Source of Earliest Record: Shennong Bencao Jing

Part Used & Method for Pharmaceutical Preparations: The fruit is gathered in summer, dried in the shade and baked until yellow or black.

Properties & Taste: Pungent, bitter and neutral

Meridians: Liver, stomach and urinary bladder.

Functions: 1. To disperse wind and clear heat; 2. To clear and benefit the head and eyes

Indications & Combinations:

1. Headache and unilateral headache due to invasion by exogenous wind and heat. Chastetree fruit (Manjingzi) is used with Ledebouriella root (Fangfeng), Chrysanthemum flower (Juhua) and Chuanxiong rhizome (Chuanxiong).

2. Upper disturbance of liver-*yang* manifested as red, painful and swelling eyes, excessive tearing, dizziness and blurred vision. Chastetree fruit (Manjingzi) is used with Chrysanthemum flower (Juhua), Cicada slough (Chantui) and Tribulus fruit (Baijili).

3. Wind-damp *bi* syndrome manifested as joint pain and cramping or heaviness of limbs. Chastetree fruit (Manjingzi) is used with Ledebouriella root (Fangfeng), Large-leaf gentian root (Qinjiao) and Chaenomeles fruit (Mugua).

Dosage: 6-12 g

Cautions & Contraindications: This herb should be used with caution for headaches or eye problems due to deficient *yin* or blood.

23a. Pueraria root (Gegen)

Pharmaceutical Name: Radix Puerariae

Botanical Name: 1. Pueraria lobata (willd.) Ohwi; 2. Pueraria thomsonii Benth.

Common Name: Pueraria root

Source of Earliest Record: Shennong Bencao Jing

Part Used & Method for Pharmaceutical Preparations: The roots are dug in spring or autumn. They are cut into slices and dried in the shade, or the slices are baked.

Properties & Taste: Pungent, sweet and cool

Meridians: Spleen and stomach

Functions: 1. To release the exterior; 2. To bring measles rash to the surface; 3. To cause *yang* to ascend so as to alleviate diarrhea; 4. To clear heat and promote production of body fluids

Indications & Combinations:

1. Exterior syndrome due to invasion by exogenous wind and cold manifested as stiffness of upper back or neck, absence of sweating, aversion to wind, fever and headache. Pueraria root (Gegen) is used with Ephedra (Mahuang), Cinnamon twigs (Guizhi) and White peony root (Baishao) in the formula Gegen Tang.

2. Exterior syndrome due to invasion by exogenous wind and heat manifested as headache, fever, painful eyes and dry throat. Pueraria root (Gegen) is used with Bupleurum root (Chaihu) and Scutellaria root (Huangqin) in the formula Chai Ge Jieji Tang.

3. Early stage of measles with incomplete expression of the rash, fever and chills. Pueraria root (Gegen) is used with Cimicifuga rhizome (Shengma) in the formula Shengma Gegen Tang.

4. Damp-heat dysentery. Pueraria root (Gegen) is used with Coptis root (Huanglian) and Scutellaria root (Huangqin) in the formula Gegen Huangqin Huanglian Tang.

5. Diarrhea due to deficient spleen. Pueraria root (Gegen) is used with Pilose asiabell root (Dangshen), White atractylodes (Baizhu) and Costus root (Muxiang) in the formula Qiwei Baishu San.

6. Thirst in febrile diseases or diabetes. Pueraria root (Gegen) is used with Ophiopogon root (Maidong), Trichosanthes root (Tianhuafen) and Fresh rehmannia root (Shengdihuang).

Dosage: 10-20 g

Cautions & Contraindications: To treat diarrhea, the herb is first baked.

23b. Pueraria flower (Gehua)

The pueraria flower is sweet and neutral in property. Its main function is to relieve alcoholic poisoning manifested as headache, dizziness, thirst, fullness and distension in the abdominal and gastric regions and vomiting. The combination used includes Pueraria flower (Gehua), Pilose asiabell root (Dangshen), Round cardamom seed (Baidoukou) and Tangerine peel (Chenpi). The dosage of the herb can be 3-12 g.

24. Bupleurum root (Chaihu)

Pharmaceutical Name: Radix bupleuri
Botanical Name: Bupleurum scorzoneraefollium wild; 2. Bupleurum chinense DC.

Common Name: Bupleurum root
Source of Earliest Record: Shennong Bencao Jing
Part Used & Method for Pharmaceutical Preparations: The roots are dug in spring or autumn, dried in the sun and cut into short pieces. The raw root can be used, or it can be baked with wine or vinegar.
Properties & Taste: Bitter, pungent and slightly cold
Meridians: Pericardium, liver, gall bladder and triple *jiao*
Functions: 1. To release the exterior and clear heat; 2. To pacify the liver so as to relieve stagnation; 3. To elevate *yang-qi*
Indications & Combinations:

1. Fever due to invasion by exogenous pathogenic factors. Bupleurum root (Chaihu) is used with Licorice root (Gancao).

2. Alternating chills and fever in lesser *yang*-syndrome. Bupleurum root (Chaihu) is used with Scutellaria root (Huangqin).

3. *Qi* stagnation in the liver manifested as distension and pain in the chest and costal regions and irregular menstruation. Bupleurum root (Chaihu) is used with Cyperus tuber (Xiangfu), Bitter orange (Zhiqiao) and Green tangerine peel (Qingpi) in the formula Chaihu Sugan San.

4. *Qi* stagnation of the liver and deficient blood. Bupleurum root (Chaihu) is used with Chinese angelica root (Danggui) and White peony root (Baishao) in the formula Xiaoyao San.

5. Sinking of *qi* in the spleen and stomach manifested as chronic diarrhea, prolapse of rectum, gastroptosis and uterine prolapse. Bupleurum root (Chaihu) is used with Ginseng (Renshen), Scutellaria root (Huangqin) and White atractylodes (Baizhu) in the formula Buzhong Yiqi Tang.
Dosage: 3-10 g
Cautions & Contraindications: This herb is contraindicated during syndromes due to hyperactivity of liver *yang* or deficiency of *yin*.

25. Cimicifuga rhizome (Shengma)

Pharmaceutical Name: Rhizoma Cimicifugae
Botanical Name: 1. Cimicifuga foetida L.; 2. Cimicifuga dahurica (Turcz) Maxim.; 3. Cimicifuga heracleifolia Kom.
Common Name: Cimicifuga rhizome, Bugbane rhizome
Source of Earliest Record: Shennong Bencao Jing
Part Used & Method for Pharmaceutical Preparations: The roots, or rhizomes, are dug in summer or autumn and dried in the sun. After

removing the fibrous roots, they are soaked in water and cut into pieces.

Properties & Taste: Pungent, sweet and slightly cold

Meridians: Spleen, lung, large intestine and stomach

Functions: 1. To release the exterior and bring measle rash to the surface; 2. To clear heat and toxins; 3. To raise the *yang-qi*

Indications & Combinations:

1. Early stage of measles with incomplete expression of the rash. Cimicifuga rhizome (Shengma) is used with Pueraria root (Gegen) in the formula Shengma Gegen Tang.

2. Excessive heat in the stomach meridian manifested as headache, swelling of gums, painful gums, painful teeth and ulceration of tongue and mouth. Cimicifuga rhizome (Shengma) is used with Coptis root (Huanglian), Fresh rehmannia root (Shengdihuang), Gypsum (Shigao) and Moutan bark (Mudanpi) in the formula Qingwei San.

3. Sore throat caused by invasion of exogenous wind and heat. Cimicifuga rhizome (Shengma) is used with Scrophularia (Xuanshen), Platycodon root (Jiegeng), Arctium fruit (Niubangzi) in the formula Niubang Tang.

4. Sinking of *qi* in the spleen and stomach manifested as chronic diarrhea, prolapse of rectum, uterine prolapse and gastroptosis. Cimicifuga rhizome (Shengma) is used with Ginseng (Renshen), Scutellaria root (Huangqin) and White atractylodes (Baizhu) in the formula Buzhong Yiqi Tang.

5. Boils, carbuncles, furuncles and skin disease. Cimicifuga rhizome (Shengma) is used with Dandelion herb (Pugongying), Honeysuckle flower (Jinyinhua), Forsythia fruit (Lianqiao) and Rcd peony (Chishao).

Dosage: 3-10 g

Cautions & Contraindications: This herb is contraindicated in patients who have difficulty breathing, who have measles with complete rashes, or who have deficient *yin* syndrome with heat.

26. Spirodela (Fuping)

Pharmaceutical Name: Herba spirodelae

Botanical Name: Spirodela polyrrhiza (L.) Schield.

Common Name: Spirodela, Duckweed

Source of Earliest Record: Shennong Bencao Jing

Part Used & Method for Pharmaceutical Preparations: The whole plant is gathered in summer, cleaned and dried in the sun.

Properties & Taste: Pungent and cold

Meridions: Lung and urinary bladder

Functions: 1. To promote sweating and release the exterior; 2. To bring measles rash to the surface and relieve itching; 3. To remove water and reduce swelling

Indications & Combinations:

1. Wind-heat type of exterior syndrome. Spirodela (Fuping) is used with Schizonepeta (Jingjie), Mentha (Bohe) and Forsythia fruit (Lianqiao).

2. Measles without full expression of rash. Spirodela (Fuping) is used with Mentha (Bohe), Arctium fruit (Niubangzi) and Cicada slough (Chantui).

3. Wind-heat type of incomplete rashes and itching of the skin. Spirodela (Fuping) is used with Mentha (Bohe) and Arctium fruit (Niubangzi).

4. Edema and difficult urination accompanied by exterior syndrome. Spirodela (Fuping) can be mashed and taken alone.

Dosage: 3-10 g

Cautions & Contraindications: This herb is contraindicated in cases with weak constitution and spontaneous sweating.

27. Shave grass (Muzei)

Pharmaceutical Name: Herba Equiseti hiemalis

Botanical Name: Equisetum hiemale L.

Common Name: Shave grass, Scouring rush

Source of Earliest Record: Jiayou Bencao

Part Used & Method for Pharmaceutical Preparations: The whole plant is gathered in summer and cut into pieces after the fibrous roots have been removed.

Properties & Taste: Sweet and bitter and neutral

Meridians: Lung and liver

Functions: 1. To dispel wind and clear heat; 2. To brighten eyes and remove visual obstruction; 3. To stop bleeding

Indications & Combinations:

1. Wind-heat exterior syndrome or wind and heat in the liver meridian manifested as red eyes, excessive tearing, blurred vision and corneal opacity. Shave grass (Muzei) is used with Cicada slough (Chantui), Pipewort (Gujingcao), Prunella spike (Xiakucao) and Tribulus fruit

(Baijili).

2. Hemorrhoidal bleeding. Shave grass (Muzei) is used with Scutellaria root (Huangqin) and Burnet root (Diyu).

Dosage: 3-10 g

Cautions & Contraindications: This herb should be used with caution during pregnancy.

II. Herbs That Clear Heat

Herbs that clear heat mainly remove interior heat. Generally speaking, interior heat syndrome excludes exterior syndrome due to invasion by exogenous pathogenic factors and heat syndrome caused by retention of food in the interior. Based on the functions and indications of the herbs, herbs that clear interior heat can be classified as follows:

a. Herbs that clear heat and reduce fire

Herbs that clear heat and reduce fire are mainly indicated for syndromes of heat in the *qi* level.

b. Herbs that clear heat and dispel dampness

Herbs that clear heat and dispel dampness are bitter and dry in property, and are mainly indicated for interior syndromes of excessive heat without consumption of body fluids.

c. Herbs that cool blood

Herbs that cool blood are used to cool heat in the blood.

d. Herbs that clear heat and remove toxins

Herbs that clear heat and remove toxins are mainly indicated for syndromes of excessive toxic heat, such as epidemic diseases, toxic dysentery, boils and carbuncles.

e. Herbs that clear heat caused by deficiency of *yin*

Herbs that clear heat caused by deficiency of *yin* are indicated for syndromes of interior heat due to deficient *yin*, such as afternoon tidal fever.

In general, herbs that clear heat are cool and cold in property. This action may impair the normal function of the spleen and stomach; therefore, they should be used with caution in cases with poor appetite, weakness of the spleen and stomach, or diarrhea. In addition, they serve as auxillary herbs in combination with toxic herbs, or with herbs that nourish *yin*.

a) Herbs That Clear Heat and Reduce Fire

Herbs that clear heat and reduce fire are mainly indicated for syndromes of heat in the *qi* level due to exogenous pathogenic heat invasion manifested as high fever, sweating, thirst, delirium, irritability, scanty and brown urine, yellow and dry tongue coating, surging and forceful pulse, excessive heat in the lungs, excessive heat in the stomach and excessive heat in the heart.

28. Gypsum (Shigao)

Pharmaceutical Name: Gypsum Fibrosum
Mineral Name: Calcium sulphate
Common Name: Gypsum
Source of Earliest Record: Shennong Bencao Jing
Part Used & Method for Pharmaceutical Preparations: The mineral is ground into powder.
Properties & Taste: Sweet, pungent and very cold
Meridians: Lung and stomach
Functions: 1. To clear heat and sedate fire; 2. To relieve irritability and thirst
Indications & Combinations:

1. Excessive heat at the *qi* level due to invasion by exogenous pathogenic heat manifested as high fever, irritability, thirst, profuse sweating and surging, rapid and forceful pulse. Gypsum (Shigao) is used with Anemarrhena rhizome (Zhimu) in the formula Baihu Tang.

2. Excessive heat at both *qi* and blood levels due to invasion by exogenous pathogenic heat manifested as continual high fever and maculopapule. Gypsum (Shigao) is used with Scrophularia (Xuanshen) and Rhinoceros horn (Xijiao).

3. Cough and asthma caused by heat in the lungs manifested as cough and asthma accompanied by fever, thirst and desire to drink. Gypsum (Shigao) is used with Ephedra (Mahuang) and Apricot seed (Xingren) in the formula Ma Xing Shi Gan Tang.

4. Flaring up of stomach fire manifested as toothache, swollen and painful gums and headache. Gypsum (Shigao) is used with Fresh rehmannia root (Shengdihuang) and Anemarrhena rhizome (Zhimu) in the formula Yunü Jian.

5. Eczema, burns and abscess. Gypsum (Shigao) is used with Natural indigo (Qingdai) and Phellodendron bark (Huangbai).

Dosage: 15-60 g.

Cautions & Contraindications: This herb is contraindicated in cases with a weak stomach.

29. Anemarrhena rhizome (Zhimu)

Pharmaceutical Name: Rhizoma Anemarrhenae
Botanical Name: Anemarrhena asphodeloides Bge.
Common Name: Anemarrhena rhizome
Source of Earliest Record: Shennong Bencao Jing
Part Used & Method for Pharmaceutical Preparations: The rhizomes are gathered in spring or autumn. After the fibrous roots have been removed, the rhizomes are cleaned, dried and soaked in water. Finally, the skin is peeled off, cut into slices and baked with salt.

Properties & Taste: Sweet, bitter and cold
Meridians: Lung, stomach and kidney
Functions: 1. To clear heat and reduce fire; 2. To nourish *yin* and moisten dryness

Indications & Combinations:

1. Excessive heat at the *qi* level. Anemarrhena rhizome (Zhimu) is used with Gypsum (Shigao) in the formula Baihu Tang.

2. Cough due to heat in the lungs or dry cough due to deficient *yin*. Anemarrhena rhizome (Zhimu) is used with Tendrilled fritillary bulb (Chuanbeimu) in the formula Ermu San.

3. Deficient *yin* of the lungs and kidneys with heat signs manifested as afternoon fever, night sweating and feverish sensation of the palms, soles and chest. Anemarrhena rhizome (Zhimu) is used with Phellodendron bark (Huangbai).

4. Diabetes manifested as extreme thirst and hunger and profuse urine. Anemarrhena rhizome (Zhimu) is used with Trichosanthes root (Tianhuafen), Schisandra fruit (Wuweizi), Ophiopogon root (Maidong) and Pueraria root (Gegen) in the formula Yuye Tang.

Dosage: 6-12 g

Cautions & Contraindications: This herb is contraindicated in diarrhea due to weakness of the spleen.

30. Reed root (Lugen)

Pharmaceutical Name: Rhizoma Phragmitis
Botanical Name: Phragmites communis Trin.

Common Name: Phragmites, Reed root
Source of Earliest Record: Mingyi Bielu
Part Used & Method for Pharmaceutical Preparations: The rhizomes are dug at the end of spring, in the beginning of summer or in autumn. After the fibrous roots have been removed, the skin is peeled off and cleaned and dried in the sun.
Properties & Taste: Sweet and cold
Functions: 1. To clear heat and relieve irritability; 2. To promote the production of body fluids and relieve thirst; 3. To stop vomiting
Meridians: Lung and stomach
Indications & Combinations:

1. Febrile diseases manifested as thirst, irritability and fever. Reed root (Lugen) is used with Gypsum (Shigao), Ophiopogon root (Maidong) and Trichosanthes root (Tianhuafen).

2. Heat in the stomach with vomiting and belching. Reed root (Lugen) is used with the juice of Fresh ginger (Shengjiang), Bamboo shavings (Zhuru) and Loquat leaf (Pipaye).

3. Heat in the lungs manifested as cough, expectoration of thick, yellow sputum and pulmonary abscess. Reed root (Lugen) is used with Honeysuckle flower (Jinyinhua), Houttuynia (Yuxingcao) and Benincasa seed (Dongguaren).

Dosage: 15-30 g
Cautions & Contraindications: This herb should be used with caution in cases with cold and deficient spleen and stomach.

31. Trichosanthes root (Tianhuafen)

Pharmaceutical Name: Radix Trichosanthis
Botanical Name: 1. Trichosanthes kirilowii Maxim.; 2. Trichosanthes japonica Regel.
Common Name: Trichosanthes root, Snakegourd root
Source of Earliest Record: Shennong Bencao Jing
Part Used & Method for Pharmaceutical Preparations: The roots are dug in autumn or winter. After cleaning, the skin is peeled off. Then, the roots are cut into pieces or slices and dried in the sun.
Properties & Taste: Bitter, slightly sweet and cold
Meridians: Lung and stomach
Functions: 1. To clear heat and promote the production of body fluids; 2. To reduce swelling and dispel pus

Indications & Combinations:

1. Thirst in febrile diseases. Trichosanthes root (Tianhuafen) is used with Glehnia root (Shashen), Ophiopogon root (Maidong) and Reed root (Lugen).

2. Extreme thirst in diabetes. Trichosanthes root (Tianhuafen) is used with Pueraria root (Gegen), Schisandra fruit (Wuweizi) and Anemarrhena rhizome (Zhimu).

3. Dry cough due to lung heat. Trichosanthes root (Tianhuafen) is used with Mulberry bark (Sangbaipi), Tendrilled fritillary bulb (Chuanbeimu) and Platycodon root (Jiegeng).

4. Boils and carbuncles. Trichosanthes root (Tianhuafen) is used with Forsythia fruit (Lianqiao), Dandelion herb (Pugongying), Tendrilled fritillary bulb (Chuanbeimu) and Honeysuckle flower (Jinyinhua).

Dosage: 10-15 g

Cautions & Contraindications: This herb should be used with caution during pregnancy.

32. Bamboo leaf (Zhuye)

Pharmaceutical Name: Folium bambusae

Botanical Name: Phyllostachy nigra (Lodd.) Munro var. henonis (Mitf.) Stapf ex Rendle

Common Name: Bamboo leaf, Bambusa

Source of Earliest Record: Mingyi Bielu

Part Used & Method for Pharamceutical Preparations: The leaves are picked at any time. It is best to prepare fresh leaves for use.

Properties & Taste: Sweet and cold

Meridians: Heart, lung and stomach

Functions: 1. To clear heat and relieve irritability; 2. To promote urination

Indications & Combinations:

1. Thirst in febrile disease. Bamboo leaf (Zhuye) is used with Gypsum (Shigao) and Ophiopogon root (Maidong) in the formula Zhuye Shigao Tang.

2. Flaring up of heart fire manifested as ulceration in the mouth or on the tongue; or heart fire shifting to the small intestine manifested as dribbling urination. Bamboo leaf (Zhuye) is used with Clematis stem (Mutong) and Fresh rehmannia root (Shengdihuang) in the formula

Daochi San.
  Dosage: 6-15 g

33. Lophatherum (Danzhuye)

Pharmaceutical Name: Herba Lophatheri
Botanical Name: Lophatherum gracile Brongn.
Common Name: Lophatherum
Source of Earliest Record: Bencao Gangmu
Part Used & Method for Pharmaceutical Preparations: The leaves are gathered in summer, dried in the sun and cut into pieces.
Properties & Taste: Sweet or no taste and cold
Meridians: Heart, stomach and small intestine
Functions: 1. To clear heat and benefit urination; 2. To clear heat in the heart and lessen irritability
Indications & Combinations:

1. Febrile diseases manifested as irritability, thirst and fever. Lophatherum (Danzhuye) is used with Gypsum (Shigao) and Anemarrhena rhizome (Zhimu).

2. Heat in heart, stomach and small intestine manifested as ulcerations of the mouth and tongue and scanty, painful urination. Lophatherum (Danzhuye) is used with Fresh rehmannia root (Shengdihuang) and Clematis stem (Mutong).
  Dosage: 5-10 g
  Cautions & Contraindications: The herb should be used with caution during pregnancy.

34. Capejasmine (Zhizi)

Pharmaceutical Name: Pructus Gardeniae
Botanical Name: Gardenia jaminoides Ellis
Common Name: Gardenia fruit, Capejasmine fruit
Source of Earliest Record: Shennong Bencao Jing
Part Used & Method for Pharmaceutical Preparations: The fruit is gathered in autumn or winter when it is ripe. Either the raw herb or the carbonized herb is used.
Properties & Taste: Bitter and cold
Meridians: Heart, liver, lung, stomach and triple *jiao*
Functions: 1. To clear heat and reduce fire; 2. To cool blood and release toxins; 3. To eliminate dampness

Indications & Combinations:

1. Febrile diseases manifested as high fever, irritability, delirium and loss of consciousness. Capejasmine (Zhizi) is used with Prepared soybean (Douchi), Forsythia fruit (Lianqiao) and Scutellaria root (Huangqin).

2. Jaundice with fever and dysuria. Capejasmine (Zhizi) is used with Oriental wormwood (Yinchenhao), Rhubarb (Dahuang) and Phellodendron bark (Huangbai).

3. Extravasation caused by heat in the blood manifested as vomiting blood, epistaxis and hematuria. Capejasmine (Zhizi) is used with Imperata rhizome (Baimaogen), Fresh rehmannia root (Shengdihuang) and Scutellaria root (Huangqin).

4. Boils and carbuncles. Capejasmine (Zhizi) is used with Coptis root (Huanglian), Scutellaria root (Huangqin) and Honeysuckle flower (Jinyinhua).

Dosage: 3-10 g

Cautions & Contraindications: The herb is contraindicated in cases with weakness of the spleen and diarrhea.

35. Prunella spike (Xiakucao)

Pharmaceutical Name: Spica Prunellae
Botanical Name: Prunella vulgaris L.
Common Name: Prunella spike, Selfheal spike
Source of Earliest Record: Shennong Bencao Jing
Part Used & Method for Pharmaceutical Preparations: The spikes are gathered in summer and dried in the sun.
Properties & Taste: Bitter, pungent and cold
Meridians: Liver and gall bladder
Functions: 1. To clear the fire in the liver; 2. To dissipate accumulation of nodules
Indications & Combinations:

1. Flaring up of liver fire manifested as red, painful, swollen and watery eyes, headache and dizziness. Prunella spike (Xiakucao) is used with Sea-ear shell (Shijueming) and Chrysanthemum flower (Juhua).

2. Accumulation of phlegm-fire manifested as scrofula, lipoma, swollen glands or goiter. Prunella spike (Xiakucao) is used with Oyster shell (Muli), Scrophularia (Xuanshen) and Laminaria (Kunbu).

Dosage: 10-15 g

Cautions & Contraindications: This herb should be used with caution in cases with a weak stomach and spleen.

36. Pipewort (Gujingcao)

Pharmaceutical Name: Flos Eriocauli
Botanical Name: Eriocaulon buergerianum koern.
Common Name: Pipewort
Source of Earliest Record: Kaibao Bencao
Part Used & Method for Pharmaceutical Preparations: The whole plant is gathered in autumn, dried in the sun and cut into pieces for use.
Properties & Taste: Sweet, neutral
Meridians: Liver and stomach
Functions: 1. To clear heat and disperse wind; 2. To brighten the eyes
Indications & Combinations: Wind-heat in the liver meridian manifested as red, painful and swollen eyes, excessive tearing, photophobia and corneal opacity. Pipewort (Gujingcao) is used with Schizonepeta (Jingjie), Chinese gentian (Longdancao) and Red peony (Chishao).
Dosage: 6-15 g
Cautions & Contraindications: This herb is contraindicated in cases with deficiency of blood.

37. Butterflybush flower (Mimenghua)

Pharmaceutical Name: Flos Buddlejae
Botanical Name: Buddleja officinalis Maxim.
Common Name: Buddleja, Butterflybush flower
Source of Earliest Record: Kaibao Bencao
Part Used & Method for Pharmaceutical Preparations: The flower buds are gathered in spring and dried in the sun.
Properties & Taste: Sweet and slightly cold
Meridian: Liver
Functions: 1. To clear heat in the liver; 2. To brighten the eyes and reduce corneal opacity
Indications & Combinations:
1. Heat in the liver manifested as red, painful and swollen eyes, photophobia, excessive tearing and corneal opacity. Butterflybush flow-

er (Mimenghua) is used with Chrysanthemum flower (Juhua), Sea-ear shell (Shijueming) and Tribulus fruit (Baijili).

2. Deficient *yin* in the liver with *yang* attacking upward manifested as dizziness, blurred vision, dry eyes and corneal opacity. Butterflybush flower (Mimenghua) is used with Wolfberry fruit (Gouqizi) and Flattened milkvetch seed (Shayuanzi).

Dosage: 6-10 g

38. Celosia seed (Qingxiangzi)

Pharmaceutical Name: Semen Celosiae
Botanical Name: 1. Celosia argentea L.; 2. Celosia cristata L.
Common Name: Celosia seed
Source of Earliest Record: Shennong Bencao Jing
Part Used & Method for Pharmaceutical Preparations: The seeds are gathered in autumn when ripe and dried in the sun.
Properties & Taste: Bitter and slightly cold
Meridian: Liver
Functions: 1. To clear heat in the liver; 2. To brighten the eyes and reduce corneal opacity

Indications & Combinations: Flaring up of liver fire manifested as red, painful and swollen eyes, blurred vision and corneal opacity. Celosia seed (Qingxiangzi) is used with Cassia seed (Juemingzi), Chrysanthemum flower (Juhua) and Plantain seed (Cheqianzi).

Dosage: 3-15 g

b) Herbs That Clear Heat and Dry Dampness

Herbs which clear heat and dry dampness are characterized as bitter and cold. They are indicated in damp-heat disorders manifested as fever, sticky tongue coating, scanty urine, jaundice, dysentery and diarrhea, furuncles, eczema, abnormal vaginal discharge and turbid urine. The herbs in this category are likely to weaken the stomach and consume *yin*. They should be used with caution in cases with weakness of the spleen and stomach, or deficient body fluids. If necessary, the herbs can be combined with herbs that nourish *yin*.

39. Scutellaria root (Huangqin)

Pharmaceutical Name: Radidx Scutellariae
Botanical Name: Scutellaria baicalensis Georgi

Common Name: Scutellaria root, Scute, Skullcap

Source of Earliest Record: Shennong Bencao Jing

Part Used & Method for Pharmaceutical Preparations: The roots are dug in spring or autumn. The fibrous roots are removed and dried in the sun.

Properties & Taste: Bitter and cold

Meridians: Lung, gall bladder, stomach and large intestine

Functions: 1. To clear heat and dry dampness; 2. To reduce fire and release toxins; 3. To stop bleeding and calm fetus

Indications & Combinations:

1. Damp-heat syndromes: a) damp-heat febrile disease—Scutellaria root (Huangqin) is used with Talc (Huashi) and Rice paper pith (Tongcao); b) jaundice—Scutellaria root (Huangqin) is used with Cape-jasmine (Zhizi), Oriental wormwood (Yinchenhao) and Bamboo leaf (Zhuye); c) dysentery or diarrhea—Scutellaria root (Huangqin) is used with Coptis root (Huanglian); d) boils, carbuncles and furuncles—Scutellaria root (Huangqin) is used with Honeysuckle flower (Jinyinhua) and Trichosanthes root (Tianhuafen).

2. Cough due to heat in the lungs. Scutellaria root (Huangqin) is used with Mulberry bark (Sangbaipi) and Anemarrhena rhizome (Zhimu).

3. Hemorrhage due to heat in the blood manifested as vomiting with blood, epistaxis, hematuria and uterine bleeding. The carbonized Scutellaria root (Huangqin) is prepared and used with Fresh rehmannia root (Shengdihuang), Imperata rhizome (Baimaogen) and Biota tops (Cebaiye).

4. Threatened abortion (restless fetus). Scutellaria root (Huangqin) is used with Chinese angelica root (Danggui) and White atractylodes (Baizhu).

Dosage: 3-10 g

Cautions & Contraindications: This herb is contraindicated in cases with deficiency cold of the spleen and stomach. The raw herb is used to calm the fetus by clearing heat, the herb stir-baked in wine is used to stop bleeding, and the carbonized herb clears heat in the upper *jiao*.

40. Coptis root (Huanglian)

Pharmaceutical Name: Rhizoma Coptidis

Botanical Name: 1. Coptis chinensis Franch. C.; 2. Coptis diltoidea C.

Y. Cheng et Hsiao; 3. Coptis teetoides C. Y. Cheng

Common Name: Coptis root

Source of Earliest Record: Shennong Bencao Jing

Part Used & Method for Pharmaceutical Preparations: Five to seven year old roots, or rhizomes, are dug and gathered in autumn and dried for use, or fried with ginger juice.

Properties & Taste: Bitter and cold

Meridians: Heart, liver, stomach and large intestine

Functions: 1. To clear heat and dry dampness; 2. To reduce fire and dispel toxins

Indications & Combinations:

1. Damp-heat syndromes: a) damp-heat blocking the middle *jiao* manifested as a full sensation in the epigastric region and vomiting —Coptis root (Huanglian) is used with Scutellaria root (Huangqin), Pinellia tuber (Banxia) and Dried ginger (Ganjiang); b) damp-heat accumulated in the intestines manifested as diarrhea or dysentery —Coptis root (Huanglian) is used with Scutellaria root (Huangqin) and Pueraria root (Gegen); if the resulting manifestation is tenesmus, Coptis root (Huanglian) is used with Costus root (Muxiang) in the formula Xiang Lian Wan.

2. Liver fire attacking the stomach manifested as vomiting. Coptis root (Huanglian) is used with Evodia fruit (Wuzhuyu). If it is heat in the stomach which causes vomiting, Coptis root (Huanglian) is used with Bamboo shavings (Zhuru).

3. Febrile diseases manifested as high fever, irritability, loss of consciousness and delirium. Coptis root (Huanglian) is used with Gypsum (Shigao) and Capejasmine (Zhizi).

4. Boils, carbuncles and furuncles. Coptis root (Huanglian) is used with Scutellaria root (Huangqin), Honeysuckle flower (Jinyinhua), Forsythia fruit (Lianqiao) and Capejasmine (Zhizi).

5. Excessive fire in the stomach. If the manifestation is hunger after consuming sufficient food, Coptis root (Huanglian) is used with Fresh rehmannia root (Shengdihuang) and Trichosanthes root (Tianhuafen). If the manifestation is a toothache, Coptis root (Huanglian) is used with Cimicifuga rhizome (Shengma) and Fresh rehmannia root (Shengdihuang).

Dosage: 2-10 g

Cautions & Contraindications: This herb should be used with caution; large dosages may weaken the stomach.

41. Phellodendron bark (Huangbai)

Pharmaceutical Name: Cortex Phellodendri

Botanical Name: 1. Phellodendron amurense Rupr.; 2. Phellodendron chinense Schneid.

Common Name: Phellodendron bark

Source of Earliest Record: Shennong Bencao Jing

Part Used & Method for Pharmaceutical Preparations: The bark should be gathered during Pure Brightness (fifth solar term). After the coarse bark is peeled off, it is dried in the sun and cut into slices. The raw bark is used, or it can be fried with salt.

Properties & Taste: Bitter and cold

Meridians: Kidney, urinary bladder and large intestine

Functions: 1. To clear heat and dry dampness; 2. To reduce fire and release toxins

Indications & Combinations:

1. Damp-heat syndrome: a) damp-heat accumulated in intestines manifested as diarrhea and dysentery—Phellodendron bark (Huangbai) is used with Pulsatilla root (Baitouweng), Coptis root (Huanglian) and Scutellaria root (Huangqin); b) internal accumulation of damp-heat manifested as jaundice—Phellodendron bark (Huangbai) is used with Capejasmine (Zhizi) and Oriental wormwood (Yinchenhao); c) downward flowing of damp-heat, turbid urination and yellow, thick leukorrhea—Phellodendron bark (Huangbai) is used with Plantain seed (Cheqianzi), Bamboo leaf (Zhuye) and Clematis stem (Mutong); d) boils caused by dampness in the lower part of the body—Phellodendron bark (Huangbai) is used with Atractylodes rhizome (Cangzhu).

2. General boils, carbuncles, furuncles and eczema. Phellodendron bark (Huangbai) is used with Scutellaria root (Huangqin) and Capejasmine (Zhizi). For external use, Phellodendron bark (Huangbai) is pounded into a powder mixed with Talc (Huashi).

3. Deficiency of *yin* with heat manifested as noturnal emissions and night sweating. Phellodendron bark (Huangbai) is used with Anemarrhena rhizome (Zhimu) and Fresh rehmannia root (Shengdihuang).

Dosage: 3-10 g

Cautions & Contraindications: This herb is contraindicated in cases with weakness and cold in the spleen and stomach.

42. Chinese gentian (Longdancao)

Pharmaceutical Name: Radix Gentianae
Botanical Name: 1. Gentiana scabra Bge.; 2. Gentiana triflora Pall.; 3. Gentiana manshurica Kitag.
Common Name: Chinese gentian
Source of Earliest Record: Shennong Bencao Jing
Part Used & Method for Pharmaceutical Preparations: The roots, or rhizomes, are gathered in autumn, dried in the sun and cut into pieces.
Properties & Taste: Bitter and cold
Meridians: Liver, gall bladder and stomach
Functions: 1. To clear heat and dry dampness; 2. To reduce fire in the liver
Indications & Combinations:

1. Damp-heat syndrome: a) damp-heat jaundice—Chinese gentian (Longdancao) is used with Oriental wormwood (Yinchenhao) and Capejasmine (Zhizi); b) damp-heat leukorrhea manifested as pain and swelling in the genitals and eczema—Chinese gentian (Longdancao) is used with Phellodendron bark (Huangbai), Flavescent sophora root (Kushen) and Plantain seed (Cheqianzi).

2. Upward attack of liver fire manifested as headache, distending sensation in the head, red eyes, deafness and pain in the costal regions. Chinese gentian (Longdancao) is used with Scutellaria root (Huangqin), Capejasmine (Zhizi), Bupleurum root (Chaihu) and Clematis stem (Mutong).

3. Fever, spasms and convulsions. Chinese gentian (Longdancao) is used with Uncaria stem (Gouteng) and Ox gallstone (Niuhuang).

Dosage: 3-10 g
Cautions & Contraindications: This herb is contraindicated in cases with weakness and cold in the spleen and stomach.

43. Flavescent sophora root (Kushen)

Pharmaceutical Name: Radix Sophorae flavescentis
Botanical Name: Sophora flavescens Ait.
Common Name: Flavescent sophora root
Source of Earliest Record: Shennong Bencao Jing
Part Used & Method for Pharmaceutical Preparations: The roots are dug in spring or autumn. After the fibrous roots have been removed, the roots are cleaned, cut into slices and dried in the sun.

Properties & Taste: Bitter and cold

Meridians: Heart, liver, stomach, large intestine and urinary bladder

Functions: 1. To clear heat and dry dampness; 2. To promote urination; 3. To disperse wind and stop itching

Indications & Combinations:

1. Damp-heat syndrome: a) damp-heat jaundice—Flavescent sophora root (Kushen) is used with Phellodendron bark (Huangbai), Capejasmine (Zhizi), Chinese gentian (Longdancao) and Oriental wormwood (Yinchenhao); b) damp-heat diarrhea and dysentery—Flavescent sophora root (Kushen) is used with Costus root (Muxiang) and Licorice root (Gancao); c) damp-heat leukorrhea and eczema of the genitals—Flavescent sophora root (Kushen) is used with Phellodendron bark (Huangbai), Cnidium fruit (Shechuangzi) and Chinese gentian (Longdancao).

2. Skin diseases, including itching of the skin, scabies and impetigo. Flavescent sophora root (Kushen) can be used internally and externally. The herb is combined with Chinese angelica root (Danggui), Dittany bark (Baixianpi), Broom cypress fruit (Difuzi) and Red peony (Chishao).

3. Painful urination caused by damp-heat. Flavescent sophora root (Kushen) is used with Dandelion herb (Pugongying) and Pyrrosia leaf (Shiwei).

Dosage: 3-10 g

Cautions & Contraindications: This herb should never be used with the herb Black false bellebore (Lilu). It is contraindicated in cases with weakness and cold in the spleen and stomach.

c) Herbs That Clear Heat and Cool Blood

Herbs that clear heat and cool blood are indicated in syndromes due to excessive heat at the blood level. The clinical manifestations are shown in various hemorrhagic diseases, including epitaxis, bloody stool, blood in the urine, functional uterine bleeding, vomiting or spitting up blood, coughing up blood and bleeding of the gums. These herbs are also used for fever with loss of consciousness, deep red tongue and rapid pulse. This category of herbs tends to be bitter and sweet-salty in taste and cold in property.

44. Rhinoceros horn (Xijiao)

Pharmaceutical Name: Cornu Rhinoceri
Zoological Name: 1. Rhinoceros unicornis L.; 2. Rhinoceros sondai-
cus Desmarest; 3. Rhinoceros sumatrensis (Fischer)
Common Name: Rhinoceros horn
Source of Earliest Record: Shennong Bencao Jing
Part Used & Method for Pharmaceutical Preparations: The horn of
the African rhinoceros is sawn into small pieces. Then, the pieces are
steamed or boiled and cut into slices or ground into powder.
Properties & Taste: Bitter, salty and cold
Meridians: Heart, liver and stomach
Functions: 1. To clear heat and relieve convulsions; 2. To cool blood
and release toxins
Indications & Combinations:

1. Hemorrhagic disease due to extravasation of blood by heat
manifested as vomiting with blood, epistaxis and subcutaneous bleeding. Rhinoceros horn (Xijiao) is used with Fresh rehmannia root
(Shengdihuang), Moutan bark (Mudanpi) and Red peony (Chishao).

2. Fever, unconsciousness, delirium and convulsions. Rhinoceros
horn (Xijiao) is used with Isatis leaf (Daqingye), Gypsum (Shigao) and
Antelope's horn (Lingyangjiao).

Dosage: 1.5-6 g
Cautions & Contraindications: Rhinoceros horn should not be mixed
with Wild aconite root (Caowu) and Monkshood root (Chuanwu), and
it must be used with caution during pregnancy.

Note: Although rhinoceros horn is a traditional medicinal substance,
its scarcity encourages the common substitution of water buffalo's horn.

45. Fresh rehmannia root (Shengdihuang)

Pharmaceutical Name: Radix Rehmanniae
Botanical Name: Rehmannia gultinosa Libosch.
Common Name: Fresh rehmannia root
Source of Earliest Record: Shennong Bencao Jing
Part Used & Method for Pharmaceutical Preparations: The roots are
dug in spring or autumn. After the fibrous roots have been removed,
the roots are dried in the sun, and then cut into slices.
Properties & Taste: Sweet, bitter and cold
Meridians: Heart, liver and kidney

Functions: 1. To clear heat and cool blood; 2. To nourish *yin* and promote the production of body fluids

Indications & Combinations:

1. Exogenous heat invading at the nutritive and blood levels manifested as dry mouth and deep red tongue proper with scanty coating. Fresh rehmannia root (Shengdihuang) is used with Scrophularia (Xuanshen), Rhinoceros horn (Xijiao) and Ophiopogon root (Maidong).

2. *Yin* and body fluids consumed in the late stage of febrile diseases manifested as fever at night, and subsiding in the morning without presence of sweating. Fresh rehmannia root (Shengdihuang) is used with Anemarrhena rhizome (Zhimu), Sweet wormwood (Qinghao) and Turtle shell (Biejia).

3. Hemorrhaging due to extravasation of blood by heat manifested as vomiting with blood, epistaxis, blood in the urine, bloody stool and functional uterine bleeding. Fresh rehmannia root (Shengdihuang) is used with Biota tops (Cebaiye) and raw Lotus leaf (Heye).

4. Febrile disease with excessive toxic heat in the blood, epistaxis and maculopapule. Fresh rehmannia root (Shengdihuang) is used with Rhinoceros horn (Xijiao), Moutan bark (Mudanpi) and Red peony (Chishao).

5. Febrile disease with consumption of body fluids manifested as red tongue proper, dry mouth, thirst and excessive drinking. Fresh rehmannia root (Shengdihuang) is used with Fragrant solomonseal rhizome (Yuzhu), Ophiopogon root (Maidong), Glehnia root (Shashen) and Dendrobium (Shihu). If there is constipation, Fresh rehmannia root (Shengdihuang) is used with Scrophularia (Xuanshen) and Ophiopogon root (Maidong).

Dosage: 9–30 g

Cautions & Contraindications: This herb is contraindicated in cases with deficiency and excessive dampness in the spleen, full sensation in the abdominal region or diarrhea.

46. Scrophularia (Xuanshen)

Pharmaceutical Name: Radix Scrophulariae
Botanical Name: Scrophularia ningpoensiis Hemsl.
Common Name: Scrophularia root, Ningpo figwort root
Source of Earliest Record: Shennong Bencao Jing
Part Used & Method for Pharmaceutical Preparations: The roots are

dug in the period at the Beginning of Winter (nineteenth solar term) and dried in the sun until they are black on the inside, then they are cut into slices.

Properties & Taste: Bitter, sweet-salty and cold
Meridians: Lung, stomach and kidney
Functions: 1. To clear heat and nourish *yin*; 2. To release toxins and nodules

Indications & Combinations:

1. Sore throat caused by exogenous pathogenic wind. Scrophularia (Xuanshen) is used with Arctium fruit (Niubangzi), Platycodon root (Jiegeng) and Mentha (Bohe).

2. Sore throat caused by excessive interior heat. Scrophularia (Xuanshen) is used with Ophiopogon root (Maidong), Platycodon root (Jiegeng) and raw Licorice root (Gancao).

3. Boils carbuncles and furuncles. Scrophularia (Xuanshen) is used with Honeysuckle flower (Jinyinhua) and raw Licorice root (Gancao).

4. Scrofula, goiter and subcutaneous nodules. Scrophularia (Xuanshen) is used with Tendrilled fritillary bulb (Chuanbeimu) and Oyster shell (Muli).

5. Febrile disease in which pathogenic factors attack the nutritive and blood levels: a) thirst, fever, insomnia and deep red tongue proper with scanty coating—Scrophularia (Xuanshen) is used with Fresh rehmannia root (Shengdihuang) and Ophiopogon root (Maidong); b) high fever, unconsciousness and maculopapule—Scrophularia (Xuanshen) is used with Anemarrhena rhizome (Zhimu), Gypsum (Shigao) and Rhinoceros horn (Xijiao).

6. Constipation due to dryness in the intestines. Scrophularia (Xuanshen) is used with Fresh rehmannia root (Shengdihuang) and Ophiopogon root (Maidong).

Dosage: 10-15 g

Cautions & Contraindications: Scrophularia (Xuanshen) is contraindicated in cases with weakness of the spleen and stomach and should not be combined with Black false bellebore (Lilu).

47. Moutan bark (Mudanpi)

Pharmaceutical Name: Cortex Moutan
Botanical Name: Paeonia suffruticosa Andr.
Common Name: Moutan bark, Tree peony bark

Source of Earliest Record: Shennong Bencao Jing

Part Used & Method for Pharmaceutical Preparations: The roots are dug and gathered in autumn. After the fibrous roots have been removed, the roots are dried in the sun.

Properties & Taste: Bitter, pungent and slightly cold

Meridians: Heart, liver and kidney

Functions: 1. To clear heat and cool blood; 2. To invigorate blood and resolve blood stagnation

Indications & Combinations:

1. Febrile disease in which pathogenic heat enters the blood level manifested as fever, vomiting with blood, epistaxis, blood in the urine, maculopapule and deep red tongue proper. Moutan bark (Mudanpi) is used with Fresh rehmannia root (Shengdihuang), Rhinoceros horn (Xijiao) and Red peony (Chishao).

2. Late stage of febrile diseases with exhaustion of body fluids or *yin* deficiency manifested as fever at night, and subsiding in the morning, without presence of sweating, red tongue proper with scanty coating and thready, rapid pulse. Moutan bark (Mudanpi) is used with Anemarrhena rhizome (Zhimu), Fresh rehmannia root (Shengdihuang), Turtle shell (Biejia) and Sweet wormwood (Qinghao).

3. Blood stagnation manifested as amenorrhea, dysmenorrhea, hard masses, lumps, tumors and modules. Moutan bark (Mudanpi) is used with Peach seed (Taoren), Cinnamon twigs (Guizhi), Red peony (Chishao) and Poria (Fuling) in the formula Guizhi Fuling Wan.

4. Boil, carbuncles and furuncles. Moutan bark (Mudanpi) is used with Honeysuckle flower (Jinyinhua) and Forsythia fruit (Lianqiao).

Dosage: 6-12 g

Cautions & Contraindications: Care should be paid when it is used during excessive menstruation or pregnancy.

48. Red peony (Chishao)

Pharmaceutical Name: Radix Paeoniae Rubra

Botanical Name: 1. Paeonia lactiflora pall.; 2. Paeonia veitchii Lynch

Common Name: Red peony root

Source of Earliest Record: Shennong Bencao Jing

Part Used & Method for Pharmaceutical Preparations: The roots are dug in autumn. After the fibrous roots and rough bark have been removed, the roots are dried in the sun, soaked in water and cut into slices.

Properties & Taste: Bitter and slightly cold

Meridians: Liver

Functions: 1. To clear heat and cool blood; 2. To remove stagnant blood and reduce swelling

Indications & Combinations:

1. Febrile diseases in which exogenous pathogenic heat enters into the nutritive and blood levels manifested as maculopapule, vomiting with blood, epistaxis, and deep red tongue proper. Red peony (Chishao) is used with Fresh rehmannia root (Shengdihuang) and Moutan bark (Mudanpi).

2. Blood stagnation manifested as dysmenorrhea, amenorrhea, acute inflammation with red swelling and pain from external injury. Red peony (Chishao) is used with Chuanxiong rhizome (Chuanxiong), Chinese angelica root (Danggui), Peach seed (Taoren) and Safflower (Honghua).

3. Boils, carbuncles and furuncles. Red peony (Chishao) is used with Honeysuckle flower (Jinyinhua) and Forsythia fruit (Lianqiao).

Dosage: 3-10 g

Cautions & Contraindications: This herb should not be combined with Black false bellebore (Lilu).

49. Arnebia (Zicao)

Pharmaceutical Name: Radix Lithospermi seu Arnebiae

Botanical Name: 1. Lithospermun erythrorhizon sieb. et zucc; 2. Arnebia euchroma (Royle Johnst); 3. Macrotomia euchroma

Common Name: Lithospermun root, Arnebia root, Groomwell root

Source of Earliest Record: Shennong Bencao Jing

Part Used & Method for Pharmaceutical Preparations: The roots are dug in spring or autumn, dried in the sun, soaked in water and cut into slices.

· *Properties & Taste:* Sweet and cold

Meridians: Heart and liver

Functions: 1. To cool blood and invigorate blood; 2. To release toxins and bring the rash to the surface; 3. To promote bowel movement and moisten the intestines

Indications & Combinations:

1. Incomplete expression of rash in measles due to toxic heat in the

blood. Arnebia (Zicao) is used with Cicada slough (Chantui), Arctium fruit (Niubangzi).

2. Maculopapule in febrile disease. Arnebia (Zicao) is used with Red peony (Chishao), Moutan bark (Mudanpi), Honeysuckle flower (Jinyinhua) and Forsythia fruit (Lianqiao).

3. Prevention of measles. Arnebia (Zicao) is used with Licorice root (Gancao).

4. Boils, carbuncles, burns and injury due to cold. Arnebia (Zicao) is used with Chinese angelica root (Danggui), Dahurian angelica root (Baizhi) and Dragon's blood (Xuejie) as an external application in the formula Shengji Yuhong Gao.

Dosage: 3-10 g

Cautions & Contraindications: This herb is contraindicated during weakness of the spleen accompanied by diarrhea.

d) Herbs That Clear Heat and Release Toxins

The category of herbs that clear heat and release toxins is indicated in syndromes caused by excessive toxic heat, including boils, carbuncles, furuncles, maculopapule, erysipelas, sore throat and dysentery. Some of these herbs may help arrest cancerous growth and release the poison from snake bites.

50a. Honeysuckle flower (Jinyinhua)

Pharmaceutical Name: Flos Lonicerae

Botanical Name: 1. Lonicera japonica Thunb. L.; 2. Lonicera hypoglauca Miq.; 3. Lonicera confusa DC.; 4. Lonicera dsystyla Rehd.

Common Name: Honeysuckle flower, Lonicera flower

Source of Earliest Record: Mingyi Bielu

Part Used & Method for Pharmaceutical Preparations: The flower buds are gathered in the beginning of summer and dried in the shade.

Properties & Taste: Sweet and cold

Meridians: Lung, stomach and large intestine

Functions: To clear heat and release toxins

Indications & Combinations:

1. Febrile diseases: a) exogenous pathogenic heat at the defensive and *qi* levels manifested as fever, thirst, slight aversion to wind and cold and sore throat—Honeysuckle flower (Jinyinhua) is used with Forsythia fruit (Lianqiao) and Arctium fruit (Niubangzi); b) exogenous patho-

54

genic heat at the *qi* level manifested as high fever, extreme thirst and surging, big pulse—Honeysuckle flower (Jinyinhua) is used with Gypsum (Shigao) and Anemarrhena rhizome (Zhimu); c) exogenous pathogenic heat at the nutritive and blood levels manifested as maculopapule that appears as a dull, deep red and dry tongue, irritability and insomnia. Honeysuckle flower (Jinyinhua) is used with Moutan bark (Mudanpi) and Fresh rehmannia root (Shengdihuang).

2. Boils, carbuncles and furuncles. Honeysuckle flower (Jinyinhua) is used alone or is combined with Dandelion herb (Pugongying), Chrysanthemum flower (Juhua) and Forsythia fruit (Lianqiao).

3. Toxic heat diarrhea. Honeysuckle flower (Jinyinhua) is used with Coptis root (Huanglian) and Pulsatilla root (Baitouweng).

Dosage: 10-15 g

Cautions & Contraindications: This herb can be applied externally.

50b. Honeysuckle stem (Rendongteng)

The tender stems of lonicera japonica thunb have properties and taste similar to that of the flower, and are gathered in autumn or winter. The combination of Honeysuckle stem (Rendongteng), Forsythia fruit (Lianqiao) and Dandelion herb (Pugongying) is indicated for boils, carbuncles and furuncles. The combination of Honeysuckle stem (Rendongteng), Mulberry twigs (Sangzhi) and Chaenomeles fruit (Mugua) is used for wind-heat-damp arthralgia manifested as red, hot, painful and swollen joints with motor impairment. The dosage for medical use is 16-20 g.

51. Forsythia fruit (Lianqiao)

Pharmaceutical Name: Fructus Forsythiae
Botanical Name: Forsythia suspensa (Thunb.) Vahl
Common Name: Forsythia fruit
Source of Earliest Record: Shennong Bencao Jing
Part Used & Method for Pharmaceutical Preparations: The green fruit gathered in the period of White Dew (fifteenth solar term) is better than the yellow fruit picked in the period of Cold Dew (seventeenth solar term). The fruit is steamed, dried in the sun, and its seeds separated from the flesh.
Properties & Taste: Bitter and slightly cold

Meridians: Heart, lung and gall bladder

Functions: 1. To clear heat and release toxins; 2. To relieve carbuncles and disperse nodules

Indications & Combinations:

1. Febrile disease: a) exogenous pathogenic heat at the defensive *qi* level manifested as headache, fever, thirst and sore throat—Forsythia fruit (Lianqiao) is used with Arctium fruit (Niubangzi) and Mentha (Bohe); b) exogenous pathogenic heat entering the pericardium manifested as high fever, irritability and loss of consciousness—Forsythia fruit (Lianqiao) is used with Rhinoceros horn (Xijiao) and Lotus seed (Lianzi).

2. Boils, carbuncles and furuncles. Forsythia fruit (Lianqiao) is used with Wild chrysanthemum flower (Yejuhua) and Honeysuckle flower (Jinyinhua).

3. Scrofula. Forsythia fruit (Lianqiao) is used with Prunella spike (Xiakucao), Scrophularia (Xuanshen) and Tendrilled fritillary bulb (Chuanbeimu).

Dosage: 6-10 g

Cautions & Contraindications: This herb is contraindicated during heat in the blood due to deficient *yin*, diarrhea due to weakness of the spleen.

52. Dandelion herb (Pugongying)

Pharmaceutical Name: Herba taraxaci

Botanical Name: 1. Taraxacum mongolicum Hand.-Mazz.; 2. Taraxacum sinicum Kitag.

Common Name: Dandelion herb

Source of Earliest Record: Xinxiu Bencao

Part Used & Method for Pharmaceutical Preparations: The whole plant is gathered in summer or autumn, cleaned in water and then dried in the sun.

Properties & Taste: Bitter, sweet and cold

Meridians: Stomach and liver

Functions: 1. To clear heat and release toxins; 2. To resolve dampness

Indications & Combinations:

1. Boils, carbuncles and furuncles. Dandelion herb (Pugongying) is used with Viola (Zihuadiding), Wild chrysanthemum flower (Yejuhua)

and Honeysuckle flower (Jinyinhua).

2. Damp-heat jaundice. Dandelion herb (Pugongying) is used with Oriental wormwood (Yinchenhao).

3. Turbid urination. Dandelion herb (Pugongying) is used with Lysimachia (Jinqiancao) and Imperata rhizome (Baimaogen).

Dosage: 10-30 g

Cautions & Contraindications: Overdosing of this herb may cause mild diarrhea.

53. Viola (Zihuadiding)

Pharmaceutical Name: Herba violae

Botanical Name: 1. Viola yedoensis Mak.; 2. Viola prionantha Bge.; 3. Viola patrini DC.

Common Name: Viola herb, Yedoens violet

Source of Earliest Record: Bencao Gangmu

Part Used & Method for Pharmaceutical Preparations: The entire plant is gathered in summer, cleaned in water, dried in the sun and cut into pieces.

Properties & Taste: Bitter, pungent and cold

Meridians: Heart and liver

Functions: To clear heat and release toxins

Indications & Combinations:

1. Boils, carbuncles and furuncles. Viola (Zihuadiding) is used with Dandelion herb (Pugongying), Wild chrysanthemum flower (Yejuhua) and Honeysuckle flower (Jinyinhua).

2. Snake bite. The juice of the fresh herb is taken orally and externally.

Dosage: 10-16 g

Cautions & Contraindications: This herb is contraindicated in cases with deficient cold syndrome.

54. Isatis leaf (Daqingye)

Pharmaceutical Name: Folium Isatidis

Botanical Name: Isatis indigotia Fort.

Common Name: Isatis leaf

Source of Earliest Record: Mingyi Bielu

Part Used & Method for Pharmaceutical Preparations: The leaves are gathered in summer or autumn and dried in the sun.

Properties & Taste: Bitter and very cold
Meridians: Heart, lung and stomach
Functions: To clear heat and release toxins
Indications & Combinations:

1. Sore throat, erysipelas, boils, carbuncles and furuncles. Isatis leaf (Daqingye) is used with Scrophularia (Xuanshen) and Honeysuckle flower (Jinyinhua).

2. High fever with maculopapule. Isatis leaf (Daqingye) is used with Moutan bark (Mudanpi).

Dosage: 10-15 g

Cautions & Contraindications: This herb is contraindicated in cases with weakness and cold in the spleen and stomach.

55. Ox gallstone (Niuhuang)

Pharmaceutical Name: Calculus Bovis
Zoological Name: Bos taurus domesticus Gmelin
Common Name: Ox gallstone, Bos calculus
Source of Earliest Record: Shennong Bencao Jing
Part Used & Method for Pharmaceutical Preparations: The gallstone of an ox is collected in any season, or the bile of an ox or pig is used instead. After gathering, the material is dried and made into powder or pills.

Properties & Taste: Bitter and cool
Meridians: Liver and heart
Functions: 1. To clear heat and release toxins; 2. To eliminate endogenous wind and stop convulsions; 3. To resolve phlegm and promote resuscitation

Indications & Combinations:

1. Loss of consciousness and convulsions caused by high fever. Ox gallstone (Niuhuang) is used with Coptis root (Huanglian), Rhinoceros horn (Xijiao) and Musk (Shexiang) in the formula Angong Niuhuang Wan.

2. Sore throat or ulcers and boils due to accumulation of toxic heat. Ox gallstone (Niuhuang) is used with Natural indigo (Qingdai) and Honeysuckle flower (Jinyinhua).

Dosage: 0.2-0.5 g

Cautions & Contraindications: This substance is contraindicated during pregnancy.

56. Houttuynia (Yuxingcao)

Pharmaceutical Name: Herba Houttuyniae
Botanical Name: Houttuynia cordate Thunb.
Common Name: Houttuynia
Source of Earliest Record: Mingyi Bielu
Part Used & Method for Pharmaceutical Preparations: The entire plant is gathered in the time between summer and autumn. After gathering, it is cleaned and dried in the sun.
Properties & Taste: Pungent and slightly cold
Meridian: Lung
Functions: To clear heat and release toxins
Indications & Combinations:

1. Lung abscess manifested as cough with bloody and pus-like sputum. Houttuynia (Yuxingcao) is used with Platycodon root (Jiegeng) and Coix seed (Yiyiren).
2. Heat in the lungs manifested as cough with yellow and thick sputum. Houttuynia (Yuxingcao) is used with Mulberry bark (Sangbaipi) and Trichosanthes fruit (Gualou).
3. Boils and swelling due to toxic heat. Houttuynia (Yuxingcao) is used with Dandelion herb (Pugongying) and Forsythia fruit (Lianqiao).
Dosage: 15-30 g

57. Dittany bark (Baixianpi)

Pharmaceutical Name: Cortex Dictamni radicis
Botanical Name: Dictamnus dasycarpus Turcz.
Common Name: Dittany bark, Fraxinella
Source of Earliest Record: Shennong Bencao Jing
Part Used & Method for Pharmaceutical Preparations: The roots are dug in spring or autumn. After the fibrous roots have been removed, the bark is peeled off, cut into slices and dried in the sun.
Properties & Taste: Bitter and cold
Meridians: Spleen and stomach
Functions: 1. To clear heat and release toxins; 2. To remove damp and stop itching
Indications & Combinations: Boils and ulcers or itching of the skin. Dittany bark (Baixianpi) is used with Flavescent sophora root (Kushen), Phellodendron bark (Huangbai) and Atractylodes rhizome (Cangzhu).
Dosage: 6-10 g

58. Globethistle (Loulu)

Pharmaceutical Name: Radix Rhapontici seu Echinopsis
Botanical Name: 1. Rhaponticum uniflorum (L.) DC.; 2. Echinops latifolius Tausch.
Common Name: Globethistle
Source of Earliest Records: Shennong Bencao Jing
Part Used & Method for Pharmaceutical Preparations: The roots are dug in autumn. After the fibrous roots have been removed, the roots are cleaned, dried in the sun and cut into slices.
Properties & Taste: Bitter and cold
Meridian: Stomach
Functions: 1. To clear heat and release toxins; 2. To reduce swelling; 3. To promote lactation
Indications & Combinations:

1. Boils, carbuncles and swelling or swelling and pain in the breast area. Globethistle (Loulu) is used with Dandelion herb (Pugongying), Trichosanthes fruit (Gualou) and Forsythia fruit (Lianqiao).

2. Postpartum galactostasis with distension in the breasts. Globethistle (Loulu) is used with Vaccaria seed (Wangbuliuxing), Pangolin scales (Chuanshanjia) and Rice-paper pith (Tongcao).
Dosage: 3-12 g

59. Natural indigo (Qingdai)

Pharmaceutical Name: Indigo Naturalis
Botanical Name: A blue powder prepared from: 1. Baphicacanthus cusia (Acanthaceae); 2. Indigofera suffruticosa Mill. (Leguminosae); 3. Polygonum tinctorium Ait. (Polygonaceae); 4. Isatis indigotica Fort. (Cruciferae)
Common Name: Natural indigo
Source of Earliest Record: Yaoxing Lun
Part Used & Method for Pharmaceutical Preparations: The combination of pigments from Baphicacanthus cusia, Indigofera suffruticosa, Polygonum tinctorium and Isatis tinctoria is prepared and dried into a blue powder.
Properties & Taste: Salty and cold
Meridians: Liver, lung and stomach
Functions: 1. To clear heat and release toxins; 2. To cool blood and reduce swelling

60

Indications & Combinations:

1. Eruptions due to toxic heat in the blood. Natural indigo (Qingdai) is used with Gypsum (Shigao) and Fresh rehmannia root (Shengdihuang) in the formula Qingdai Shigao Tang.

2. Hemorrhagic disease due to extravasation of the blood by heat manifested as vomiting of blood, epistaxis and cough with blood and sputum. Natural indigo (Qingdai) is used with Biota tops (Cebaiye) and Imperata rhizome (Baimaogen).

3. Infantile convulsions due to high fever. Natural indigo (Qingdai) is used with Ox gallstone (Niuhuang) and Uncaria stem (Gouteng) in the formula Liang Jing Wan.

4. Heat in the lungs manifested as cough, asthma and cough with thick yellow sputum. Natural indigo (Qingdai) is used with Trichosanthes fruit (Gualou), Tendrilled fritillary bulb (Chuanbeimu) and Costazia bone (Haifushi) in the formula Qingdai Haishi Wan.

5. Acute mumps, boils and carbuncles. Natural indigo (Qingdai) is used with Scrophularia (Xuanshen), Honeysuckle flower (Jinyinhua) and Forsythia fruit (Lianqiao).

Dosage: 1.5-3 g

Cautions & Contraindications: This substance is contraindicated during a cold in the stomach.

60. Pulsatilla root (Baitouweng)

Pharmaceutical Name: Radix Pulsatillae
Botanical Name: Pulsatilla chinensis (Bge.) Regel
Common Name: Pulsatilla root, Anemone
Source of Earliest Record: Shennong Bencao Jing
Part Used & Method for Pharmaceutical Preparations: The roots are dug in spring or late autumn, cleaned and dried in the sun.
Properties & Taste: Bitter and cold
Meridian: Large intestine
Functions: 1. To clear heat and release toxins; 2. To cool the blood and stop dysentery

Indications & Combinations: Dysentery, manifested as fever, abdominal pain, bloody and pus-like stool and tenesmus. Pulsatilla root (Baitouweng) is used with Phellodendron bark (Huangbai) and Coptis root (Huanglian) in a formula such as Baitouweng Tang.

Dosage: 6-15 g

61. Portulaca (Machixian)

Pharmaceutical Name: Herba portulacae
Botanical Name: Portulaca oleracea L.
Common Name: Purslane, Portulaca
Source of Earliest Record: Xinxiu Bencao
Part Used & Method for Pharmaceutical Preparations: The entire plant is gathered in summer, steamed or boiled and then dried in the sun.
Properties & Taste: Sour and cold
Meridians: Large intestine and liver
Functions: 1. To clear heat and release toxins; 2. To cool the blood and stop dysentery
Indications & Combinations: Dysentery manifested as fever, abdominal pain, blood and pus in the stool and tenesmus. Portulaca (Machixian) is used with Scutellaria root (Huangqin) and Coptis root (Huanglian). Also, Portulaca (Machixian) can be taken alone as treatment for these symptoms.
Dosage: 30–60 g (double dosage for the fresh herb)

62. Green chiretta (Chuanxinlian)

Pharmaceutical Name: Herb Andrographitis
Botanical Name: Andrographis paniculata (Burm. f.) Nees
Common Name: Green chiretta, Kariyat
Source of Earliest Record: Lingnan Caoyao Lu
Part Used & Method for Pharmaceutical Preparations: The aerial parts of the plant are gathered in the early autumn when the plant begins to flower. Then it is cut into pieces and dried.
Properties & Taste: Bitter and cold
Meridians: Lung, stomach, large and small intestines
Functions: 1. To clear heat and release toxins; 2. To dry dampness
Indications & Combinations:

1. The beginning of warm febrile disease manifested as fever, headache and sore throat. Green chiretta (Chuanxinlian) is used with Honeysuckle flower (Jinyinhua), Platycodon root (Jiegeng) and Arctium fruit (Niubangzi).

2. Heat in the lungs manifested as cough and asthma or cough with yellow sputum. Green chiretta (Chuanxinlian) is used with Houttuynia (Yuxingcao), Platycodon root (Jiegeng) and Trichosanthes fruit (Gua-

lou).

3. Dysentery due to dampness and heat. Green chiretta (Chuanxin-lian) is used with Portulaca (Machixian).

Dosage: 6-15 g

Cautions & Contraindications: Prolonged overdosing of this herb may impair stomach *qi*.

e) Herbs That Clear Heat Caused by *Yin* Deficiency

Herbs that clear heat caused by *yin* deficiency are indicated in deficiency of *yin* with heat syndrome manifested as fever, afternoon fever, feverish sensation in the palms, soles and chest, night sweating, red tongue proper with scanty coating and thready, rapid pulse.

These herbs are often combined with herbs that nourish *yin* to strengthen the function of clearing heat caused by *yin* deficiency. In addition, some of these herbs are indicated in the late stage of febrile disease caused by invasion of exogenous pathogenic heat, in which *yin* and body fluids are damaged and pathogenic factors remain inside. The commonly seen manifestations are fever, fever at night, and fever subsiding in the morning without presence of sweating.

In general, these herbs are not suitable for fever due to common cold and cases of deficiency of *yin* and blood without heat signs.

63. Sweet wormwood (Qinghao)

Pharmaceutical Name: Herba artemisiae annuae
Botanical Name: Artemisia annua L.
Common Name: Sweet wormwood
Source of Earliest Record: Shennong Bencao Jing
Part Used & Method for Pharmaceutical Preparations: The entire plant is gathered in summer or autumn, dried in the shade and cut into pieces.

` *Properties & Taste:* Bitter, pungent and cold
Meridians: Liver, gall bladder and kidney
Functions: 1. To reduce heat caused by deficient *yin*; 2. To cool blood and release summer heat; 3. To relieve malaria
Indications & Combinations:

1. Malaria. Sweet wormwood (Qinghao) is used alone or with Scutellaria root (Huangqin) and Pinellia tuber (Banxia) in the formula Hao Qin Qingdan Tang.

2. Late stage of febrile disease, with pathogenic heat damaging *yin* and body fluids, manifested as fever, fever at night, and subsiding in the morning without presence of sweating, red tongue proper with scanty coating and thready, rapid pulse. Sweet wormwood (Qinghao) is used with Turtle shell (Biejia), Moutan bark (Mudanpi) and Fresh rehmannia root (Shengdihuang) in the formula Qinghao Biejia Tang.

3. Heat signs due to deficient *yin* manifested as afternoon fever and night sweating. Sweet wormwood (Qinghao) is used with Large-leaf gentian root (Qinjiao), Turtle shell (Biejia) and Anemarrhena rhizome (Zhimu).

4. Invasion by summer-heat manifested as fever, dizziness and headache. Sweet wormwood (Qinghao) is used with Mung bean (Ludou) and Lotus leaf (Heye).

Dosage: 3-10 g

Cautions & Contraindications: This herb should not be boiled for a long time.

64. Swallowwort root (Baiwei)

Pharmaceutical Name: Radix Cynanchi

Botanical Name: 1. Cynanchum atratum Bge.; 2. Cynanchum versicolor Bge.

Common Name: Swallowwort root

Source of Earliest Record: Shennong Bencao Jing

Part Used & Method for Pharmaceutical Preparations: The roots, or rhizomes, are gathered in autumn and dried in the sun.

Properties & Taste: Bitter, salty and cold

Meridians: Stomach and liver

Functions: 1. To clear heat and cool blood; 2. To benefit urination and relieve urinary tract infection

Indications & Combinations:

1. Internal heat and deficient *yin* manifested as afternoon fever and night sweating or as febrile disease due to exogenous pathogenic heat at the nutritive and blood levels and accompanied by sustained fever. Swallowwort root (Baiwei) is used with Wolfberry bark (Digupi) and Fresh rehmannia root (Shengdihuang).

2. Postpartum fever caused by deficient *yin*. Swallowwort root (Baiwei) is used with Ginseng (Renshen) and Chinese angelica root (Danggui).

3. Urinary tract infection manifested as heat syndrome or bloody urine. Swallowwort root (Baiwei) is used with Lophatherum (Danzhuye), Clematis stem (Mutong) and Talc (Huashi).

4. Boils, carbuncles, sore throat and snake bite. Swallowwort root (Baiwei) is used externally and internally.

Dosage: 3-12 g

65. Wolfberry bark (Digupi)

Pharmaceutical Name: Cortex Lycii
Botanical Name: 1. Lycium chinensis Mill.; 2. Lycium barbarum L.
Common Name: Wolfberry bark, Lycium bark
Source of Earliest Record: Shennong Bencao Jing
Part Used & Method for Pharmaceutical Preparations: The roots are dug in spring or autumn. The bark is peeled off the roots, dried in the sun and cut into pieces.
Properties & Taste: Sweet or tasteless and cold
Meridians: Lung and kidney
Functions: 1. To cool blood; 2. To clear heat in the lungs
Indications & Combinations:

1. Heat in the blood and deficient *yin* manifested as afternoon fever and night sweating. Wolfberry bark (Digupi) is used with Anemarrhena rhizome (Zhimu) and Turtle shell (Biejia).

2. Heat in the lungs and deficient *yin* manifested as cough, asthma and cough with blood. Wolfberry bark (Digupi) is used with Imperata rhizome (Baimaogen) and Biota tops (Cebaiye).

Dosage: 6-15 g

Cautions & Contraindications: This herb is contraindicated in cases with fever due to common cold or weakness of the spleen accompanied by diarrhea.

66. Stellaria root (Yinchaihu)

Pharmaceutical Name: Radix Stellariae
Botanical Name: Stellaria dichotoma L. var. lanceolata Bge.
Common Name: Stellaria root
Source of Earliest Record: Bencao Gangmu Shiyi
Part Used & Method for Pharmaceutical Preparations: The roots are dug in autumn or the Beginning of Spring (first solar term). After the fibrous roots are removed, the roots are cleaned in water, dried in the

sun and cut into slices.

Properties & Taste: Sweet and slightly cold

Meridians: Liver and stomach

Functions: 1. To reduce heat caused by deficient *yin*; 2. To clear heat in infants caused by malnutrition

Indications & Combinations:

1. Heat signs due to deficiency of *yin* manifested as afternoon fever and night sweating. Stellaria root (Yinchaihu) is used with Sweet wormwood (Qinghao), Turtle shell (Biejia) and Wolfberry bark (Digupi) in the formula Qinggu San.

2. Infantile malnutrition manifested as swollen abdomen and emaciation. Stellaria root (Yinchaihu) is used with Capejasmine (Zhizi), Pilose asiabell root (Dangshen) and Scutellaria root (Huangqin) in the formula Chaihu Qinggan Tang.

Dosage: 3-10 g

Cautions & Contraindications: This herb is contraindicated in fever due to invasion by exogenous pathogenic wind and cold, or in cases with deficient blood syndrome but no signs of heat.

III. Purgative Herbs

Purgative herbs either stimulate or lubricate the large intestine to promote bowel movement. They are mainly indicated in constipation. Through the function of purgation, impacted feces and fluid remaining in the intestines are discharged, pathogenic heat or cold dispelled and edema relieved.

Based on their functions and indications, the herbs are divided into three classes: herbs that purge feces, herbs that lubricate intestines and herbs that transform water.

Notes in application:

a) When interior syndrome occurs with exterior syndrome, these herbs are used with herbs that release the exterior syndrome. Alternatively, herbs that release the exterior are given first, then the herbs that treat the interior syndrome.

b) When body resistance (anti-pathogenic factor) is weak, these herbs are used with tonifyiny herbs.

c) These herbs should be used with caution during weakness of the body due to chronic disease, during menstruation, pregnancy and after delivery.

d) Since the herbs induce diarrhea, they should not be used once the bowel movement has become normal.

a) Herbs That Purge

Herbs that purge cause diarrhea. They are bitter and cold in property, and function to reduce fire and promote bowel movement. They are indicated in retention of feces due to accumulation of excessive heat in the stomach and intestines. They are often used with herbs that promote *qi* circulation and with herbs that clear heat and drain feces downward.

67. Rhubarb (Dahuang)

Pharmaceutical Name: Radix et Rhizoma rhei
Botanical Name: 1. Rheum palmatum L.; 2. Rheum officinale Baill.; 3. Rheum tanguticum Maxim. ex Balf.
Common Name: Rhubarb
Source of Earliest Record: Shennong Bencao Jing
Part Used & Method for Pharmaceutical Preparations: The roots, or rhizomes, are dug in autumn or spring. After the fibrous roots and bark have been removed, the roots are cut into pieces and dried in the sun.
Properties & Taste: Bitter and cold
Meridians: Spleen, stomach, large intestine and liver
Functions: 1. To promote bowel movement; 2. To reduce fire and release toxins; 3. To invigorate blood
Indications & Combinations:

1. Constipation: a) heat accumulated in constipation—Rhubarb (Dahuang) is used with Glauber's salt (Mangxiao) in the formula Da Chengqi Tang; b) cold accumulation in constipation—Rhubarb (Dahuang) is used with Prepared aconite root (Fuzi) and Dried ginger (Ganjiang) in the formula Wenpi Tang; c) constipation with heat accumulation and damage to *yin*—Rhubarb (Dahuang) is used with Fresh rehmannia root (Shengdihuang), Scrophularia (Xuanshen) and Ophiopogon root (Maidong) in the formula Zengye Chengqi Tang.

2. Extravasation due to heat in the blood manifested as vomiting with blood and epistaxis, or upward attack by pathogenic fire manifested as red, painful and swollen eyes, sore throat and painful and swollen gums. These two syndromes are treated by combining Rhubarb (Da-

huang), Coptis root (Huanglian) and Scutellaria root (Huangqin) in the formula Xiexin Tang.

3. Boils, carbuncles and furuncles. Rhubarb (Dahuang) is used with Peach seed (Taoren) and Moutan bark (Mudanpi).

4. Stagnation of blood manifested as amenorrhea, postpartum retention of lochia, postpartum abdominal pain, abdominal masses and traumatic injury. Rhubarb (Dahuang) is used with Chuanxiong rhizome (Chuanxiong), Peach seed (Taoren), Safflower (Honghua) and Moutan bark (Mudanpi).

Dosage: 3-12 g

Cautions & Contraindications: The raw herb is strong in moving feces. Fried with wine, the herb is good for invigorating blood. The carbonized herb is applied during hemorrhagic disease. Overboiling of the herb weakens the function of purgation. This herb is contraindicated during menstruation and pregnancy.

68. Glauber's salt (Mangxiao)

Pharmaceutical Name: Natrii Sulfas
Mineral Name: 1. Mirabilite; 2. Glauber's salt; 3. Sodium sulfate
Common Name: Mirabilite, Glauber's salt
Source of Earliest Record: Mingyi Bielu
Part Used & Method for Pharmaceutical Preparations: Sodium sulfate
Properties & Taste: Salty, bitter and cold
Meridians: Stomach and large intestine
Functions: 1. To purge feces downward; 2. To soften hardness; 3. To clear heat
Indications & Combinations:

1. Constipation. Glauber's salt (Mangxiao) is used with Rhubarb (Dahuang) in the formula Dachengqi Tang.

2. Sore throat, ulcerated mouth, red eyes or boils. Glauber's salt (Mangxiao) is used with Sodium borate (Pengsha) and Borneol (Bingpian) for external use.

Dosage: 10-15 g

Cautions & Contraindications: This herb is contraindicated during pregnancy.

69. Senna leaf (Fanxieye)

Pharmaceutical Name: Folium Sennae

Botanical Name: 1. Cassia angustifolia Vahl; 2. Cassia acutifolia Delile
Common Name: Senna leaf
Source of Earliest Record: Yaoxue Dacidian
Part Used & Method for Pharmaceutical Preparations: The leaves are gathered in September and cleaned and dried in the sun.
Properties & Taste: Sweet, bitter and cold
Meridian: Large intestine
Functions: To purge feces downward
Indications & Combinations: Constipation. Senna leaf (Fanxieye) is used alone, or it is used with Immature bitter orange (Zhishi) and Magnolia bark (Houpo).
Dosage: 1.5–3 g for mild constipation; 3–10 g for severe constipation
Cautions & Contraindications: This herb is contraindicated during menstruation, lactation and pregnancy.

70. Aloes (Luhui)

Pharmaceutical Name: Aloe
Botanical Name: 1. Aloe vera L.; 2. Aloe ferox Mill.
Common Name: Aloes
Source of Earliest Record: Yaoxing Lun
Part Used & Method for Pharmaceutical Preparations: The leaves are gathered all year round. The juice is squeezed out of the leaves, boiled until it makes a thick soup and then put into a container and stored in a cool place.
Properties & Taste: Bitter and cold
Meridians: Liver and large intestine
Functions: 1. To purge feces; 2. To clear heat in the liver; 3. To kill worms
Indications & Combinations:

1. Constipation accompanied by excessive fire in the liver meridian manifested as constipation, dizziness, headache and irritability. Aloes (Luhui) is used with Chinese gentian (Longdancao), Capejasmine (Zhizi), Natural indigo (Qingdai) and Chinese angelica root (Danggui) in the formula Danggui Luhui Wan.

2. Abdominal pain caused by accumulation of worms manifested as sallow complexion and emaciation. Aloes (Luhui) is used with herbs that kill worms, in a formula such as Feier Wan.
Dosage: 1-2 g

Cautions & Contraindications: This herb is combined with other herbs in pills or powder, but should not be used in a decoction. It is contraindicated during pregnancy and in cases with weakness of the spleen and stomach manifested as poor appetite or diarrhea.

b) Herbs That Lubricate the Intestines

These herbs are mostly seeds of plants which contain oil that lubricates the intestines and moves the stool. They are indicated in constipation due to deficient body fluids in an aged person or weakness of the body due to chronic disease. This category of herbs is often used in combination with herbs that nourish blood or promote circulation of *qi*, so as to strengthen the function of lubricating intestines for normal bowel movement.

71. Hemp seed (Huomaren)

Pharmaceutical Name: Fructus Cannabis
Botanical Name: Cannabis sativa L.
Common Name: Cannabis seed, Hemp seed
Source of Earliest Record: Shennong Bencao Jing
Part Used & Method for Pharmaceutical Preparations: The ripe seeds are gathered in autumn, cleaned and dried in the sun. This herb must be ground in a mortar and pestle before use.
Properties & Taste: Sweet and neutral
Meridians: Spleen and large intestine
Functions: To lubricate intestines and move feces
Indications & Combinations:

1. Constipation due to dryness in the intestines. Hemp seed (Huomaren) is used with Chinese angelica root (Danggui), Prepared rehmannia root (Shudihuang) and Apricot seed (Xingren) in the formula Yixue Runchang Wan.

2. Constipation with hemorrhoids due to dryness and heat in the large intestine. Hemp seed (Huomaren) is used with Rhubarb (Dahuang) and Magnolia bark (Houpo) in the formula Maziren Wan.

Dosage: 10-30 g
Cautions & Contraindications: This herb is contraindicated in cases with diarrhea.

72. Bush-cherry seed (Yuliren)

Pharmaceutical Name: Semen pruni
Botanical Name: 1. Prunus japonica Thunb.; 2. Prunus humilis Bge.;
3. Prunus tomentosa Thunb.
Common Name: Bush-cherry seed
Source of Earliest Record: Shennong Bencao Jing
Part Used & Method for Pharmaceutical Preparations: The ripe seeds
from the fruit are gathered in autumn and dried in the sun. The seeds
are then ground in a mortar and pestle.
Properties & Taste: Pungent, bitter and neutral
Meridians: Small and large intestines
Functions: 1. To lubricate intestines and move feces; 2. To promote
urination and reduce edema
Indications & Combinations:

1. Constipation due to dryness in the intestines. Bush-cherry seed
(Yuliren) is used with Apricot seed (Xingren), Peach seed (Taoren) and
Arborvitae seed (Baiziren) in the formula Wuren Wan.

2. Edema. Bush-cherry seed (Yuliren) is used with Mulberry bark
(Sangbaipi), Phaseolus seed (Chixiaodou) and Imperata rhizome (Bai-
maogen) in the formula Yuliren Tang.
Dosage: 5-12 g
Cautions & Contraindications: This herb is contraindicated in cases
with depletion of body fluids, or during pregnancy.

c) Herbs That Transform Water

These herbs purge water. They cause the discharge of water,
together with feces, from the body. Some of these herbs promote
urination and are indicated in cases with edema in the limbs, ascites,
fullness in the chest and asthma due to phlegm-dampness.

These herbs are toxic; overdosing or prolonged administration is
very harmful to the health. When symptoms are relieved, the herbs
should be stopped.

73. Genkwa flower (Yuanhua)

Pharmaceutical Name: Flos Genkwa
Botanical Name: Daphne genkwa Sieb. et Zucc.
Common Name: Genkwa flower

Source of Earliest Record: Shennong Bencao Jing

Part Used & Method for Pharmaceutical Preparations: The flower buds are gathered in spring and dried in the sun, baked or fried with vinegar.

Properties & Taste: Pungent, bitter, warm and toxic

Meridians: Lung, kidney and large intestine

Functions: 1. To transform water and stop cough; 2. To resolve phlegm and stop cough; 3. To kill worms

Indications & Combinations:

1. Edema in the face or body, ascites and retention of fluid in the chest. Genkwa flower (Yuanhua) is used with Kansui root (Gansui) and Peking spurge root (Daji) in the formula Shizao Tang.

2. Sudden cough and cold-damp type of chronic bronchitis. Genkwa flower (Yuanhua) is used with Jujube (Dazao).

3. Scabs, white ringworm and stubborn ringworm. Genkwa flower (Yuanhua) is ground into powder and combined with powdered Realgar (Xionghuang) and pig fat oil for external application.

Dosage: 1.5-3 g

Cautions & Contraindications: This herb must not be used with Licorice root (Gancao) as it counteracts it, and Genkwa flower (Yuanhua) is contraindicated during pregnancy.

74. Kansui root (Gansui)

Pharmaceutical Name: Radix kansui

Botanical Name: Euphorbia kansui T. N. Liou ex T. P. Wang

Common Name: Kansui root

Source of Earliest Record: Shennong Bencao Jing

Part Used & Method for Pharmaceutical Preparations: The tuberous root is dug in late autumn or early spring. The root bark is peeled off, and the root is dried in the sun. Then it is soaked in vinegar.

Properties & Taste: Bitter, sweet, cold and toxic

Meridians: Lung, kidney and large intestine

Functions: 1. To transform water and reduce edema; 2. To disperse nodules and relieve swelling

Indications & Combinations:

1. Edema and full sensation in abdominal region. Kansui root (Gansui) is used with Pharbitis seed (Qianniuzi) in the formula Erqi Tang.

2. Ascites. Kansui root (Gansui) is used with Peking spurge root (Daji) and Genkwa flower (Yuanhua) in the formula Shizao Tang.

3. Retention of water or fluid in the chest. Kansui root (Gansui) is used with Rhubarb (Dahuang) and Glauber's salt (Mangxiao) in the formula Da Xianxiong Tang.

4. Boils, carbuncles and furuncles. Kansui root (Gansui) is ground into powder and mixed with water for external application.

Dosage: 0.5-1 g

Cautions & Contraindications: This herb is best used in pill and powder form. It should not be used with the herb Licorice root (Gancao) and is contraindicated during pregnancy.

75. Peking spurge root (Daji)

Pharmaceutical Name: Radix Euphorbiae seu Knoxiae

Botanical Name: 1. Euphorbia pekinesis Rupr.; 2. Knoxia valerianoides Thorel et Pitard

Common Name: Euphorbia root, Peking spurge root

Source of Earliest Record: Shennong Bencao Jing

Part Used & Method for Pharmaceutical Preparations: The roots are dug in autumn or spring. After the fibrous roots have been removed, the roots are cleaned and dried in the sun, and then they are soaked in vinegar.

Properties & Taste: Bitter, pungent, cold and poisonous

Meridians: Lung, kidney and large intestine

Functions: 1. To transform water and reduce edema; 2. To disperse nodules and relieve swelling

Indications & Combinations:

1. Edema of the face and the body, retention of fluid in the chest and ascites. Peking spurge root (Daji) is used with Jujube (Dazao), Kansui root (Gansui) and Genkwa flower (Yuanhua) in the formula Shizao Tang.

2. Boils, carbuncles, scrofula and subcutaneous nodules. Peking spurge root (Daji) is used with Pleione rhizome (Shancigu) and Moleplant seed (Qianjinzi) for internal and external use in the formula Zijin Ding.

Dosage: 1.5-3 g

Cautions & Contraindications: This herb should not be mixed with Licorice root (Gancao), and it is contraindicated during pregnancy.

76. Croton seed (Badou)

Pharmaceutical Name: Semen Crotonis
Botanical Name: Croton tiglium L.
Common Name: Croton seed
Source of Earliest Record: Shennong Bencao Jing
Part Used & Method for Pharmaceutical Preparations: The ripe seeds are gathered in autumn, dried in the sun and ground into powder.
Properties & Taste: Pungent and very toxic
Meridians: Stomach and large intestine
Functions: 1. To drain accumulated cold downward; 2. To transform water and reduce edema; 3. To resolve phlegm and benefit throat
Indications & Combinations:

1. Abdominal pain and constipation due to cold or retention of food in the intestines. Croton seed (Badou) is used with Rhubarb (Dahuang) and Dried ginger (Ganjiang) in the formula Sanwu Beiji Wan.

2. Retention of milk in babies, profuse sputum and infantile convulsions. Croton seed (Badou) is used with Medicated leaven (Shenqu), Arisaema tuber with bile (Dannanxing) and Cinnabar (Zhusha) in the formula Baochi San.

3. Ascites. Croton seed (Badou) is used with Apricot seed (Xingren).

4. Pharyngitis, excessive sputum blocking the windpipe, rapid breathing and even suffocation. The powder of Croton seed (Badou) is blown into the throat to cause vomiting.

5. Boils and carbuncles. Croton seed (Badou) is used externally.
Dosage: 0.1-0.3 g
Cautions & Contraindications: This herb is contraindicated during pregnancy. It must not be mixed with the herb Pharbitis flower (Qianniuhua). No hot food or drinks should be consumed while administering the herb.

IV. Herbs That Expel Wind and Dampness

These herbs expel wind and dampness from skin, muscles, channels and collaterals. They relax tendons, promoting circulation of channels and collaterals, stopping pain and strengthening joints and bones. Their main indications are wind-damp obstruction pain, migrating pain, spasm of tendons, numbness of muscles, hemiplegia, soreness and pain in the lower back and knees and flaccid lower limbs.

The selection of herbs for obstruction-type pain is based on the nature and location of the obstruction. For example, if the exterior is attacked by pathogenic factors, these herbs are used with herbs that expel wind and release exterior syndrome. If the collaterals are affected by pathogenic factors, these herbs are used with herbs that invigorate circulation of *qi* and blood. In excessive cold and dampness, these herbs are used with herbs that warm the channels. For a patient with heat due to prolonged accumulation of pathogenic factors, these herbs are taken with herbs that clear heat.

As some herbs in this category are pungent, warm and dry in taste and properties, they are apt to consume *yin* and blood; therefore, care should be taken in their use when a person suffers from deficiency of *yin* and blood.

77. Pubescent angelica root (Duhuo)

Pharmaceutical Name: Radix Angelicae pubescentis
Botanical Name: Angelica pubescens Maxim. f. biserrata Shan et Yuan
Common Name: Pubescent angelica root
Source of Earliest Record: Shennong Bencao Jing
Part Used & Method for Pharmaceutical Preparations: The roots are dug in spring or autumn and then baked and cut into slices after the fibrous parts have been removed.
Properties & Taste: Pungent, bitter and warm
Meridians: Liver, kidney and urinary bladder
Functions: 1. To expel wind and dampness; 2. To stop pain; 3. To release the exterior and disperse cold
Indications & Combinations:

1. Wind-damp obstruction syndrome (rheumatic pain). Pubescent angelica root (Duhuo) is used with Large-leaf gentian root (Qinjiao), Ledebouriella root (Fangfeng) and Mulberry mistletoe (Sangjisheng) in the formula Duhuo Jisheng Tang.

2. Wind-cold type of exterior syndrome. Pubescent angelica root (Duhuo) is used with Notopterygium root (Qianghuo) in the formula Qianghuo Shengshi Tang.

Dosage: 3-10 g

Cautions & Contraindications: This herb is contraindicated in cases with syndromes of deficient *yin* or blood with heat and pain.

78. Clematis root (Weilingxian)

Pharmaceutical Name: Radix Clematidis
Botanical Name: 1. Clematis chinensis Osbeck; 2. Clematis hexapetala Pall.
Common Name: Clematis root
Source of Earliest Record: Xinxiu Bencao
Part Used & Method for Pharmaceutical Preparations: The roots, or rhizomes, are dug and gathered in autumn and then cleaned and dried in the sun.
Properties & Taste: Pungent, salty and warm
Meridians: Urinary bladder
Functions: 1. To dispel wind and damp; 2. To promote the circulation of meridians
Indications & Combinations:

1. Wind-damp obstruction syndrome manifested as rheumatic pain, soreness, pain and numbness in the joints and motor impairment. Clematis root (Weilingxian) is used with Pubescent angelica root (Duhuo), Mulberry mistletoe (Sangjisheng) and Chinese angelica root (Danggui).

2. Fish bone stuck in the throat. The decoction of the herb is taken orally with vinegar.

Dosage: 5-10 g

Cautions & Contraindications: This herb is contraindicated in a person with a weak constitution.

79. Tetrandra root (Fangji)

Pharmaceutical Name: Radix Stephaniae tetrandrae
Botanical Name: 1. Stephania tetrandra S. Moore; 2. Cocculus trilobus (Thunb.) DC.; 3. Aristolochia fangchi Wu et L. D. Chou et S. M. Hwang
Common Name: Stephania root, Tetrandra root
Source of Earliest Record: Shennong Bencao Jing
Part Used & Method for Pharmaceutical Preparations: The roots are dug in autumn. After the root bark has been removed, the roots are

cleaned, dried in the sun and cut into pieces or slices.

Properties & Taste: Bitter, pungent and cold

Meridians: Urinary bladder, kidney and spleen

Functions: 1. To dispel wind and dampness; 2. To stop pain; 3. To relieve edema

Indications & Combinations:

1. Wind-damp obstruction syndrome or damp-heat obstruction syndrome. Tetrandra root (Fangji) is used with Coix seed (Yiyiren), Talc (Huashi), Silkworm excrement (Cansha) and Chaenomeles fruit (Mugua).

2. Cold-damp obstruction syndrome. Tetrandra root (Fangji) is used with Cinnamon twigs (Guizhi) and Prepared aconite root (Fuzi).

3. Edema: a) edema with heat signs—Tetrandra root (Fangji) is used with Lepidium seed (Tinglizi) and Zanthoxylum (Jiaomu) in the formula Ji Jiao Li Huang Wan; b) edema with signs of weakness of the spleen—Tetrandra root (Fangji) is used with Astragalus root (Huangqi) and White atractylodes (Baizhu) in the formula Fangji Huangqi Tang.

Dosage: 5-10 g

Cautions & Contraindications: This herb is contraindicated in cases with deficient *yin.*

80. Large-leaf gentian root (Qinjiao)

Pharmaceutical Name: Radix Gentianae macrophyllae

Botanical Name: 1. Gentiana macrophylla pall.; 2. Gentiana crassicaulis Duthie ex Burkill; 3. Gentiana dahurica Fisch.; 4. Gentiana straminea Maxim.

Common Name: Large-leaf gentian root

Source of Earliest Record: Shennong Bencao Jing

Part Used & Method for Pharmaceutical Preparations: The roots are dug in spring or autumn. After the fibrous root bark has been removed, the roots are cleaned, dried in the sun and cut into slices.

Properties & Taste: Bitter, pungent and slightly cold

Meridians: Stomach, liver and gall bladder

Functions: 1. To dispel wind and dampness; 2. To clear heat caused by *yin* deficiency

Indications & Combinations:

1. Wind-damp obstruction syndrome: a) pain with heat signs —Large-leaf gentian root (Qinjiao) is used with Tetrandra root (Fangji)

and Honeysuckle stem (Rendongteng); b) pain with cold signs—Large-leaf gentian root (Qinjiao) is used with Notopterygium root (Qianghuo), Pubescent angelica root (Duhuo), Cinnamon twigs (Guizhi) and Prepared aconite root (Fuzi).

2. Afternoon fever caused by deficient *yin*. Large-leaf gentian root (Qinjiao) is used with Sweet wormwood (Qinghao), Turtle shell (Biejia), Anemarrhena rizome (Zhimu) and Wolfberry bark (Digupi) in the formula Qinjiao Biejia Tang.

3. Damp-heat jaundice. Large-leaf gentian root (Qinjiao) is used with Oriental wormwood (Yinchenhao) and Capejasmine (Zhizi).

Dosage: 5-10 g

Cautions & Contraindications: This herb is contraindicated for a person with a weak constitution or in cases suffering from diarrhea.

81. Siegesbeckia (Xixiancao)

Pharmaceutical Name: Herba Siegesbeckiae

Botanical Name: 1. Siegesbeckia pubescens Mak.; 2. Siegesbeckia orientalis L.; 3. Siegesbeckia glabrescens Mak.

Common Name: Siegesbeckia herb

Source of Earliest Record: Xinxiu Bencao

Part Used & Method for Pharmaceutical Preparations: The aerial parts of the herb can be gathered in summer or autumn. They are then cleaned, dried in the sun and cut into small pieces.

Properties & Taste: Bitter and cold

Meridians: Liver and kidney

Functions: 1. To dispel wind and dampness; 2. To clear the meridians; 3. To clear heat and release toxins

Indications & Combinations:

1. Wind-damp obstruction syndrome manifested as rheumatic pain. Siegesbeckia (Xixiancao) can be used singly or with Glorybower leaf (Chouwutong) in the formula Xi Tong Wan.

2. Boils, carbuncles, furuncles, eczema and measles. The herb is used both internally and externally.

3. Hypertension. Siegesbeckia (Xixiancao) can be used singly or with Glorybower leaf (Chouwutong) and Uncaria stem (Gouteng).

Dosage: 10-15 g

Cautions & Contraindications: This herb is contraindicated in cases with deficient blood syndromes.

82. Glorybower leaf (Chouwutong)

Pharmaceutical Name: Folium Clerodentri trichotomi
Botanical Name: Clerodendron trichotomum Thunb.
Common Name: Glorybower leaf, Clerodendron leaf
Source of Earliest Record: Bencao Tujing
Part Used & Method for Pharmaceutical Preparations: The leaves are gathered before the plant bears fruit in summer. They are then dried in the sun.
Properties & Taste: Pungent, bitter, sweet and cool
Meridian: Liver
Functions: To dispel wind and dampness
Indications & Combinations:

1. Wind-damp obstruction syndrome manifested as rheumatic pain, numbness of limbs and hemiplegia. Glorybower leaf (Chouwutong) is used with Siegesbeckia (Xixiancao), Uncaria stem (Gouteng) and Mulberry mistletoe (Sangjisheng).

2. Eczema. The decoction of the herb is used for external washing.
Dosage: 5-15 g
Cautions & Contraindications: This herb should not be boiled for a long time.

83. Chaenomeles fruit (Mugua)

Pharmaceutical Name: Fructus chaenomelis
Botanical Name: Chaenomeles speciosa (Sweet) Nakai
Common Name: Chaenomeles fruit, Flowering quince fruit, Chinese quince
Source of Earliest Record: Mingyi Bielu
Part Used & Method for Pharmaceutical Preparations: The fruit is gathered in summer or autumn when it is ripe. Then it is halved, soaked in hot water, dried in the sun and cut into slices.
Properties & Taste: Sour and warm
Meridians: Liver and spleen
Functions: 1. To promote blood circulation in the channels and collaterals; 2. To relax muscles and tendons; 3. To transform dampness and harmonize the stomach
Indications & Combinations:

1. Convulsions and spasms. Chaenomeles fruit (Mugua) is used with Frankincense (Ruxiang) and Myrrh (Moyao) in the formula Mugua Jian.

79

2. Painful and swollen legs with irritability. Chaenomeles fruit (Mugua) is used with Evodia fruit (Wuzhuyu) and Areca seed (Binglang) in the formula Jiming San.

3. Wind-damp obstruction syndrome manifested as rheumatic pain, numbness of limbs and joint pain. Chaenomeles fruit (Mugua) is used with Tetrandra root (Fangji), Clematis root (Weilingxian) and Chinese angelica root (Danggui).

Dosage: 6-12 g

84. Chinese starjasmine (Luoshiteng)

Pharmaceutical Name: Calilis trachelospermi
Botanical Name: Tranchelospermun jasminoides (Lindl.) Lem.
Common Name: Chinese starjasmine
Source of Earliest Record: Shennong Bencao Jing
Part Used & Method for Pharmaceutical Preparations: The foliated stems are gathered in winter or spring, cleaned, dried in the sun and cut into small pieces. The raw stems can be steamed with yellow wine.
Properties & Taste: Bitter and slightly cold
Meridians: Heart and liver
Functions: 1. To dispel wind and dampness and clear the collaterals; 2. To cool the blood and reduce swelling
Indications & Combinations:

1. Wind-damp obstruction syndrome manifested as rheumatic pain, spasm of the muscles and contraction of tendons. Chinese starjasmine (Luoshiteng) is used with Acanthopanax bark (Wujiapi) and Cyathula root (Niuxi).

2. Sore throat and abscess. Chinese starjasmine (Luoshiteng) is used with Honeylocust thorn (Zaojiaoci), Trichosanthes fruit (Gualou), Frankincense (Ruxiang) and Myrrh (Moyao) in the formula Zitong Linbao San.

Dosage: 6-15 g

85. Paniculate swallowwort root (Xuchangqing)

Pharmaceutical Name: Radix Cynanchi paniculati
Botanical Name: Cynanchum paniculatum (Bge.) Kitag.
Common Name: Cynanchum paniculatum, Paniculate swallowwort root
Source of Earliest Record: Shennong Bencao Jing

Part Used & Method for Pharmaceutical Preparations: The roots, or rhizomes, are dug and gathered in autumn, cleaned, dried in the shade and cut into slices.

Properties & Taste: Pungent and warm

Meridians: Liver and stomach

Functions: 1. To dispel wind and dampness; 2. To stop pain and itching

Indications & Combinations:

1. Wind-damp obstruction syndrome manifested as rheumatic joint pain, lower back pain, abdominal pain, toothache and pain due to external injuries. Paniculate swallowwort root (Xuchangqing) is used alone, or with other herbs in accordance with clinical manifestations.

2. Eczema and measles. Paniculate swallowwort root (Xuchangqing) is used with Flavescent sophora root (Kushen), Broom cypress fruit (Difuzi) and Dittany bark (Baixianpi).

Dosage: 3-10 g

Cautions & Contraindications: This herb should not be boiled too long.

86. Mulberry twigs (Sangzhi)

Pharmaceutical Name: Ramulus Mori

Botanical Name: Morus alba L.

Common Name: Morus branch, Mulberry twigs

Source of Earliest Record: Bencao Tujing

Part Used & Method for Pharmaceutical Preparations: The tender branches are gathered at the end of spring or the beginning of summer; then they are dried in the sun and cut into slices.

Properties & Taste: Bitter and neutral

Meridian: Liver

Functions: 1. To dispel wind and dampness; 2. To clear the collaterals

Indications & Combinations: Wind-damp obstruction syndrome manifested as rheumatic pain and spasm of the limbs. Mulberry twigs (Sangzhi) is used alone or with Tetrandra root (Fangji), Chaenomeles fruit (Mugua) and Chinese starjasmine (Luoshiteng).

Dosage: 10-30 g

Cautions & Contraindications: This herb should be used cautiously in cases with deficient *yin* syndrome.

81

87. Mulberry mistletoe (Sangjisheng)

Pharmaceutical Name: Ramulus Taxilli
Botanical Name: Taxillus chinensis (DC.) Danser
Common Name: Loranthus, Mulberry mistletoe
Source of Earliest Record: Shennong Bencao Jing
Part Used & Method for Pharmaceutical Preparations: The foliated stems and branches are gathered in winter or spring, cut into pieces and dried in the sun.
Properties & Taste: Bitter and neutral
Meridians: Liver and kidney
Functions: 1. To dispel wind and dampness; 2. To tonify the liver and kidney, and strengthen the tendons and combinations; 3. To calm the fetus and prevent miscarriage
Indications & Combinations:

1. Wind-damp obstruction syndrome manifested as rheumatic pain and soreness and pain of the lower back and knees. Mulberry mistletoe (Sangjisheng) is used with Pubescent angelica root (Duhuo), Cyathula root (Niuxi), Eucommia bark (Duzhong) and Cibot rhizome (Gouji) in the formula Duhuo Jisheng Tang.

2. Restless fetus, threatened abortion caused by deficient liver and kidney and dysfunction of Chong and Ren meridians. Mulberry mistletoe (Sangjisheng) is used with Mugwort leaf (Aiye), Donkey hide gelatin (Ejiao), Eucommia bark (Duzhong) and Teasel root (Xuduan).

3. Hypertension. Mulberry mistletoe (Sangjisheng) is used with Uncaria stem (Gouteng), Chrysanthemum flower (Juhua), Wolfberry fruit (Gouqizi) and Glorybower leaf (Chouwutong).
Dosage: 10-20 g

88. Acanthopanax bark (Wujiapi)

Pharmaceutical Name: Cortex Acanthopanacis
Botanical Name: Acanthopanax gracilistylus W. W. Smith
Common Name: Acanthopanax bark
Source of Earliest Record: Shennong Bencao Jing
Part Used & Method for Pharmaceutical Preparations: The bark of the root is gathered in summer or autumn and then dried in the sun.
Properties & Taste: Pungent, bitter and warm
Meridians: Liver and kidney
Functions: 1. To dispel wind and dampness; 2. To strengthen the

tendons and bones; 3. To benefit urination

Indications & Combinations:

1. Wind-damp obstruction syndrome manifested as rheumatic pain and spasm of the limbs. Acanthopanax bark (Wujiapi) is used alone or with Clematis root (Weilingxian), Pubescent angelica root (Duhuo), Mulberry twigs (Sangzhi) and Chaenomeles fruit (Mugua).

2. Deficient liver and kidney manifested as soreness, weakness and pain in the lumbar region and the knees. Acanthopanax bark (Wujiapi) is used with Eucommia bark (Duzhong), Cyathula root (Niuxi), Mulberry mistletoe (Sangjisheng) and Teasel root (Xuduan).

3. Edema. Acanthopanax bark (Wujiapi) is used with Poria peel (Fulingpi) and Areca nut shell (Dafupi) in the formula Wupi Yin.

Dosage: 5-10 g

89. Tiger's bone (Hugu)

Pharmaceutical Name: Os tigris

Zoological Name: Panthera tigris L.

Common Name: Tiger's bone

Source of Earliest Record: Mingyi Bielu

Part Used & Method for Pharmaceutical Preparations: The fresh bone is dried in the shade, and then pounded into small pieces or soaked in wine or made into pills or powder.

Properties & Taste: Pungent and warm

Meridians: Liver and kidney

Functions: 1. To dispel wind and dampness and stop pain; 2. To strengthen tendons and bones

Indications & Combinations:

1. Wind-damp obstruction syndrome manifested as rheumatic pain, spasm of the limbs and motor impairment of joints. Tiger's bone (Hugu) is used with Chaenomeles fruit (Mugua), Cyathula root (Niuxi), Acanthopanax bark (Wujiapi), Mulberry twigs (Sangzhi) and Teasel root (Xuduan) in the formula Hugu Mugua Jiu.

2. Deficient liver and kidney manifested as fragile bones and tendons and weakness of the limbs. Tiger's bone (Hugu) is used with Prepared rehmannia root (Shudihuang) and Cyathula root (Niuxi) in the formula Hu Qian Wan.

Dosage: 3-6 g

90. Erythrina bark (Haitongpi)

Pharmaceutical Name: Coxtex Erythrinae
Botanical Name: Erythrina variegata L. var. orientalis (L.) Merr.
Common Name: Erythrina bark, Coralbean bark
Source of Earliest Record: Haiyao Bencao
Part Used & Method for Pharmaceutical Preparations: The thorny bark is gathered in the early summer, then dried in the sun.
Properties & Taste: Bitter, pungent and neutral
Meridian: Liver
Functions: 1. To dispel wind and dampness; 2. To clear the meridians
Indications & Combinations: Wind-damp obstruction syndrome manifested as rheumatic joint pain, spasm of the limbs and lower back and knee pain. Erythrina bark (Haitongpi) is used with other herbs which have the similar functions, such as Tetrandra root (Fangji), Clematis root (Weilingxian) and Futokadsura stem (Haifengteng).
Dosage: 6-12 g

91. Silkworm excrement (Cansha)

Pharmaceutical Name: Excrementum Bombycis mori
Zoological Name: Bombys mori L.
Common Name: Silkworm excrement
Source of Earliest Record: Mingyi Bielu
Part Used & Method for Pharmaceutical Preparations: Silkworm excrement is collected from June to August, then dried in the sun.
Properties & Taste: Pungent, sweet and warm
Meridians: Liver, spleen and stomach
Functions: 1. To dispel wind and dampness; 2. To harmonize the stomach and transform dampness
Indications & Combinations:

1. Damp-heat obstruction syndrome. Silkworm excrement (Cansha) is used with Tetrandra root (Fangji), Coix seed (Yiyiren) and Talc (Huashi) in the formula Xuanbi Tang.

2. Eczema. The decoction of the herb is used for external washing.

3. Turbid dampness blocking the spleen and stomach manifested as vomiting, diarrhea, cramps and abdominal pain. Silkworm excrement (Cansha) is used with Scutellaria root (Huangqin), Chaenomeles fruit (Mugua) and Evodia fruit (Wuzhuyu) in the formula Canshi Tang.

Dosage: 5-10 g

92. Hairy birthwort (Xungufeng)

Pharmaceutical Name: Herba Aristolochiae Mollissimae
Botanical Name: Aristolochia mollissima Hance
Common Name: Hairy birthwort
Source of Earliest Record: Zhiwu Mingshi Tukao
Part Used & Method for Pharmaceutical Preparations: The whole plant is gathered in summer or autumn, cleaned and dried.
Properties & Taste: Pungent, bitter and neutral
Meridian: Liver
Functions: 1. To dispel wind and dampness; 2. To clear the channels and collaterals; 3. To stop pain
Indications & Combinations: Wind-damp obstruction syndrome manifested as joint pain, numbness of the limbs, tendon and muscle spasms and pain from external injury. Hairy birthwort (Xungufeng) may be used alone in decoction or soaked in wine, or used with other herbs that dispel wind and dampness.
Dosage: 10-15 g

93. Futokadsura stem (Haifengteng)

Pharmaceutical Name: Caulis Piperis futokadsurae
Botanical Name: 1. Piper futokadsura Sieb. et Zucc.; 2. Piper hancei Maxim.
Common Name: Kasura stem, Futokadsura stem
Source of Earliest Record: Bencao Zaixin
Part Used & Method for Pharmaceutical Preparations: The stems are gathered in summer or autumn, dried in the sun and cut into slices.
Properties & Taste: Pungent, bitter and slightly warm
Meridian: Liver
Functions: 1. To dispel wind and dampness; 2. To clear the channels and collaterals
Indications & Combinations: Wind-damp obstruction syndrome manifested as painful and stiff joints, tendon and muscle spasms, lower back pain, painful knees and pain from external injury. Futokadsura stem (Haifengteng) is used with other herbs that dispel wind and invigorate the circulation of blood in channels and collaterals, such as Erythrina bark (Haitongpi), Large-leaf gentian root (Qinjiao) and Mul-

berry twigs (Sangzhi).
Dosage: 5-10 g

94. Homalomena rhizome (Qiannianjian)

Pharmaceutical Name: Rhizoma Homalomenae
Botanical Name: Homalomena occulta (Lour.) Schott
Common Name: Homalomena rhizome
Source of Earliest Record: Bencao Gangmu Shiyi
Part Used & Method for Pharmaceutical Preparations: The rhizomes are dug in spring or autumn. After the fibrous roots have been removed, the rhizomes are cleaned, dried in the sun and cut into slices.
Properties & Taste: Bitter, pungent and warm
Meridians: Liver and kidney
Functions: 1. To dispel wind and dampness; 2. To strengthen tendons and bones
Indications & Combinations: Wind-damp obstruction syndrome manifested as cold sensation and pain in the lower back and knees and spasms or numbness of the lower limbs. Homalomena rhizome (Qiannianjian) is soaked in wine with Tiger's bone (Hugu), Cyathula root (Niuxi) and Wolfberry fruit (Gouqizi).
Dosage: 5-10 g

95. Pine nodular branch (Songjie)

Pharmaceutical Name: Lignum Pini Nodi
Botanical Name: 1. Pinus tabulaeformis Carr.; 2. Pinus massoniana Lamb.
Common Name: Knotty pine wood, Pine nodular branch
Source of Earliest Record: Mingyi Bielu
Part Used & Method for Pharmaceutical Preparations: Pine wood knots are collected and dried in either sun or shade. The knots are then soaked in water, cut into slices and dried in the sun again.
Properties & Taste: Bitter and warm
Meridian: Liver
Functions: 1. To dispel wind and dry dampness; 2. To stop pain
Indications & Combinations:
1. Wind-damp obstruction syndrome. Pine nodular branch (Songjie) is used with herbs that dispel wind and dampness. In acute arthritis with severe pain, Pine nodular branch (Songjie) is soaked in

wine for drinking.

2. External injury pain. Pine nodular branch (Songjie) is used with herbs that invigorate blood circulation, including Peach seed (Tao-ren), Safflower (Honghua), Frankincense (Ruxiang) and Myrrh (Mo-yao).

Dosage: 10-15 g

V. Aromatic Herbs That Transform Dampness

These herbs transform dampness and are mostly spicy-pungent, fragrant, warm and dry. They promote *qi*, transform turbid dampness and strengthen the spleen and stomach in its functions of transforming and transporting. The main indications of dampness are a full sensation in the epigastric and abdominal regions, vomiting, sour regurgitation, poor appetite, lassitude, diarrhea, sweet taste in the mouth and sticky and moist tongue coating. In addition, these herbs are indicated for damp-heat syndrome and summer-heat associated with dampness syndrome.

Aromatic herbs can be used with other herbs that warm the interior. For cold-damp syndrome and damp-heat syndrome, the aromatic herbs are combined with herbs that clear heat and dry dampness. Since dampness is characterized by viscosity and stagnation, aromatic herbs that transform dampness are often combined with herbs that promote *qi* circulation. If dampness is due to spleen deficiency, aromatic herbs are combined with herbs that tonify the spleen. Caution is advised in patients with deficiency of *yin*.

96. Atractylodes rhizome (Cangzhu)

Pharmaceutical Name: Rhizoma atractylodis

Botanical Name: 1. Atractylodes lancea (Thunb.) DC.; 2. A. chinensis (DC.) Koidz.; 3. Atractylodes japonica koidz. ex Kitam.

Common Name: Atractylodes rhizome

Source of Earliest Record: Shennong Bencao Jing

Part Used & Method for Pharmaceutical Preparations: The rhizomes are dug in spring or autumn; those gathered in autumn are better. After the fibrous roots have been removed, the rhizomes are cleaned and dried in the sun, soaked in water and cut into slices. The raw slices are then fried until yellowish in color.

Properties & Taste: Pungent, bitter and warm

Meridians: Spleen and stomach

Functions: 1. To dry dampness and strengthen the spleen; 2. To expel wind and dampness; 3. To promote sweating

Indications & Combinations:

1. Dampness blocking the spleen and stomach manifested as epigastric distension and fullness, poor appetite, nausea or vomiting, lassitude and sticky tongue coating. Atractylodes rhizome (Cangzhu) is used with Magnolia bark (Houpo) and Tangerine peel (Chenpi) in the formula Pingwei San.

2. Wind-cold-damp obstruction syndrome manifested as swollen and painful knee joints and weakness of the lower limbs. Atractylodes rhizome (Cangzhu) is used with Chaenomeles fruit (Mugua), Mulberry twigs (Sangzhi) and Pubescent angelica root (Duhuo).

3. Exterior syndrome due to invasion by exogenous pathogenic wind, cold and dampness manifested as soreness and heaviness of the limbs, chills, fever, headache and heavy sensation in the head. Atractylodes rhizome (Cangzhu) is used with Ledebouriella root (Fangfeng) and Asarum herb (Xixin).

4. Downward flow of damp-heat manifested as swollen and painful knees and legs and weakness of the lower limbs. Atractylodes rhizome (Cangzhu) is used with Phellodendron bark (Huangbai) and Cyathula root (Niuxi) in the formula Sanmiao Wan.

Dosage: 5-10 g

97. Magnolia bark (Houpo)

Pharmaceutical Name: Cortex Magnoliae officinalis

Botanical Name: 1. Magnolia officinalis Rehd. et wils.; 2. Magnolia officinalis Rhed. et Wills. var. biloba Rhed. et Wills.

Common Name: Magnolia bark

Source of Earliest Record: Shennong Bencao Jing

Part Used & Method for Pharmaceutical Preparations: Between April and June, the bark is peeled off and dried in the shade. After a process of boiling, piling, steaming and drying, the herb is ready for use.

Properties & Taste: Bitter, pungent and warm

Meridians: Spleen, stomach, lung and large intestine

Functions: 1. To promote *qi* circulation; 2. To dry dampness; 3. To descend rebellious *qi* and relieve asthma; 4. To resolve retention of food

Indications & Combinations:

1. Disharmony of spleen and stomach due to stagnation of dampness and retention of food manifested as epigastric distension and fullness. Magnolia bark (Houpo) is used with Atractylodes rhizome (Cangzhu) and Tangerine peel (Chenpi) in the formula Pingwei San. If dampness blocks the spleen and stomach causing retention of food, abdominal distension and pain and constipation, Magnolia bark (Houpo) is used with Rhubarb (Dahuang) and Immature bitter orange (Zhishi) in the formula Da Chengqi Tang.

2. Cough and asthma. Magnolia bark (Houpo) is used with Apricot seed (Xingren) in the formula Guizhi Jia Houpo Xingzi Tang.

Dosage: 3-10 g

98. Agastache (Huoxiang)

Pharmaceutical Name: Herba agastachis seu, Herba pogastemonis

Botanical Name: 1. Pogostemon cablin Blanco; 2. Agastache rugosa (Fisch. et Mey.) O. Ktze.

Common Name: Agastache, Pogostemon cablin

Source of Earliest Record: Mingyi Bielu

Part Used & Method for Pharmaceutical Preparations: The aerial parts of the plant are gathered in summer or autumn, cut into pieces and dried in the shade.

Properties & Taste: Pungent and slightly warm

Meridians: Spleen, stomach and lung

Functions: 1. To transform dampness; 2. To dispel summer-heat; 3. To stop vomiting

Indications & Combinations:

1. Dampness blocking the spleen and stomach manifested as epigastric and abdominal distension, nausea, vomiting and poor appetite. Agastache (Huoxiang) is used with Atractylodes rhizome (Cangzhu), Magnolia bark (Houpo) and Pinellia tuber (Banxia) in the formula Buhuanjin Zhenqi San.

2. Internal injury caused by raw and cold food and invasion by exogenous wind and cold in summer manifested as chills, fever, headache, epigastric fullness, nausea, vomiting and diarrhea. Agastache (Huoxiang) is used with Perilla leaf (Zisuye), Pinellia tuber (Banxia),

Magnolia bark (Houpo) and Tangerine peel (Chenpi) in the formula Huoxiang Zhengqi San.

3. Vomiting: a) vomiting caused by turbid dampness in the spleen and stomach—Agastache (Huoxiang) is used alone or with Pinellia tuber (Banxia) and Fresh ginger (Shengjiang); b) vomiting caused by damp-heat in the spleen and stomach—Agastache (Huoxiang) is used with Coptis root (Huanglian), Bamboo shavings (Zhuru) and Loquat leaf (Pipaye); c) vomiting caused by weakness in the spleen and stomach—Agastache (Huoxiang) is used with Pilose asiabell root (Dangshen) and Licorice root (Gancao); d) vomiting caused by pregnancy—Agastache (Huoxiang) is used with Amomum fruit (Sharen) and Pinellia tuber (Banxia).

Dosage: 5-10 g

99. Eupatorium (Peilan)

Pharmaceutical Name: Herba Eupatorii
Botanical Name: Eupatorium fortunei Turcz.
Common Name: Eupatorium
Source of Earliest Record: Shennong Bencao Jing
Part Used & Method for Pharmaceutical Preparations: The aerial parts of the plant are harvested either in summer or autumn, with autumn being preferable. They are cut into pieces and dried in the sun.
Properties & Taste: Pungent and neutral
Meridians: Spleen and stomach
Functions: 1. To transform dampness; 2. To release summer-heat
Indications & Combinations:

1. Dampness blocking spleen and stomach manifested as epigastric and abdominal distension and fullness, nausea, vomiting and poor appetite. Eupatorium (Peilan) is used with Agastache (Huoxiang), Atractylodes rhizome (Cangzhu), Magnolia bark (Houpo) and Round cardamom seed (Baidoukou).

2. Invasion by exogenous summer-heat and dampness or early stage of damp-heat febrile diseases manifested as stifling sensation in the chest, absence of hunger, low-grade fever and sallow complexion. Eupatorium (Peilan) is used with Agastache (Huoxiang), Sweet wormwood (Qinghao), Talc (Huashi) and Coix seed (Yiyiren).

Dosage: 5-10 g

100a. Amomum fruit (Sharen)

Pharmaceutical Name: Fructus Amomi

Botanical Name: 1. Amomum vilosum Lour.; 2. Amomum longiligulare T. L. Wu; 3. A. xanthioides Wall.

Common Name: Amomum fruit

Source of Earliest Record: Kaibao Bencao

Part Used & Method for Pharmaceutical Preparations: The fruit is gathered in summer or autumn, whenever it ripens. It is dried in the sun or in a low-temperature room and then mashed.

Properties & Taste: Pungent and warm

Meridians: Spleen and stomach

Functions: 1. To promote *qi* circulation and transform dampness; 2. To calm fetus

Indications & Combinations:

1. Dampness blocking spleen and stomach or *qi* stagnation in the spleen manifested as distension and pain, no appetite, vomiting, nausea and diarrhea. Amomum fruit (Sharen) is used with Atractylodes rhizome (Cangzhu), Round cardamom seed (Baidoukou) and Magnolia bark (Houpo) for cases of dampness blocking the spleen and stomach. Amomum fruit (Sharen), Costus root (Muxiang) and Immature bitter orange (Zhishi) in the formula Xiang Sha Zhi Shu Wan are used for cases of *qi* stagnation due to retention of food. Amomum fruit (Sharen), Tangerine peel (Chenpi), Pilose asiabell root (Dangshen) and White atractylodes (Baizhu) in the formula Xiang Sha Liujunzi Wan are used for *qi* stagnation caused by weakness of the spleen.

2. Morning sickness or restless fetus. Amomum fruit (Sharen) is used with White atractylodes (Baizhu) and Perilla stem (Sugeng).

Dosage: 3-6 g

100b. Amomum shell (Sharenqiao)

The shell of Amomum fruit (Sharen) has similar properties and functions to the Amomum fruit (Sharen), however, the warming property of Amomum shell (Sharenqiao) is less strong and its ability to transform dampness and promote circulation of *qi* is weaker. This herb is indicated in *qi* stagnation in the spleen and stomach, epigastric and abdominal distension and fullness, nausea, vomiting and poor appetite.

91

101. Round cardamom seed (Baidoukou)

Pharmaceutical Name: Fructus Amomi kravanh

Botanical Name: 1. Amomum kravanh Pierre ex Gagnep. 2. Amomum compactum Soland. ex Maton

*Common Name:*Round cardamom seed

Source of Earliest Record: Kaibao Bencao

Part Used & Method for Pharmaceutical Preparations: The yellow fruit is gathered from October to December, dried in the sun and broken into pieces.

Properties & Taste: Pungent and warm

Meridians: Lung, spleen and stomach

Functions: 1. To promote *qi* circulation and transform dampness; 2. To warm the spleen and stomach and stop vomiting

Indications & Combinations:

1. Dampness blocking spleen and stomach or *qi* stagnation in the spleen manifested as distension, fullness and no appetite. Round cardamom seed (Baidoukou) is used with Magnolia bark (Houpo), Atractylodes rhizome (Cangzhu) and Tangerine peel (Chenpi).

2. Early stage of damp-heat febrile diseases manifested as stifling sensation in the chest, absence of hunger and sticky tongue coating. Round cardamom seed (Baidoukou) is used with Talc (Huashi), Coix seed (Yiyiren) and Amomum fruit (Sharen) in the formula Sanren Tang. For cases of excess heat, Round cardamom seed (Baidoukou) is used with Scutellaria root (Huangqin), Coptis root (Huanglian) and Talc (Huashi) in the formula Huangqin Huashi Tang.

3. Vomiting due to cold in the stomach. Round cardamom seed (Baidoukou) is used with Agastache (Huoxiang) and Pinellia tuber (Banxia).

4. Infantile vomiting due to cold in the stomach. Round cardamom seed (Baidoukou) is used with Amomum fruit (Sharen) and Licorice root (Gancao).

Dosage: 3-6 g

102. Katsumadai seed (Caodoukou)

Pharmaceutical Name: Semen Alpiniae katsumadai

Botanical Name: Alpinia katsumadai Hayata

Common Name: Katsumadai seed

Source of Earliest Record: Mingyi Bielu

Part Used & Method for Pharmaceutical Preparations: The yellow fruit is gathered in summer or autumn and dried in the sun. The seeds are smashed after the flesh of the fruit has been peeled off.

Properties & Taste: Pungent and warm

Meridians: Spleen and stomach

Functions: 1. To dry dampness and warm the spleen and stomach; 2. To promote *qi* circulation

Indications & Combinations: Cold-damp blocking and stagnating spleen and stomach manifested as epigastric and abdominal distension and fullness, cold pain, vomiting and diarrhea. In cases of excessive dampness, Katsumadai seed (Caodoukou) is used with Magnolia bark (Houpo), Atractylodes rhizome (Cangzhu) and Pinellia tuber (Banxia). In cases of excessive cold, Katsumadai seed (Caodoukou) is used with Cinnamon bark (Rougui) and Dried ginger (Ganjiang).

Dosage: 3–6 g

103. Tsaoko (Caoguo)

Pharmaceutical Name: Fructus Tsaoko

Botanical Name: Amomum tsao-ko Crevost et Lemaire

Common Name: Tsaoko, Amomum seed

Source of Earliest Record: Yinshan Zhenyao

Part Used & Method for Pharmaceutical Preparations: The ripe fruit is gathered in autumn and dried in the sun. The seeds are collected after the carbonized fruit is broken into pieces.

Properties & Taste: Pungent and warm

Meridians: Spleen and stomach

Functions: 1. To dry dampness and warm spleen and stomach; 2. To relieve malaria

Indications & Combinations:

1. Cold-damp blocking and stagnating spleen and stomach manifested as epigastric and abdominal distension and fullness, cold pain, vomiting and diarrhea. Tsaoko (Caoguo) is used with Magnolia bark (Houpo), Atractylodes rhizome (Cangzhu) and Pinellia tuber (Banxia).

2. Malaria. Tsaoko (Caoguo) is used with Dichroa root (Changshan) and Bupleurum root (Chaihu).

Dosage: 3–6 g

VI. Herbs That Benefit Urination and Drain Dampness

Herbs that benefit urination and drain dampness transform accumulated dampness or fluid into urine. Some of these herbs also clear heat and drain dampness. These herbs are sweet or tasteless, neutral or slightly cold, and are indicated in dysuria, edema, urinary tract disorders, phlegm-damp, jaundice and eczema. All of these herbs should be used with caution in cases with deficiency of *yin* and body fluids.

104. Poria (Fuling)

Pharmaceutical Name: Poria
Botanical Name: Poria cocos (schw.) wolf
Common Name: Poria, Tuckahoe, Indian bread, Hoelen
Source of Earliest Record: Shennong Bencao Jing
Part Used & Method for Pharmaceutical Preparations: The fungus is gathered, cut into pieces and dried in the shade.
Properties & Taste: Sweet or no taste and neutral
Meridians: Heart, spleen and kidney
Functions: 1. To transform dampness and strengthen spleen; 2. To calm the mind
Indications & Combinations:

1. Dysuria and edema. Poria (Fuling) is used with Umbellate porefungus (Zhuling), Alismatis rhizome (Zexie) and White atractylodes (Baizhu) in the formula Wuling San.

2. Retention of phlegm and fluids manifested as dizziness, palpitations and cough. Poria (Fuling) is used with White atractylodes (Baizhu) and Cinnamon twigs (Guizhi) in the formula Ling Gui Zhu Gan Tang.

3. Excessive dampness and deficiency of the spleen manifested as poor appetite, diarrhea and lassitude. Poria (Fuling) is used with Pilose asiabell root (Dangshen) and White atractylodes (Baizhu) in the formula Sijunzi Tang.

4. Palpitations and insomnia. Poria (Fuling) is used with Wild jujube seed (Suanzaoren) and Polygala root (Yuanzhi).
Dosage: 10-15 g

105. Umbellate pore-fungus (Zhuling)

Pharmaceutical Name: Polyporus
Botanical Name: Polyporus umbellarus (pers.) Fr.
Common Name: Polyporus grifolia, Umbellate pore-fungus
Source of Earliest Record: Shennong Bencao Jing
Part Used & Method for Pharmaceutical Preparations: The fungus is gathered in spring or autumn, cleaned, dried in the sun and cut into slices.
Properties & Taste: Sweet or no taste and neutral
Meridians: Kidney and urinary bladder
Functions: To transform dampness and promote water metabolism
Indications & Combinations: Dysuria, turbid urine, edema, diarrhea and profuse leukorrhea. Umbellate pore-fungus (Zhuling) is used with Poria (Fuling) and Alismatis rhizome (Zexie) in the formula Siling San.
Dosage: 5-10 g

106. Alismatis rhizome (Zexie)

Pharmaceutical Name: Rhizoma Alismatis
Botanical Name: Alisma orientalis (Sam.) Juzep.
Common Name: Alismatis rhizome, Water plantain tuber
Source of Earliest Record: Shennong Bencao Jing
Part Used & Method for Pharmaceutical Preparations: The rhizomes are dug in winter. After the fibrous roots and bark have been removed, the rhizomes are soaked in water, cut into slices and dried in the sun.
Properties & Taste: Sweet or no taste and cold
Meridians: Kidney and urinary bladder
Functions: To transform dampness and promote water metabolism
Indications & Combinations: Dysuria, turbid urine, edema, diarrhea and profuse leukorrhea, or retention of phlegm and fluids, leading to dizziness, vertigo, palpitation and cough. Alismatis rhizome (Zexie) is used with Poria (Fuling), Umbellate pore-fungus (Zhuling) and White atractylodes (Baizhu) in the formula Wuling San.
Dosage: 5-10 g

107. Coix seed (Yiyiren)

Pharmaceutical Name: Semen Coicis
Botanical Name: Coix lachryma-jobi L. var. ma-yuen (Roman.) Stapf
Common Name: Coix seed, Job's tears seed

Source of Earliest Record: Shennong Bencao Jing

Part Used & Method for Pharmaceutical Preparations: The seeds are obtained by removing the hard husk of the fruit, which is gathered in autumn.

Properties & Taste: Sweet or no taste and slightly cold

Meridians: Spleen, stomach and lung

Functions: 1. To transform dampness and promote water metabolism; 2. To strengthen the spleen; 3. To clear heat and eliminate pus

Indications & Combinations:

1. Deficiency of spleen manifested as edema, dysuria and diarrhea. Coix seed (Yiyiren) is used with Alismatis rhizome (Zexie) and White atractylodes (Baizhu).

2. Beginning stage of damp-heat febrile diseases when the pathogenic factor is at the *qi* level. Coix seed (Yiyiren) is used with Talc (Huashi), Bamboo leaf (Zhuye) and Rice paper pith (Tongcao) in the formula Sanren Tang.

3. Accumulation of damp-heat or stagnation of *qi* and blood manifested as lung abscess and intestinal abscess. Coix seed (Yiyiren), Reed stem (Weijing), Benincasa seed (Dongguaren) and Peach seed (Taoren) in the formula Qianjin Weijing Tang is used for lung abscess with cough, sputum and pus. Coix seed (Yiyiren) and Patrinia herb (Baijiangcao) in the formula Yiyi Fuzi Baijiang San is used for intestinal abscess.

Dosage: 10-30 g

Caution & Contraindications: To tonify and strengthen the spleen, this herb is dry-fried.

108. Plantain seed (Cheqianzi)

Pharmaceutical Name: Semen plantaginis

Botanical Name: 1. Plantago asiatice L.; 2. Plantago depressa willd.

Common Name: Plantain seed, Plantain herb

Source of Earliest Record: Shennong Bencao Jing

Part Used & Method for Pharmaceutical Preparations: The seeds, gathered in summer or autumn when they are ripe, are dry-fried or fried with salt water.

Properties & Taste: Sweet and cold

Meridians: Kidney, liver and lung

Functions: 1. To promote water metabolism and relieve abnormal urination; 2. To stop diarrhea; 3. To clear heat in the liver and brighten eyes; 4. To clear the lung and resolve phlegm

Indications & Combinations:

1. Damp-heat flowing into the urinary bladder manifested as dysuria, painful urination, frequent urination and distending and full sensation in the lower abdominal region. Plantain seed (Cheqianzi) is used with Clematis stem (Mutong), Capejasmine (Zhizi) and Talc (Huashi) in the formula Bazheng San.

2. Damp-heat diarrhea. Plantain seed (Cheqianzi) is used with Poria (Fuling), White atractylodes (Baizhu) and Alismatis rhizome (Zexie).

3. Heat in the liver manifested as red, painful and swollen eyes. Plantain seed (Cheqianzi) is used with Chrysanthemum flower (Juhua), Chinese gentian (Longdancao) and Scutellaria root (Huangqin).

4. Deficiency of *yin* in the liver and kidney manifested as blurred vision and cataracts. Plantain seed (Cheqianzi) is used with Fresh rehmannia root (Shengdihuang), Ophiopogon root (Maidong) and Wolfberry fruit (Gouqizi).

5. Cough with profuse sputum due to heat in the lungs. Plantain seed (Cheqianzi) is used with Trichosanthes fruit (Gualou), Scutellaria root (Huangqin) and Tendrilled fritillary bulb (Chuanbeimu).

Dosage: 5-10 g

Cautions & Contraindications: This herb should be wrapped in cloth for decoctions if a strainer is not used.

109. Talc (Huashi)

Pharmacutical Name: Pulvus Talci

Mineral Name: 1. Talcum; 2. Hydrous magnesium silicate

Common Name: Talc, Talcum

Source of Earliest Record: Shennong Bencao Jing

Part Used & Method for Pharmaceutical Preparations: The mineral is ground into powder for use.

Properties & Taste: Sweet or no taste and cold

Meridians: Stomach and urinary bladder

Functions: 1. To promote water metabolism and relieve abnormal urination; 2. To clear heat and release summer-heat

Indications & Combinations:

1. Damp-heat in the urinary bladder manifested as painful urination, urgency of micturition, frequent urination, lower abdominal distention

and fever. Talc (Huashi) is used with Clematis stem (Mutong), Plantain seed (Cheqianzi), Common knotgrass (Bianxu) and Capejasmine (Zhizi) in the formula Bazheng San.

2. Summer-heat and dampness syndrome manifested as thirst, stifling sensation in the chest, vomiting and diarrhea. Talc (Huashi) is used with Licorice root (Gancao) in the formula Liu Yi San.

3. Boils, eczema, miliaria and skin diseases. Talc (Huashi) is used with Gypsum (Shigao) and Calamine Colamina (Luganshi) externally.

Dosage: 10-15 g

110. Clematis stem (Mutong)

Pharmaceutical Name: Caulis Aristolochiae seu Clematis

Botanical Name: 1. Aristolochia manshuriensis Kom.; 2. Clematis armandii Franch.; 3. C. Montana Buch.-Ham.

Common Name: Akebia, Clematis stem

Source of Earliest Record: Shennong Bencao Jing

Part Used & Method for Pharmaceutical Preparations: The stems are gathered in spring or autumn. The bark is removed, and the stems are dried in the sun.

Properties & Taste: Bitter and cold

Meridians: Heart, small intestine and urinary bladder

Functions: 1. To promote water metabolism and relieve abnormal urination; 2. To clear heat and promote lactation

Indications & Combinations:

1. Damp-heat in the urinary bladder manifested as dysuria, painful urination, frequent urination, urgency of micturition and abdominal distension and fullness, or flaring up of heart fire manifested as ulceration of the mouth and tongue, irritability and blood in the urine. Clematis stem (Mutong) is used with Bamboo leaf (Zhuye), Licorice root (Gancao) and Fresh rehmannia root (Shengdihuang) in the formula Daochi San.

2. Insufficient lactation. Clematis stem (Mutong) is used with Vaccaria seed (Wangbuliuxing) and Pangolin scales (Chuanshanjia), or Clematis stem (Mutong) is cooked with pig's feet.

Dosage: 3-6 g

Cautions & Contraindications: Avoid giving overdosages of the herb. It is contraindicated during pregnancy.

111. Ricepaper pith (Tongcao)

Pharmaceutical Name: Medulla tetrapanacis
Botanical Name: Tetrapanax papyriferus (Hook.) K. Koch
Common Name: Ricepaper pith
Source of Earliest Record: Bencao Shiyi
Part Used & Method for Pharmaceutical Preparations: The stems are gathered in autumn, cut into pieces and the bark is removed. The stems are dried in the sun and cut into thin slices.
Properties & Taste: Sweet or no taste and slightly cold
Meridians: Lung and stomach
Functions: 1. To clear heat and promote water metabolism; 2. To promote lactation
Indications & Combinations:

1. Damp-heat in the urinary bladder manifested as dysuria, painful urination, frequent urination and urgency of micturition. Ricepaper pith (Tongcao) is used with herbs that transform damp and clear heat, such as Talc (Huashi) and Plantain seed (Cheqianzi).

2. Insufficient lactation. Ricepaper pith (Tongcao) is used with Vaccaria seed (Wangbuliuxing) and Pangolin scales (Chuanshanjia), or Ricepaper pith (Tongcao) is cooked with pig's feet.

Dosage: 2-5 g
Cautions & Contraindications: This herb should be used with caution during pregnancy.

112. Lysimachia (Jinqiancao)

Pharmaceutical Name: 1. Herba Lysimachiae; 2. Herba Desmodii
Botanical Name: 1. Lysimachia christinae Hance (primulaceae); 2. Dessmodium styracifolium (Osbeck) Merr. (Leguminosae)
Common Name: Lysimachia, Dessmodium
Source of Earliest Record: Bencao Gangmu Shiyi
Part Used & Method for Pharmaceutical Preparations: The whole plant is gathered in summer or autumn, cleaned and dried in the sun.
Properties & Taste: Sweet or no taste and neutral
Meridians: Liver, gall bladder, kidney and urinary bladder
Functions: 1. To promote water metabolism and relieve abnormal urination; 2. To transform dampness and relieve jaundice
Indications & Combinations:

1. Damp-heat in the urinary bladder manifested as hot urination,

urinary tract stones, painful urination, frequent urination, urgency of micturition, abdominal pain and biliary stones. Lysimachia (Jinqiancao) is used with Lygodium spores (Haijinsha) and Chicken's gizzard skin (Jineijin) in the formula Sanjin Tang.

2. Damp-heat jaundice. Lysimachia (Jinqiancao) is used with Oriental wormwood (Yinchenhao) and Capejasmine (Zhizi).

Dosage: 30-60 g

113. Lygodium spores (Haijinsha)

Pharmaceutical Name: Spora Lygodii
Botanical Name: Lygodium japonicum (Thunb.) Sw.
Common Name: Lygodium spores, Japanese fern spores
Source of Earliest Record: Jiayou Bencao
Part Used & Method for Pharmaceutical Preparations: The spores are gathered in autumn and dried in the sun.
Properties & Taste: Sweet and cold
Meridians: Urinary bladder and small intestine
Functions: To promote water metabolism and regulate abnormal urination
Indications & Combinations: Damp-heat in the urinary bladder manifested as various abnormal urinary symptoms including hot urine, urinary tract stones, bloody urine, turbid urine, dysuria, painful urination, urgency of micturition and frequent urination. Lygodium spores (Haijinsha) is used with Talc (Huashi), Lysimachia (Jinqiancao), Plantain seed (Cheqianzi) and Amber (Hupo).
Dosage: 6-12 g
Cautions & Contraindications: The herb should be wrapped with a cloth for decoction, or decoction should be put through a strainer.

114. Pyrrosia leaf (Shiwei)

Pharmaceutical Name: Folium Pyrrosiae
Botanical Name: 1. Pyrrosia shearei (Bak.) Ching; 2. Pyrrosia petiolosa (Christ) Ching; 3. P. Lingua (Thunb.) Farwell
Common Name: Pyrrosia leaf
Source of Earliest Record: Shennong Bencao Jing
Part Used & Method for Pharmaceutical Preparations: The leaves are gathered all year round. They are cleaned, dried in the sun and cut into small pieces.

Properties & Taste: Bitter or sweet and slightly cold
Meridians: Lung and urinary bladder
Functions: To promote water metabolism and regulate abnormal urination
Indications & Combinations: Damp-heat in the urinary bladder manifested as dysuria, painful urination, hot urine, urinary tract stones, blood in the urine, turbid urine, urgency of micturition and frequent urination. Pyrrosia leaf (Shiwei) is used with Talc (Huashi), Lygodium spores (Haijinsha) and Plantain seed (Cheqianzi).
Dosage: 5-10 g

115. Hypoglauca yam (Bixie)

Pharmaceutical Name: Rhizoma Dioscoreae hypoglaucae
Botanical Name: 1. Dioscorea hypoglauca Palib; 2. Dioscorea septemloba Thunb.; 3. Dioscorea futschauensis Uline
Common Name: Hypoglauca yam
Source of Earliest Record: Shennong Bencao Jing
Part Used & Method for Pharmaceutical Preparations: The rhizomes are dug in spring or autumn. After the fibrous roots have been removed, the rhizomes are cleaned, dried in the sun and cut into slices.
Properties & Taste: Bitter and neutral
Meridians: Liver, stomach and urinary bladder
Functions: 1. To resolve turbid urine; 2. To expel wind and transform dampness
Indications & Combinations:

1. Turbid urine caused by cold-damp in the urinary bladder. Hypoglauca yam (Bixie) is used with Bitter cardamom (Yizhiren), Grass-leaved sweetflag (Shicangpu) and Lindera root (Wuyao) in the formula Bixie Fenqing Yin.

2. Mild urinary problem due to damp-heat flowing down to the urinary bladder. Hypoglauca yam (Bixie) is used with Phellodendron bark (Huangbai) and Plantain seed (Cheqianzi).

3. Wind-damp obstruction syndrome manifested as joint pain, numbness of the lower limbs and lower back pain. Hypoglauca yam (Bixie) is taken alone.

4. Cold-damp obstruction syndrome. Hypoglauca yam (Bixie) is used with Cinnamon twigs (Guizhi) and Prepared aconite root (Fuzi).

5. Damp-heat obstruction syndrome. Hypoglauca yam (Bixie) is

used with Mulberry twigs (Sangzhi), Large-leaf gentian root (Qinjiao) and Coix seed (Yiyiren).

Dosage: 10-15 g

116. Oriental wormwood (Yinchenhao)

Pharmaceutical Name: Herba Artemisiae Scopariae
Botanical Name: 1. Artemisia capillaris Thunb.; 2. Artemisia scoparia Waldst. et Kit.
Common Name: Capillaris, Oriental wormwood
Source of Earliest Record: Shennong Bencao Jing
Part Used & Method for Pharmaceutical Preparations: The young shoots are gathered in spring, when they are three inches high, and then dried in the sun.
Properties & Taste: Bitter and slightly cold
Meridians: Spleen, stomach, liver and gall bladder
Functions: 1. To clear heat and transform dampness; 2. To relieve jaundice
Indications & Combinations: Jaundice: a) damp-heat *yang* jaundice —Oriental wormwood (Yinchenhao) is used with Capejasmine (Zhizi) and Rhubarb (Dahuang) in the formula Yinchenhao Tang; b) cold-damp *yin* jaundice—Oriental wormwood (Yinchenhao) is used with Prepared aconite root (Fuzi) and Dried ginger (Ganjiang) in the formula Yinchen Sini Tang.
Dosage: 10-30 g

117. Broom cypress fruit (Difuzi)

Pharmaceutical Name: Fructus kochiae
Botanical Name: Kochia scoparia (L.) Schrad.
Common Name: Kochia fruit, Broom cypress fruit
Source of Earliest Record: Shennong Bencao Jing
Part Used & Method for Pharmaceutical Preparations: When the fruit ripens in autumn, it is gathered and dried in the sun.
Properties & Taste: Bitter and cold
Meridian: Urinary bladder
Functions: 1. To clear heat and transform dampness; 2. To stop itching
Indications & Combinations:
1. Damp-heat in the urinary bladder manifested as dysuria, painful

urination, frequent urination and urgency of micturition. Broom cypress fruit (Difuzi) is used with herbs that clear heat and promote urination, including Talc (Huashi) and Plantain seed (Cheqianzi).

2. Eczema and scabies. Broom cypress fruit (Difuzi) is used with Phellodendron bark (Huangbai), Flavescent sophora root (Kushen) and Dittany bark (Baixianpi).

Dosage: 10-15 g

118a. Benincasa peel (Dongguapi)

Pharmaceutical Name: Exocarpium Benincasae
Botanical Name: Benincasa hispida (Thunb.) Cogn.
Common Name: Benincasa peel, Chinese wax gourd
Source of Earliest Record: Kaibao Bencao
Part Used & Method for Pharmaceutical Preparations: The peel of the gourd is dried in the sun.
Properties & Taste: Sweet and slightly cold
Meridians: Lung and small intestine
Functions: To promote water metabolism and reduce edema
Indications & Combinations: Edema. Benincasa peel (Dongguapi) is used with Phaseolus seed (Chixiaodou), Imperata rhizome (Baimaogen) and Poria (Fuling) in the formula Donggua Wan.
Dosage: 15-30 g

118b. Benincasa seed (Dongguaren)

The Benincasa seed (Dongguaren), or Chinese wax gourd seed, is sweet and cold in properties, and clears heat in the lungs, resolves phlegm and eliminates pus. The herb is indicated in cough due to heat in the lungs, lung abscess and intestinal abscess. The dosage is 10-15 g.

119. Calabash gourd (Hulu)

Pharmaceutical Name: Pericarpium lagenariae
Botanical Name: Lagenaria siceraria (Molina) Standl.
Common Name: Calabash gourd
Source of Earliest Record: Rihuazi Bencao
Part Used & Method for Pharmaceutical Preparations: When the calabash gourd ripens in autumn, its peel is collected and dried in the sun.
Properties & Taste: Sweet and neutral

Meridians: Lung and small intestine
Functions: To promote water metabolism and reduce edema
Indications & Combinations: Edema. Calabash gourd (Hulu) is used with herbs which promote water metabolism, such as Benincasa peel (Dongguapi).
Dosage: 15-30 g

120. Phaseolus seed (Chixiaodou)

Pharmaceutical Name: Semen Phaseoli
Botanical Name: 1. Phaseolus calcaratus Roxb.; 2. Phaseolus angularis Wight
Common Name: Phaseolus seed, Adzuki bean
Source of Earliest Record: Shennong Bencao Jing
Part Used & Method for Pharmaceutical Preparations: The seeds are gathered in autumn and dried in the sun.
Properties & Taste: Sweet or sour and neutral
Meridians: Heart and small intestine
Functions: 1. To promote water metabolism and reduce edema; 2. To relieve jaundice; 3. To dispel toxins and eliminate pus
Indications & Combinations:
1. Edema. Phaseolus seed (Chixiaodou) is used with Imperata rhizome (Baimaogen) and Mulberry bark (Sangbaipi).
2. Edema due to deficiency in spleen or kidneys. Phaseolus seed (Chixiaodou) is cooked with carp to make a soup for drinking.
3. Boils and carbuncles due to toxic heat. The decoction of Phaseolus seed (Chixiaodou) is used externally for washing.
4. Damp-heat jaundice. Phaseolus seed (Chixiaodou) is used with Oriental wormwood (Yinchenhao) and Capejasmine (Zhizi).
Dosage: 10-30 g

121. Common knotgrass (Bianxu)

Pharmaceutical Name: Herba Polygoni avicularis
Botanical Name: Polygonum aviculare L.
Common Name: Polygonum, Common knotgrass
Source of Earliest Record: Shennong Bencao Jing
Part Used & Method for Pharmaceutical Preparations: The aerial parts of the plant are gathered in summer and dried in the sun.
Properties & Taste: Bitter and slightly cold

Meridian: Urinary bladder

Functions: 1. To promote water metabolism and regulate abnormal urination; 2. To expel parasites and stop itching

Indications & Combinations:

1. Damp-heat in the urinary bladder manifested as scanty urine with blood, painful urination, urgency of micturition and frequent urination. Common knotgrass (Bianxu) is used with Pink (Qumai), Clematis stem (Mutong) and Talc (Huashi) in the formula Bazhen San.

2. Eczema and trichomonas vaginalis. The decoction of Common knotgrass (Bianxu) is used externally for washing.

Dosage: 10-15 g

122. Pink (Qumai)

Pharmaceutical Name: Herba dianthi

Botanical Name: 1. Dianthus superbus L.; 2. Dianthus chinensis L.

Common Name: Dianthus, Pink

Source of Earliest Record: Shennong Bencao Jing

Part Used & Method for Pharmaceutical Preparations: The whole plant is gathered and dried after it flowers in summer or autumn.

Properties & Taste: Bitter and cold

Meridians: Heart, small intestine and urinary bladder

Functions: 1. To promote urination and regulate abnormal urination; 2. To invigorate blood circulation

Indications & Combinations:

1. Damp-heat in the urinary bladder manifested as scanty urine with blood, painful urination, frequent urination and urgency of micturition. Pink (Qumai) is used with Clematis stem (Mutong), Talc (Huashi) and Common knotgrass (Bianxu) in the formula Bazheng San.

2. Amenorrhea from blood stagnation. Pink (Qumai) is used with herbs that invigorate blood circulation, such as Peach seed (Taoren) and Safflower (Honghua).

Dosage: 10-15 g

Cautions & Contraindications: This herb is contraindicated during pregnancy.

123. Abutilon (Dongkuizi)

Pharmaceutical Name: Semen Malvae

Botanical Name: Malva verticillata L.

Common Name: Abutilon seed

Source of Earliest Record: Shennong Bencao Jing

Part Used & Method for Pharmaceutical Preparations: After the fruit ripens in summer or autumn, the seeds are gathered and ground into powder.

Properties & Taste: Sweet and cold

Meridians: Large intestine and small intestine

Functions: 1. To promote urination and regulate abnormal urination; 2. To promote lactation; 3. To moisten intestines and move feces

Indications & Combinations:

1. Dysuria and edema. Abutilon (Dongkuizi) is used with Poria (Fuling) and White atractylodes (Baizhu).

2. Scanty urine with blood and painful urination. Abutilon (Dongkuizi) is used with Plantain seed (Cheqianzi), Lygodium spores (Haijin-sha) and Talc (Huashi).

3. Obstructed lactation and breast distension. Abutilon (Dongkuizi) is used with Amomum fruit (Sharen) and Ricepaper pith (Tongcao).

4. Constipation. Abutilon (Dongkuizi) is used with herbs that moisten intestines and move feces, such as Chinese angelica root (Danggui), Peach seed (Taoren) and Arborvitae seed (Baiziren).

Dosage: 9-15 g

VII. Herbs That Warm the Interior

Herbs that warm the interior and expel cold are pungent and hot. They warm the spleen and stomach, expel cold and stop pain in interior cold syndromes. The interior cold syndromes can be caused either by invasion of exogenous pathogenic cold leading to deficiency of *yang qi* in the spleen and stomach, or by weakness of *yang qi* giving rise to excessive *yin* and cold in the interior.

Manifestations of interior cold syndromes include: cold pain in the epigastric and abdominal regions, vomiting and diarrhea; or cold extremities, pale, profuse and clear urine, pale tongue with white coating and deep and thready pulse. In serious cases, there is collapse of *yang* with ice-cold extremities and weak-thready pulse.

Herbs that warm the interior are used in combination with herbs that release the exterior when an exterior syndrome accompanies the interior cold syndrome. Herbs that promote *qi* circulation are used with herbs that warm the interior for interior cold and stagnation syndromes. Herbs that strengthen the spleen in the transformation of dampness are combined with herbs of this category for interior cold and dampness syndromes. Herbs that tonify the spleen and kidney are added to the combination for deficiency of the spleen and kidneys. Herbs that tonify the source *qi* are used with these herbs for collapsing *yang* and *qi*.

These herbs are contraindicated during heat syndromes, *yin* deficiency with heat signs and during pregnancy.

124. Prepared aconite root (Fuzi)

Pharmaceutical Name: Radix Aconiti lateralis praeparata
Botanical Name: Aconitum carmichaeli Debx.
Common Name: Prepared aconite root
Source of Earliest Record: Shennong Bencao Jing
Part Used & Method for Pharmaceutical Preparations: The roots are dug in late July and early August. After the fibrous roots have been removed, the roots are prepared with salt.
Properties & Taste: Pungent, hot and toxic
Meridians: Heart, kidney and spleen
Functions: 1. To warm and strengthen kidney *yang*; 2. To expel cold and stop pain
Indications & Combinations:

1. Collapsing of *yang* syndrome manifested as cold extremities, spontaneous cold sweating and fading pulse. Prepared aconite root (Fuzi) is used with Dried ginger (Ganjiang) and Licorice root (Gancao) in the formula Sini Tang.

2. Collapsing of *yang qi* syndrome manifested as profuse sweating, shortness of breath and asthma. Prepared aconite root (Fuzi) is used with Ginseng (Renshen) in the formula Shen Fu Tang.

3. Deficiency of kidney *yang* and declined kidney fire manifested as chills, cold limbs, soreness and weakness of lumbar region, impotence and frequent urination. Prepared aconite root (Fuzi) is used with Cinnamon bark (Rougui), Dogwood fruit (Shanzhuyu) and Prepared rehmannia root (Shudihuang) in the formula Gui Fu Bawei Wan.

4. Weakness of spleen *yang* manifested as cold in the epigastric and abdominal regions and diarrhea. Prepared aconite root (Fuzi) is used with Ginseng (Renshen), White atractylodes (Baizhu) and Dried ginger

(Ganjiang) in the formula Fuzi Lizhong Wan.

5. Deficient *yang* in the spleen and kidneys manifested as dysuria and general edema. Prepared aconite root (Fuzi) is used with White atractylodes (Baizhu) and Poria (Fuling) in the formula Zhenwu Tang.

6. Heart *yang* deficiency manifested as palpitations, shortness of breath and stifling sensation and pain in the chest. Prepared aconite root (Fuzi) is used with Ginseng (Renshen) and Cinnamon twigs (Guizhi).

7. Weakness of defensive *yang* manifested as spontaneous sweating. Prepared aconite root (Fuzi) is used with Astragalus root (Huangqi) and Cinnamon twigs (Guizhi).

8. Invasion by wind and cold in a person with deficient *yang*. Prepared aconite root (Fuzi) is used with Ephedra (Mahuang) and Asarum herb (Xixin) in the formula Mahuang Fuzi Xixin Tang.

9. Cold-damp obstruction syndrome manifested as general joint pain and chills. Prepared aconite root (Fuzi) is used with Cinnamon twigs (Guizhi) and White atractylodes (Baizhu) in the formula Gancao Fuzi Tang.

Dosage: 3-15 g

Cautions & Contraindications: This herb is contraindicated during pregnancy.

125. Dried ginger (Ganjiang)

Pharmaceutical Name: Rhizoma zingiberis
Botanical Name: Zingiber officinale (Willd.) Rosc.
Common Name: Dried ginger
Source of Earliest Record: Shennong Bencao Jing
Part Used & Method for Pharmaceutical Preparations: The rhizomes are dug in winter. After the fibrous roots have been removed, the rhizomes are cleaned, dried in the sun and cut into slices.
Properties & Taste: Pungent and hot
Meridians: Spleen, stomach, heart and lung
Functions: 1. To warm spleen and stomach and dispel cold; 2. To prevent *yang* from collapsing; 3. To warm the lungs and resolve phlegm-damp
Indications & Combinations:

1. Cold attacking the spleen and stomach manifested as cold pain in the epigastric and abdominal regions, vomiting and diarrhea. Dried

ginger (Ganjiang) is used with Evodia fruit (Wuzhuyu) and Pinellia tuber (Banxia).

2. Weakness and cold in the spleen and stomach manifested as fullness and distension in the epigastric and abdominal regions, vomiting, nausea, loose stool, poor appetite, lassitude and deficient, weak pulse. Dried ginger (Ganjiang) is used with White atractylodes (Baizhu) and Poria (Fuling) in the formula Lizhong Wan.

3. Collapsing of *yang* manifested as cold sweating, cold extremities, spontaneous sweating, listlessness and fading pulse. Dried ginger (Ganjiang) is used with Prepared aconite root (Fuzi) in the formula Sini Tang.

4. Cold phlegm in the lungs manifested as chills, asthma, cough with clear and profuse sputum and cold feeling in the upper back. Dried ginger (Ganjiang) is used with Ephedra (Mahuang), Asarum herb (Xixin) and Pinellia tuber (Banxia) in the formula Xiao Qinglong Tang.

Dosage: 3-10 g

Cautions & Contraindications: This herb should be used with caution during pregnancy.

126. Cinnamon bark (Rougui)

Pharmaceutical Name: Cortex Cinnamomi
Botanical Name: Cinnamomum cassia presl
Common Name: Cinnamon bark, Cassia bark
Source of Earliest Record: Mingyi Bielu
Part Used & Method for Pharmaceutical Preparations: The bark is cut in the period of Great Heat (twelfth solar term) and peeled off in the period of the Beginning of Autumn (thirteenth solar term). It is dried in the shade and cut into slices.
Properties & Taste: Pungent, sweet and hot
Meridians: Kidney, spleen, heart and liver
Functions: 1. To tonify the kidneys; 2. To dispel cold and stop pain; 3. To warm the channels and promote circulation
Indications & Combinations:

1. Kidney *yang* deficiency manifested as cold limbs, soreness and weakness of the lumbar region and knees, impotence, spermatorrhea and frequent urination. Cinnamon bark (Rougui) is used with Prepared aconite root (Fuzi), Prepared rehmannia root (Shudihuang) and Dogwood fruit (Shanzhuyu) in the formula Gui Fu Bawei Wan.

109

2. Deficient *yang* of the spleen and kidneys manifested as cold pain in the epigastric and abdominal regions, poor appetite and loose stool. Cinnamon bark (Rougui) is used with Dried ginger (Ganjiang), White atractylodes (Baizhu) and Prepared aconite root (Fuzi) in the formula Gui Fu Lizhong Wan.

3. Cold stagnation in the meridians manifested as epigastric and abdominal cold pain, lower back pain, general pain, irregular menstruation and dysmenorrhea. Cinnamon bark (Rougui) is used with Dried ginger (Ganjiang), Evodia fruit (Wuzhuyu), Chinese angelica root (Danggui) and Chuanxiong rhizome (Chuanxiong).

4. *Yin* type of boils (chronic boils). Cinnamon bark (Rougui) is used with Astragalus root (Huangqi) and Chinese angelica root (Danggui) in the formula Tuoli Huangqi Tang.

Dosage: 2-5 g

Cautions & Contraindications: This herb is contraindicated during pregnancy.

127. Evodia fruit (Wuzhuyu)

Pharmaceutical Name: Fructus Evodiae
Botanical Name: Evodia rutaecarpa (Juss.) Benth.
Common Name: Evodia fruit
Source of Earliest Record: Shennong Bencao Jing
Part Used & Method for Pharmaceutical Preparations: The fruit is gathered in August or November and dried in the sun. It is then soaked in the decoction of Licorice root (Gancao).
Properties & Taste: Pungent, bitter, hot and slightly toxic
Meridians: Liver, spleen and stomach
Functions: 1. To dispel cold and stop pain; 2. To pacify the liver and direct rebellious *qi* downward; 3. To stop vomiting
Indications & Combinations:

1. Cold attacking the spleen and stomach manifested as epigastric and abdominal cold pain. Evodia fruit (Wuzhuyu) is used with Dried ginger (Ganjiang) and Costus root (Muxiang).

2. Cold stagnation in the liver meridians manifested as hernia. Evodia fruit (Wuzhuyu) is used with Fennel fruit (Xiaohuixiang) and Lindera root (Wuyao).

3. Weakness of spleen and stomach, and liver *qi* rising upward manifested as headache and vomiting. Evodia fruit (Wuzhuyu) is used

with Ginseng (Renshen) and Fresh ginger (Shengjiang) in the formula Wuzhuyu Tang.

4. Deficiency and cold of the spleen and kidneys manifested as chronic diarrhea. Evodia fruit (Wuzhuyu) is used with Schisandra fruit (Wuweizi) and Nutmeg (Roudoukou) in the formula Sishen Wan.

5. Beriberi. Evodia fruit (Wuzhuyu) is used with Chaenomeles fruit (Mugua) for external application.

6. Vomiting and acid regurgitation: a) cold in the stomach—Evodia fruit (Wuzhuyu) is used with Fresh ginger (Shengjiang) and Pinellia tuber (Banxia); b) fire transformed from prolonged liver *qi* stagnation —Evodia fruit (Wuzhuyu) is used with Coptis root (Huanglian) in the formula Zuojin Wan.

Dosage: 1.5-5 g

128. Asarum herb (Xixin)

Pharmaceutical Name: Herba asari cum Radice

Botanical Name: 1. Asarum hetrotropoides Fr. var. mandshuricum (Maxim.) Kitag. 2. A. sieboldii Miq.

Common Name: Asarum herb, Wild ginger

Source of Earliest Record: Shennong Bencao Jing

Part Used & Method for Pharmaceutical Preparations: The entire plant is gathered in summer and dried in the shade.

Properties & Taste: Pungent and warm

Meridians: Lung and kidney

Functions: 1. To dispel cold and stop pain; 2. To warm the lungs and resolve phlegm-damp; 3. To relieve nasal congestion

Indications & Combinations:

1. Headache, toothache and obstruction pain: a) wind-cold headache—Asarum herb (Xixin) is used with Chuanxiong rhizome (Chuanxiong) in the formula Chuanxiong Cha Tiao San; b) wind-cold toothache—Asarum herb (Xixin) is used with Dahurian angelica root (Baizhi); c) toothache due to excessive heat in the stomach—Asarum herb (Xixin) is used with Gypsum (Shigao) and Scutellaria root (Huangqin); d) wind-cold-damp obstruction syndrome (joint pain) —Asarum herb (Xixin) is used with Notopterygium root (Qianghuo), Ledebouriella root (Fangfeng) and Cinnamon twigs (Guizhi).

2. Wind-cold exterior syndromes manifested as chills, fever, headache and general pain. Asarum herb (Xixin) is used with Notoptery-

gium root (Qianghuo) and Ledebouriella root (Fangfeng) in the formula Jiuwei Qianghuo Tang.

3. Cold phlegm fluid attacking the lungs manifested as asthma and cough with profuse, clear sputum. Asarum herb (Xixin) is used with Ephedra (Mahuang) and Dried ginger (Ganjiang) in the formula Xiao Qinglong Tang.

4. Rhinorrhea manifested as copiously running nose, nasal congestion and headache. Asarum herb (Xixin) is used with Angelica root (Baizhi), Magnolia flower (Xinyi) and Mentha (Bohe).

Dosage: 1-3 g

Cautions & Contraindications: This herb is contraindicated in headache due to deficient *yin* and hyperactivity of *yang*, or cough caused by heat in the lungs.

129. Prickly ash peel (Huajiao)

Pharmaceutical Name: Pericarpium Zanthoxyli

Botanical Name: 1. Zanthoxylum bungeanum Maxim; 2. Zathoxylum schinifolium Sieb. et Zucc.

Common Name: Chinese pepper, Prickly ash peel, Zanthoxylum

Source of Earliest Record: Xinxiu Bencao

Part Used & Method for Pharmaceutical Preparations: The prickly ash peel is gathered in autumn and dried in the sun.

Properties & Taste: Pungent, hot and slightly toxic

Meridians: Spleen, stomach and kidney

Functions: 1. To warm the spleen and stomach; 2. To stop pain; 3. To kill parasites

Indications & Combinations:

1. *Yang* deficiency of the spleen and stomach manifested as epigastric and abdominal cold pain, vomiting and diarrhea. Prickly ash peel (Huajiao) is used with Pilose asiabell root (Dangshen), Dried ginger (Ganjiang) and Malted barley (Yitang) in the formula Da Jianzhong Tang.

2. Roundworm manifested as abdominal pain and vomiting. Prickly ash peel (Huajiao) is used with Black plum (Wumei), Dried ginger (Ganjiang) and Coptis root (Huanglian) in the formula Wumei Wan.

Dosage: 2-5 g

130. Cloves (Dingxiang)

Pharmaceutical Name: Flos Caryophylatae
Botanical Name: Eugenia caryophyllata Thunb.
Common Name: Cloves
Source of Earliest Record: Yaoxing Lun
Part Used & Method for Pharmaceutical Preparations: The flower buds are gathered in September or March, when the buds turn bright red. Then, they are dried.
Properties & Taste: Pungent and warm
Meridians: Spleen, stomach and kidney
Functions: 1. To warm the spleen and stomach and direct rebellious *qi* downward; 2. To warm the kidneys and tonify the *yang*
Indications & Combinations:

1. Cold in the stomach manifested as belching and vomiting. Cloves (Dingxiang) is used with Pinellia tuber (Banxia) and Fresh ginger (Shengjiang).

2. Weakness and cold in the spleen and stomach manifested as poor appetite, vomiting and diarrhea. Cloves (Dingxiang) is used with Amomum fruit (Sharen) and White atractylodes (Baizhu).

3. Weakness and cold in the stomach manifested as belching and vomiting. Cloves (Dingxiang) is used with Ginseng (Renshen) or Pilose asiabell root (Dangshen) and Fresh ginger (Shengjiang).

4. Kidney *yang* deficiency manifested as impotence. Cloves (Dingxiang) is used with Prepared aconite root (Fuzi), Cinnamon bark (Rougui), Morinda root (Bajitian) and Epimedium (Yinyanghuo).

Dosage: 2-5 g
Cautions & Contraindications: This herb should not be combined with the herb Curcuma root (Yujin).

131. Galangal rhizome (Gaoliangjiang)

Pharmaceutical Name: Rhizome Alpinia officinarum
Botanical Name: Alpinia officinarum Hance
Common Name: Galanga rhizome, Lesser Galangal
Source of Earliest Record: Mingyi Bielu
Part Used & Method for Pharmaceutical Preparations: The four to six year old rhizomes are dug in late summer or at the beginning of autumn. After the fibrous roots have been removed, the rhizomes are cut into pieces and dried in the sun.

Properties & Taste: Spleen and stomach
Meridians: Spleen and stomach
Functions: To warm the spleen and stomach and stop pain
Indications & Combinations:

1. Cold and *qi* stagnation manifested as epigastric and abdominal pain. Galangal rhizome (Gaoliangjiang) is used with Cyperus tuber (Xiangfu) in the formula Liang Fu Wan.

2. Cold in the stomach manifested as vomiting. Galangal rhizome (Gaoliangjiang) is used with Pinellia tuber (Banxia) and Fresh ginger (Shengjiang).

Dosage: 3-10 g

132. Fennel fruit (Xiaohuixiang)

Pharmaceutical Name: Fructus Foeniculi
Botanical Name: Foeniculum vulgare Mill.
Common Name: Fennel fruit
Source of Earliest Record: Xinxiu Bencao
Part Used & Method for Pharmaceutical Preparations: The fruit is gathered in late summer or early autumn and dried in the sun.
Properties & Taste: Pungent and warm
Meridians: Liver, kidney, spleen and stomach
Functions: 1. To dispel cold and stop pain; 2. To regulate *qi* and harmonize the stomach
Indications & Combinations:

1. Cold stagnation in the liver meridian manifested as hernia. Fennel fruit (Xiaohuixiang) is used with Cinnamon bark (Rougui) and Lindera root (Wuyao) in the formula Nuangan Jian.

2. Cold in the stomach manifested as vomiting and epigastric distension and pain. Fennel fruit (Xiaohuixiang) is used with Dried ginger (Ganjiang) and Costus root (Muxiang).

Dosage: 3-8 g

VIII. Herbs That Regulate *Qi*

Herbs that regulate *qi* are aromatic, pungent and bitter. They are good for promoting the free flow of *qi*, and are indicated in *qi* stagnation and *qi* perversion. *Qi* stagnation may be manifested as stifling distension and pain, while *qi* perversion as nausea, vomiting, belching, asthma and cough.

Several manifestations may appear depending on the organs involved. If the lungs fail their function of descending, the failure is manifested as discomfort, stifling sensation in the chest, cough and asthma. If the liver is stagnated, the manifestations are hypochondriac pain, stifling sensation in the chest, hernia pain, nodules, distension and pain in the breasts, or irregular menstruation. If *qi* stagnation in the spleen and stomach impair their normal functions of ascending and descending, the resulting symptoms include fullness, distension and pain in the epigastric and abdominal regions, belching, sour regurgitation, nausea, vomiting and diarrhea or constipation.

How these herbs are combined with other ones is determined by the complex set of pathological conditions present. For example, if excessive heat and phlegm accumulate in the lungs with the resulting manifestations of cough and asthma, these herbs should be used with herbs that clear heat and resolve phlegm.

When using these herbs, it is important to remember that most are aromatic, pungent and dry. Prolonged administration can injure *yin*. They should be used with caution in patients with deficient *qi* or deficient *yin*.

133. Tangerine peel (Chenpi)

Pharmaceutical Name: Pericarpium Citri reticulatae
Botanical Name: Citrus reticulata Blanco
Common Name: Tangerine peel
Source of Earliest Record: Shennong Bencao Jing
Part Used & Method for Pharmaceutical Preparations: After tangerines ripen in autumn, the skins are collected and dried.
Properties & Taste: Pungent, bitter and warm
Meridians: Spleen and lung
Functions: 1. To regulate *qi* in the spleen and stomach; 2. To dry dampness and resolve phlegm
Indications & Combinations:

1. *Qi* stagnation in the spleen and stomach manifested as epigastric and abdominal distension and fullness, belching, nausea and vomiting, poor appetite and diarrhea. Tangerine peel (Chenpi) is used with Bitter orange (Zhiqiao) and Costus root (Muxiang) for epigastric and abdom-

inal distension and fullness, with Fresh ginger (Shengjiang) and Bamboo shavings (Zhuru) for nausea and vomiting, and with Pilose asiabell root (Dangshen) and White atractylodes (Baizhu) for poor appetite and diarrhea.

2. Dampness blocking the spleen and stomach manifested as fullness and stifling sensation in the chest and epigastric region, poor appetite, lassitude, diarrhea and white and sticky tongue coating. Tangerine peel (Chenpi) is used with Atractylodes rhizome (Cangzhu) and Magnolia bark (Houpo) in the formula Pingwei San.

3. Excessive dampness, deficiency of the spleen and turbid phlegm blocking the lungs manifested as cough with profuse sputum. Tangerine peel (Chenpi) is used with Pinellia tuber (Banxia) and Poria (Fuling) in the formula Erchen Tang.

Dosage: 3-10 g

134. Green tangerine peel (Qingpi)

Pharmaceutical Name: Pericarpium Citri reticulatae viride
Botanical Name: Citrus reticulata blanco
Common Name: Green tangerine peel
Source of Earliest Record: Bencao Tujing
Part Used & Method for Pharmaceutical Preparations: When tangerines are still green in June or July, the green skins are removed, cleaned and dried in the sun.
Properties & Taste: Bitter, pungent and warm
Meridians: Liver, gall bladder and stomach
Functions: 1. To promote the free flow of *qi* in the liver; 2. To relieve retention of food and disperse stagnation
Indications & Combinations:

1. Stagnation of *qi* in the liver manifested as distension and pain in the breast and hypochondriac regions. Green tangerine peel (Qingpi) is used with Bupleurum root (Chaihu), Curcuma root (Yujin), Cyperus tuber (Xiangfu) and Green tangerine leaf (Qingjuye).

2. Mastitis. Green tangerine peel (Qingpi) is used with Trichosanthes fruit (Gualou), Dandelion herb (Pugongying), Honeysuckle flower (Jinyinhua) and Forsythia fruit (Lianqiao).

3. Cold stagnated in the liver meridian manifested as painful swelling of testicles or scrotum, or hernia. Green tangerine peel (Qingpi) is used with Lindera root (Wuyao), Fennel fruit (Xiaohuixiang) and

Costus root (Muxiang) in the formula Tiantai Wuyao San.

4. Retention of food manifested as fullness, distension and pain in the epigastric region. Green tangerine peel (Qingpi) is used with Hawthorn fruit (Shanzha), Germinated barley (Maiya) and Medicated leaven (Shenqu) in the formula Qingpi Wan.

Dosage: 3-10 g

135. Immature bitter orange (Zhishi)

Pharmaceutical Name: Fructus Aurantii immaturus
Botanical Name: 1. Citrus aurantium L.; 2. Citrus sinensis Osbeck
Common Name: Immature bitter orange fruit
Source of Earliest Record: Shennong Bencao Jing
Part Used & Method for Pharmaceutical Preparations: The immature fruit is gathered in July or August. The fruit is halved and dried in the sun, cleaned, soaked in water overnight, cut into slices and dried again.

Properties & Taste: Bitter, pungent and slightly cold
Meridians: Spleen, stomach and large intestine
Functions: 1. To disperse stagnant *qi* and relieve food retention; 2. To resolve phlegm and relieve fullness sensation

Indications & Combinations:

1. Retention of food manifested as epigastric and abdominal distension and fullness and belching with foul odor. Immature bitter orange (Zhishi) is used with Hawthorn fruit (Shanzha), Germinated barley (Maiya) and Medicated leaven (Shenqu).

2. Abdominal distension, fullness and constipation. Immature bitter orange (Zhishi) is used with Magnolia bark (Houpo) and Rhubarb (Dahuang).

3. Weakness of the spleen and stomach in transporting and transforming manifested as epigastric and abdominal distension and fullness after meals. Immature bitter orange (Zhishi) is used with White atractylodes (Baizhu) in the formula Zhi Zhu Wan.

4. Damp-heat stagnating in the intestines manifested as dysentery, tenesmus and abdominal pain. Immature bitter orange (Zhishi) is used with Rhubarb (Dahuang), Coptis root (Huanglian) and Scutellaria root (Huangqin) in the formula Zhishi Daozhi Wan.

5. Turbid phlegm blocking circulation of *qi* in the chest manifested as stifling sensation and pain in the chest, epigastric fullness and nausea. Immature bitter orange (Zhishi) is used Macrostem onion (Xiebai),

Cinnamon twigs (Guizhi) and Trichosanthes fruit (Gualou) in the formula Zhishi Xiebai Guizhi Tang.

6. Prolapse of the uterus, rectum and stomach. Immature bitter orange (Zhishi) is used with White atractylodes (Baizhu) and Astragalus root (Huangqi).

Dosage: 3-10 g

Cautions & Contraindications: This herb should be used with caution during pregnancy.

136. Finger citron (Foshou)

Pharmaceutical Name: Fructus Citri sarcodactylis
Botanical Name: Citrus medica L. var. Sarcodactylis Swingle
Common Name: Finger citron fruit
Source of Earliest Record: Bencao Tujing
Part Used & Method for Pharmaceutical Preparations: The ripe fruit is gathered from October to December, then cut into slices and dried in the sun.
Properties & Taste: Pungent, bitter and warm
Meridians: Liver, spleen, stomach and lung
Functions: 1. To pacify liver and regulate *qi*; 2. To harmonize the spleen and stomach and resolve phlegm
Indications & Combinations:

1. *Qi* stagnation in the liver manifested as costal pain and stifling sensation in the chest. Finger citron (Foshou) is used with Cyperus tuber (Xiangfu), Citron (Xiangyuan) and Curcuma root (Yujin).

2. *Qi* stagnation in the spleen and stomach manifested as epigastric and abdominal distension and fullness, stomach pain, poor appetite, belching, nausea and vomiting. Finger citron (Foshou) is used with Costus root (Muxiang) and Bitter orange (Zhiqiao).

3. Chest pain and cough with profuse sputum. Finger citron (Foshou) is used with Loquat leaf (Pipaye), Vegetable sponge (Sigualuo) and Apricot seed (Xingren).

Dosage: 3-10 g

137. Citron (Xiangyuan)

Pharmaceutical Name: Fructus Citri
Botanical Name: 1. Citrus medica L.; 2. Citrus wilsonii Tanaka
Common Name: Citron fruit

Source of Earliest Record: Bencao Tujing

Part Used & Method for Pharmaceutical Preparations: The ripe fruit is gathered in October, cleaned, dried in the sun and cut into slices.

Properties & Taste: Pungent, slightly bitter, sour and warm

Meridians: Liver, spleen and lung

Functions: 1. To promote the free flow of *qi* in the liver; 2. To harmonize the spleen and stomach and resolve phlegm

Indications & Combinations:

1. *Qi* stagnation in the liver manifested as costal pain and stifling sensation in the chest. Citron (Xiangyuan) is used with Curcuma root (Yujin), Finger citron (Foshou) and Cyperus tuber (Xiangfu).

2. *Qi* stagnation in the spleen and stomach manifested as epigastric and abdominal distension and pain, nausea, vomiting, poor appetite and belching. Citron (Xiangyuan) is used with Costus root (Muxiang), Finger citron (Foshou), Bitter orange (Zhiqiao) and Tangerine peel (Chenpi).

3. Cough with profuse sputum. Citron (Xiangyuan) is used with Pinellia tuber (Banxia) and Poria (Fuling).

Dosage: 3-10 g

138. Costus root (Muxiang)

Pharmaceutical Name: Radix Aucklandiae seu Vladimiriae

Botanical Name: 1. Aucklandia lappa Decne.; 2. Vladimiria souliei (Franch.) Ling

Common Name: Aucklandia root, Costus root

Source of Earliest Record: Shennong Bencao Jing

Part Used & Method for Pharmaceutical Preparations: The roots are dug in October and can be used raw or baked.

Properties & Taste: Pungent, bitter and warm

Meridians: Spleen, stomach, large intestine and gall bladder

Functions: 1. To regulate *qi* in the spleen and stomach; 2. To stop pain

Indications & Combinations:

1. *Qi* stagnation in the spleen and stomach manifested as poor appetite, epigastric and abdominal distension and pain, borborygmus and diarrhea. Costus root (Muxiang) is used with Poria (Fuling), Bitter orange (Zhiqiao) and Tangerine peel (Chenpi).

2. Damp-heat dysentery manifested as tenesmus and abdominal

pain. Costus root (Muxiang) is used with Rhubarb (Dahuang) and Areca seed (Binglang) in the formula Muxiang Binglang Wan.

Dosage: 3-10 g

Cautions & Contraindications: The raw herb is used for *qi* stagnation, and the baked herb is used for diarrhea.

139. Cyperus tuber (Xiangfu)

Pharmaceutical Name: Rhizoma Cyperi

Botanical Name: Cyperus rotundus L.

Common Name: Cyperus tuber, Nutgrass rhizome

Source of Earliest Record: Mingyi Bielu

Part Used & Method for Pharmaceutical Preparations: The rhizomes are dug in September or October. They are cleaned and dried in the sun. The fibrous roots are burned away, leaving the rhizomes ready for use.

Properties & Taste: Pungent, slightly bitter, slightly sweet and neutral

Meridians: Liver and triple *jiao*

Functions: 1. To promote the free flow of *qi* in the liver; 2. To regulate menstruation and stop pain

Indications & Combinations:

1. *Qi* stagnation in the liver manifested as costal pain and stifling sensation in the chest. Cyperus tuber (Xiangfu) is used with Bupleurum root (Chaihu), Curcuma root (Yujin) and White peony root (Baishao).

2. Liver *qi* attacking the stomach manifested as epigastric and abdominal distension and pain. Cyperus tuber (Xiangfu) is used with Costus root (Muxiang), Citron (Xiangyuan) and Finger citron (Foshou).

3. Cold and *qi* stagnation in the stomach. Cyperus tuber (Xiangfu) is used with Galangal rhizome (Gaoliangjiang) in the formula Liang Fu Wan.

4. Cold stagnation in the liver meridian manifested as painful swelling of testicles or scrotum, or hernia. Cyperus tuber (Xiangfu) is used with Fennel fruit (Xiaohuixiang) and Lindera root (Wuyao).

5. *Qi* stagnation in the liver manifested as irregular menstruation, dysmenorrhea and distension and pain in the breasts. Cyperus tuber (Xiangfu) is used with Bupleurum root (Chaihu), Chinese angelica root (Danggui) and Chuanxiong rhizome (Chuanxiong).

Dosage: 6-12 g

140. Lindera root (Wuyao)

Pharmaceutical Name: Radix Linderae
Botanical Name: Lindera strychnifolia (Sieb. et Zucc.) Vill.
Common Name: Lindera root, Spicebush root
Source of Earliest Record: Bencao Shiyi
Part Used & Method for Pharmaceutical Preparations: The roots are dug in August. After the fibrous roots and bark have been removed, the roots are cut into slices and dried in the sun.
Properties & Taste: Pungent and warm
Meridians: Lung, spleen, kidney and urinary bladder
Functions: 1. To regulate *qi* and stop pain; 2. To warm the kidneys and dispel cold
Indications & Combinations:

1. Cold and *qi* stagnation: a) manifested as stifling sensation in the chest and costal pain—Lindera root (Wuyao) is used with Trichosanthes fruit (Gualou), Curcuma root (Yujin) and Bitter orange (Zhiqiao); b) manifested as epigastric and abdominal distension and pain—Lindera root (Wuyao) is used with Costus root (Muxiang); c) manifested as painful swelling of testicles or scrotum, or hernia. Lindera root (Wuyao) is used with Fennel fruit (Xiaohuixiang) and Green tangerine peel (Qingpi) in the formula Tiantai Wuyao San; d) manifested as dysmenorrhea—Lindera root (Wuyao) is used with Cyperus tuber (Xiangfu), Chinese angelica root (Danggui) and Chuanxiong rhizome (Chuanxiong).

2. Kidney *yang* deficiency and deficiency and cold of the urinary bladder manifested as frequent urination and enuresis. Lindera root (Wuyao) is used with Bitter cardamom (Yizhiren) and Dioscorea (Shanyao) in the formula Suoquan Wan.
Dosage: 3-10 g

141. Eagle wood (Chenxiang)

Pharmaceutical Name: Lignum Aquilariae resinatum
Botanical Name: 1. Aquilaria agallocha Roxb.; 2. Aquilaria sinensis (Lour.) Gilg
Common Name: Aquilaria, Eagle wood
Source of Earliest Record: Mingyi Bielu
Part Used & Method for Pharmaceutical Preparations: The heartwood, or resinous wood, is dried in a shady place, then sawn into

powder.

Properties & Taste: Pungent, bitter and warm

Meridians: Spleen, stomach and kidney

Functions: 1. To regulate *qi* and stop pain; 2. To descend the perverse *qi* and stop vomiting; 3. To strengthen the kidneys and stop asthma

Indications & Combinations:

1. Cold and *qi* stagnation manifested as epigastric and abdominal distension and pain. Eagle wood (Chenxiang) is used with Lindera root (Wuyao) and Costus root (Muxiang).

2. Cold in the stomach manifested as belching and vomiting. Eagle wood (Chenxiang) is used with Cloves (Dingxiang) and Round cardamom seed (Baidoukou).

3. Asthma due to failure of the kidneys in receiving *qi*. Eagle wood (Chenxiang) is used with Prepared aconite root (Fuzi) and Cinnamon bark (Rougui).

Dosage: 1-1.5 g

142. Sichuan chinaberry (Chuanlianzi)

Pharmaceutical Name: Fructus Toosedan

Botanical Name: Melia toosedan Sieb. et Zucc.

Common Name: Sichuan chinaberry, Melia, Fruit of Sichuan pagoda tree

Source of Earliest Record: Shennong Bencao Jing

Part Used & Method for Pharmaceutical Preparations: The fruit is gathered in winter, cleaned and dried in the sun and broken into pieces.

Properties & Taste: Bitter, cold and slightly toxic

Meridians: Liver, stomach, small intestine and urinary bladder

Functions: To regulate *qi* and stop pain

Indications & Combinations:

1. *Qi* stagnation in the liver and stomach manifested as epigastric and abdominal distension and pain. Sichuan chinaberry (Chuanlianzi) is used with Corydalis tuber (Yanhusuo) in the formula Jinlingzi San.

2. Hernia with painful swelling of testicles or scrotum. Sichuan chinaberry (Chuanlianzi) is used with Fennel fruit (Xiaohuixiang), Costus root (Muxiang) and Evodia fruit (Wuzhuyu) in the formula Daoqi Tang.

Dosage: 3-10 g

Cautions & Contraindications: This herb is contraindicated in cases with deficiency and cold in the stomach and spleen.

143. Macrostem onion (Xiebai)

Pharmaceutical Name: Bulbus Allii macrostemi
Botanical Name: Allium macrostemon Bge.
Common Name: Macrostem onion, Bakeri, Bulb of Chinese chive
Source of Earliest Record: Shennong Bencao Jing
Part Used & Method for Pharmaceutical Preparations: The macrostem, or bulb, of the onion is dug in May, cleaned and dried in the sun.
Properties & Taste: Pungent, bitter and warm
Meridians: Lung, stomach and large intestine
Functions: 1. To promote the flow of *yang* and dissipate cold phlegm; 2. To regulate *qi* and reduce stagnation
Indications & Combinations:

1. Cold phlegm stagnated in the chest manifested as stifling sensation and pain in the chest and dyspnea. Macrostem onion (Xiebai) is used with Trichosanthes fruit (Gualou) in the formula Gualou Xiebai Baijiu Tang.

2. Dysentery manifested as tenesmus. Macrostem onion (Xiebai) is used with Immature bitter orange (Zhishi), Costus root (Muxiang) and White peony root (Baishao).
Dosage: 5-10 g

144. Sandalwood (Tanxiang)

Pharmaceutical Name: Lignum Santati albi
Botanical Name: Santatum album L.
Common Name: Santalum, Sandal wood
Source of Earliest Record: Mingyi Bielu
Part Used & Method for Pharmaceutical Preparations: The heartwood of sandalwood is cut into slices in the summer.
Properties & Taste: Pungent and warm
Meridians: Spleen, stomach and lung
Functions: 1. To regulate *qi* in the spleen and stomach; 2. To dispel cold and stop pain
Indications & Combinations:

1. Cold and *qi* stagnation manifested as epigastric and abdominal pain and vomiting with clear fluid. Sandalwood (Tanxiang) is used with

Amomum fruit (Sharen) and Lindera root (Wuyao).

2. Angina pectoris and coronary heart disease. Sandalwood (Tan-xiang) is used with Corydalis tuber (Yanhusuo) and Asarum herb (Xixin) in the formula Kuanxiong Wan.

Dosage: 1-3 g

145. Persimmon calyx (Shidi)

Pharmaceutical Name: Calyx kaki
Botanical Name: Diospyros kaki L. f.
Common Name: Kaki calyx, Persimmon calyx
Source of Earliest Record: Mingyi Bielu
Part Used & Method for Pharmaceutical Preparations: The calyx is gathered in August or September and dried in the sun.
Properties & Taste: Bitter and neutral
Meridian: Stomach
Functions: To direct *qi* downward and stop hiccups
Indications & Combinations: Hiccups: a) due to cold in the stomach —Persimmon calyx (Shidi) is used with Cloves (Dingxiang) and Fresh ginger (Shengjiang); b) due to heat in the stomach—Persimmon calyx (Shidi) is used with Reed root (Lugen) and Bamboo shavings (Zhuru).
Dosage: 6-10 g

146. Rose (Meiguihua)

Pharmaceutical Name: Flos Rosae rugosae
Botanical Name: Rosa rugosa Thunb.
Common Name: Rose
Source of Earliest Record: Shiwu Bencao
Part Used & Method for Pharmaceutical Preparations: The flowers or flower buds are gathered between April and June, then baked before using.
Properties & Taste: Sweet, slightly bitter and warm
Meridians: Liver and spleen
Functions: 1. To regulate *qi* and reduce stagnation; 2. To remove blood stagnation
Indications & Combinations:

1. *Qi* stagnation in the liver and stomach manifested as costal pain, epigastric distension and stomach pain. Rose (Meiguihua) is used with

Finger citron (Foshou), Cyperus tuber (Xiangfu) and Curcuma root (Yujin).

2. *Qi* stagnation in the liver and blood manifested as irregular menstruation and distension and pain in the breasts before the menstruation period. Rose (Meiguihua) is used with Chinese angelica root (Danggui), Chuanxiong rhizome (Chuanxiong), White peony root (Baishao) and Bugleweed (Zelan).

3. Blood stasis and pain caused by external injuries. Rose (Meiguihua) is used with Chinese angelica root (Danggui), Corydalis tuber (Yanhusuo) and Red peony (Chishao).

Dosage: 3-6 g

147. Mume flower (Lü'emei)

Pharmaceutical Name: Flos Mume
Botanical Name: Prumus mume (Sieb.) Zieb. et Zucc.
Common Name: Mume flower, Japanese apricot flower
Source of Earliest Record: Bencao Gangmu
Part Used & Method for Pharmaceutical Preparations: The flowers or flower buds are gathered in January or February and dried in the sun or baked.
Properties & Taste: Sour, astringent and neutral
Meridians: Liver and stomach
Functions: 1. To promote the free flow of *qi* in the liver and reduce stagnation; 2. To regulate *qi* and harmonize the stomach
Indications & Combinations:

1. *Qi* stagnation in the liver and stomach manifested as distension and pain in the hypochondriac regions, belching and epigastric pain. Mume flower (Lü'emei) is used with Bupleurum root (Chaihu), Cyperus tuber (Xiangfu), Green tangerine peel (Qingpi) and Costus root (Muxiang).

2. Phlegm and *qi* stagnated in the throat (globus hystericus) manifested as the sensation of a foreign body in the throat. Mume flower (Lü'emei) is used with Trichosanthes peel (Gualoupi), Tangerine peel (Chenpi), Mulberry bark (Sangbaipi), Albizia bark (Hehuanpi) and Perilla leaf (Zisuye).

Dosage: 3-6 g

IX. Herbs That Relieve Food Stagnation

Herbs that relieve food stagnation are indicated in distension and fullness in the epigastric and abdominal regions, belching, sour regurgitation, nausea, vomiting, abnormal bowel movement or indigestion due to weakness of the spleen and stomach. When food is stagnated, it is necessary to add herbs that promote *qi* in order to enhance therapeutic effects. If food stagnation is accompanied by cold manifestations, herbs that warm the spleen and stomach are added. If food stagnation is accompanied by heat manifestations, herbs that are cold and bitter in nature are added to clear heat. If food stagnation results in turbid dampness blocking the spleen and stomach, aromatic herbs that drain dampness are added. If there is weakness of the spleen and stomach in transporting and transforming, these herbs are combined with herbs that tonify the spleen and stomach.

148. Hawthorn fruit (Shanzha)

Pharmaceutical Name: Fructus Crataegi

Botanical Name: 1. Crataegus cuneata Sieb, et Zucc; 2. Crataegus pinnatifida Bge. var Major N. E. Br.; 3. Crataegus pinnatifida Bge.

Common Name: Hawthorn fruit, Crataegus fruit

Source of Earliest Record: Xinxiu Bencao

Part Used & Method for Pharmaceutical Preparations: The fruit is gathered in late autumn or in the beginning of winter, dried in the sun and fried, or raw, fruit may be used.

Properties & Taste: Sour, sweet and slightly warm

Meridians: Spleen, stomach and liver

Functions: 1. To eliminate food retention; 2. To invigorate blood circulation and remove stagnation

Indications & Combinations:

1. Food retention (especially of fatty food) accompanied by abdominal and epigastric distension, pain and diarrhea. Hawthorn fruit (Shanzha) is used with Medicated leaven (Shenqu), Germinated barley (Maiya), Costus root (Muxiang) and Bitter orange (Zhiqiao).

2. Postpartum abdominal pain and lochia due to blood stagnation. Hawthorn fruit (Shanzha) is used with Chinese angelica root (Danggui), Chuanxiong rhizome (Chuanxiong) and Motherwort (Yimucao).

Dosage: 10-15 g

149. Medicated leaven (Shenqu)

Pharmaceutical Name: Massa fermentata medicinalis
Common Name: Medicated leaven
Source of Earliest Record: Yaoxing Lun
Part Used & Method for Pharmaceutical Preparations: Medicated leaven is a fermented mixture of wheat flour, bran and the fresh aerial parts of Armented annua, Xanthium sibixicum, Polygonum hydropiper and other herbs.
Properties & Taste: Sweet, pungent and warm
Meridians: Spleen and stomach
Functions: To eliminate food retention and harmonize the stomach
Indications & Combinations: Retention of food manifested as epigastric and abdominal distension and fullness, no appetite, gurgling sound and diarrhea. Medicated leaven (Shenqu) is used with Hawthorn fruit (Shanzha) and Germinated barley (Maiya).
Dosage: 6-15 g

150. Germinated barley (Maiya)

Pharmaceutical Name: Fructus Hordei germinatus
Botanical Name: Hordeum vulgare L.
Common Name: Germinated barley
Source of Earliest Record: Mingyi Bielu
Part Used & Method for Pharmaceutical Preparations: Barley is soaked in water for a day, and then it is put into a basket. Water is sprinkled over the barley daily until it germinates.
Properties & Taste: Sweet and neutral
Meridians: Spleen, stomach and liver
Functions: 1. To eliminate retention of food and harmonize the stomach; 2. To restrain lactation; 3. To promote free flow of liver *qi* and remove stagnation
Indications & Combinations:
1. Retention of food manifested as no appetite and epigastric and abdominal distension. Germinated barley (Maiya) is used with Hawthorn fruit (Shanzha), Medicated leaven (Shenqu) and Chicken's gizzard skin (Jineijin).
2. Restrained lactation or breast distension with pain. The decoction of half raw and half fried Germinated barley (Maiya) should be taken twice a day, 30-60 g each time.

3. *Qi* stagnation in the liver and stomach manifested as distension and fullness in the chest and costal regions and epigastric pain. Germinated barley (Maiya) is used with Bupleurum root (Chaihu), Immature bitter orange (Zhishi) and Sichuan chinaberry (Chuanlianzi).

Dosage: 10-15 g

Cautions & Contraindications: This herb is contraindicated during lactation.

151. Germinated millet (Guya)

Pharmaceutical Name: 1. Fructus Oryzae germinatus; 2. Fructus Setariae germinatus

Botanical Name: 1. Oryza sativa L. 2. Setaria italica (L.) Beauv.

Common Name: Germinated millet

Source of Earliest Record: Bencao Gangmu

Part Used & Method for Pharmaceutical Preparations: The germinated rice sprouts are dried in the sun.

Properties & Taste: Sweet and neutral

Meridians: Spleen and stomach

Functions: 1. To eliminate food retention and harmonize the stomach; 2. To improve appetite

Indications & Combinations:

1. Retention of food. Germinated millet (Guya) is used with Medicated leaven (Shenqu) and Hawthorn fruit (Shanzha).

2. Weakness of the spleen and stomach manifested as poor appetite. Germinated millet (Guya) is used with Pilose asiabell root (Dangshen), White atractylodes (Baizhu) and Tangerine peel (Chenpi).

Dosage: 10-15 g

152. Radish seed (Laifuzi)

Pharmaceutical Name: Semen Raphani

Botanical Name: Raphanus sativus L.

Common Name: Radish seed

Source of Earliest Record: Rihuazi Bencao

Part Used & Method for Pharmaceutical Preparations: The ripe seeds are gathered in the beginning of summer and dried in the sun.

Properties & Taste: Pungent, sweet and neutral

Meridians: Spleen, stomach and lung

Functions: 1. To eliminate food retention; 2. To descend *qi* and resolve phlegm

Indications & Combinations:

1. Retention of food manifested as epigastric and abdominal distension and fullness, acid regurgitation, abdominal pain, diarrhea and tenesmus. Radish seed (Laifuzi) is used with Hawthorn fruit (Shanzha), Medicated leaven (Shenqu) and Tangerine peel (Chenpi) in the formula Baohe Wan.

2. Excessive phlegm manifested as cough with profuse sputum or asthma. Radish seed (Laifuzi) is used with White mustard seed (Baijiezi) and Perilla seed (Suzi) in the formula Sanzi Yangqing Tang.

Dosage: 6-10 g

153. Chicken's gizzard skin (Jineijin)

Pharmaceutical Name: Endothelium corneum gigeriae galli

Zoological Name: Gallus gallus domesticus Brisson

Common Name: Chicken's gizzard skin or lining

Source of Earliest Record: Shennong Bencao Jing

Part Used & Method for Pharmaceutical Preparations: The inside membrane of the gizzard is peeled off, cleaned and dried in the sun. Then it is ground into powder.

Properties & Taste: Sweet and neutral

Meridians: Spleen, stomach, small intestine and urinary bladder

Functions: 1. To eliminate food retention; 2. To transform stones

Indications & Combinations:

1. Indigestion, retention of food and epigastric and abdominal distension and fullness. Chicken's gizzard skin (Jineijin) is used with Hawthorn fruit (Shanzha) and Germinated barley (Maiya).

2. Infantile weakness of the spleen, including infantile malnutrition. Chicken's gizzard skin (Jineijin) is used with White atractylodes (Baizhu), Dioscorea (Shanyao) and Poria (Fuling).

3. Gallstones and urinary tract stones. Chicken's gizzard skin (Jineijin) is used with Lysimachia (Jinqiancao) and Lygodium spores (Haijinsha) in the formula Sanjin Tang.

Dosage: 3-10 g

Cautions & Contraindications: If the herb is prepared as a powder, the dosage each time is 1.5-3 g.

X. Herbs That Expel Parasites

Herbs that expel parasites are used to treat roundworm, tapeworm, pinworm, hookworm and other intestinal parasites.

Selecting the proper herb depends upon the type of parasite and the patient's body constitution. In cases of a complicated pathological condition, these herbs may be used with herbs of other categories. For example, if a patient suffers from intestinal parasites and constipation, these herbs are used with those that purge stool.

Since some of these herbs are toxic, overdosage may cause side effects. They are contraindicated during pregnancy and in persons with a weak constitution.

154. Quisqualis fruit (Shijunzi)

Pharmaceutical Name: Fructus Quisqualis

Botanical Name: Quisqualis indica L.

Common Name: Quisqualis fruit, Rangoon creeper fruit with seeds

Source of Earliest Record: Kaibao Bencao

Part Used & Method for Pharmaceutical Preparations: The fruit is gathered in September or October when its skin turns purplish. The seeds are collected after the fruit is dried in the sun.

Properties & Taste: Sweet and warm

Meridians: Spleen and stomach

Functions: To kill parasites

Indications & Combinations: Roundworm (ascariasis). Quisqualis fruit (Shijunzi) is used with Chinaberry bark (Kulianpi) and Areca seed (Binglang).

Dosage: 6-10 g

Cautions & Contraindications: Overdosage of the herb will cause hiccups, dizziness, vertigo and vomiting. Taking this herb with hot tea can also cause hiccups.

155. Chinaberry bark (Kulianpi)

Pharmaceutical Name: Cortex meliae Radicis

Botanical Name: 1. Melia azedarach L; 2. Melia Toosendam Sieb, et zucc.

Common Name: Melia bark, Chinaberry bark, Chinatree bark

Source of Earliest Record: Mingyi Bielu

Part Used & Method for Pharmaceutical Preparations: The bark is collected in spring or autumn. After drying, the bark is cut into slices.

Properties & Taste: Bitter and cold

Meridians: Spleen, stomach and liver

Functions: To kill parasites

Indications & Combinations:

1. Roundworm (ascariasis). Chinaberry bark (Kulianpi) is used alone.

2. Hookworm (ancylostoma). Chinaberry bark (Kulianpi) is used with Areca seed (Binglang).

3. Pinworm (enterobius vermicularis). Chinaberry bark (Kulianpi) is used with Stemona root (Baibu) and Black plum (Wumei). The thick decoction can be taken as an enema to wash intestines once every night. Treatment should be continued for two to four times.

Dosage: 6-15 g

Cautions & Contraindications: This herb is toxic and should not be taken for a prolonged period. It is contraindicated for a person with a weak constitution or with a liver disorder.

156. Areca seed (Binglang)

Pharmaceutical Name: Semen arecae

Botanical Name: Areca cathechu L.

Common Name: Areca seed, Betel nut

Source of Earliest Record: Mingyi Bielu

Part Used & Method for Pharmaceutical Preparations: The seeds from the ripe fruit are collected in winter or spring. They are dried in the sun, soaked in water and cut into slices.

Properties & Taste: Pungent, bitter and warm

Meridians: Stomach and large intestine

Functions: 1. To kill parasites; 2. To promote *qi* circulation; 3. To promote water metabolism

Indications & Combinations:

1. Parasites in the intestines (especially tapeworm). Areca seed (Binglang) is used with Pumpkin seed (Nanguazi).

2. Retention of food with abdominal distension and constipation or tenesmus in dysentery. Areca seed (Binglang) is used with Costus root (Muxiang), Bitter orange (Zhiqiao) and Rhubarb (Dahuang) in the formula Muxiang Binglang Wan.

3. Edema. Areca seed (Binglang) is used with Poria peel (Fulingpi) and Alismatis rhizome (Zexie).

4. Swollen and painful legs. Areca seed (Binglang) is used with Chaenomeles fruit (Mugua), Evodia fruit (Wuzhuyu) and Perilla leaf (Zisuye).

5. Side-effect of vomiting caused by intake of the herb Dichroa root (Changshan). Areca seed (Binglang) used with Dichroa root (Changshan) can lessen the latter's side-effect.

Dosage: 10-15 g

Cautions & Contraindications: This herb is contraindicated in a person with weakness of the spleen accompanied by diarrhea.

157. Pumpkin seed (Nanguazi)

Pharmaceutical Name: Semen Cucurbitae moschatae
Botanical Name: Cucurbita moschata Duch.
Common Name: Pumpkin seed and husks
Source of Earliest Record: Xiandai Shiyong Zhongyao
Part Used & Method for Pharmaceutical Preparations: After the pumpkin ripens in summer or autumn, its seeds are removed, cleaned in water, dried in the sun and crushed into powder. Fresh seeds are also used, and, when available, they are a better choice.
Properties & Taste: Sweet and neutral
Meridians: Stomach and large intestine
Functions: To kill parasites
Indications & Combinations: Tapeworm. Pumpkin seed (Nanguazi) is used with Areca seed (Binglang).
Dosage: 60-120 g
Cautions & Contraindications: In treating tapeworm, the 60-120 g of powder of the herb is taken. Two hours later, the decoction of 60-120 g Areca seed (Binglang) is taken, and then half an hour later, 15 g of Glauber's salt (Mangxiao) in decoction is taken. This method will discharge both the tapeworm and feces.

158. Agrimonia bud (Hecaoya)

Pharmaceutical Name: Germma Agrimoniae
Botanical Name: Agrimonia pilosa Ledeb.
Common Name: Agrimonia bud
Source of Earliest Record: Zhonghua Yixue Zazhi

Part Used & Method for Pharmaceutical Preparations: The buds are gathered in late winter or early spring. After removing the brown down of the bud, the buds are dried in the sun and, finally, pounded into powder.

Properties & Taste: Bitter and cool

Meridians: Liver, small and large intestines

Functions: 1. To kill parasites; 2. To purge stool

Indications & Contraindications: Tapeworm. Agrimonia bud (Hecaoya) is taken with warm boiled water in the morning before breakfast. The tapeworm should be discharged within five to six hours.

Dosage: 30-50 g

159. Omphalia (Leiwan)

Pharmaceutical Name: Omphalia

Botanical Name: Omphalia lapidescens Schroet.

Common Name: Omphalia

Source of Earliest Record: Shennong Bencao Jing

Part Used & Method for Pharmaceutical Preparations: The fungus is gathered in spring, autumn and winter. It is cleaned, dried in the sun and, finally, pounded into powder. It is also made into pill form.

Properties & Taste: Bitter, cold and slightly toxic

Meridians: Stomach and large intestine

Functions: To kill parasites

Indications & Combinations: Hookworm and roundworm. Omphalia (Leiwan) is used with Areca seed (Binglang) and Chinaberry bark (Kulianpi).

Dosage: 6-15 g

160. Carpesium fruit (Heshi)

Pharmaceutical Name: Fructus Carpesii

Botanical Name: 1. Carpesium abrotanoides L.; 2. Daucus caroto L.

Common Name: Carpesium fruit

Source of Earliest Record: Xinxiu Bencao

Part Used & Method for Pharmaceutical Preparations: The fruit is gathered in August or September and dried in the sun.

Properties & Taste: Bitter, pungent, neutral and slightly toxic

Meridians: Spleen and stomach

Functions: To kill parasites

Indications & Combinations: Parasites in the intestines, including roundworm, pinworm and tapeworm. Carpesium fruit (Heshi) is used with Quisqualis fruit (Shijunzi) and Areca seed (Binglang).

Dosage: 3-10 g

161. Torrya seed (Feizi)

Pharmaceutical Name: Semen Torreyae
Botanical Name: Torreya grandis Fort.
Common Name: Torrya seed
Source of Earliest Record: Mingyi Bielu
Part Used & Method for Pharmaceutical Preparations: The seeds are gathered in winter when the fruit is ripe and then dried in the sun.

Properties & Taste: Sweet and neutral
Meridians: Lung and large intestine
Functions: To kill parasites
Indications & Combinations: Parasites in the intestines: a) hookworm —Torrya seed (Feizi) is used with Basket fern (Guanzhong) and Areca seed (Binglang); b) tapeworm—Torrya seed (Feizi) is used with Pumpkin seed (Nanguazi) and Areca seed (Binglang); c) roundworm—Torrya seed (Feizi) is used with Quisqualis fruit (Shijunzi), Chinaberry bark (Kulianpi) and Black plum (Wumei).

Dosage: 30-50 g
Cautions & Contraindications: This herb can be taken with a decoction, but is most effective when made into a medical ball with honey and taken directly.

162. Basket fern (Guanzhong)

Pharmaceutical Name: Rhizoma Dryopteris crassirhizomae
Botanical Name: 1. Dryopteris crassirhixoma Nakai; 2. Osmunda japonica Thunb. 3. Woodwardia unigemmata (Makino) Nakai
Common Name: Dryopteris rhizome, Basket fern
Source of Earliest Record: Shennong Bencao Jing
Part Used & Method for Pharmaceutical Preparations: The rhizomes are dug in winter. After the fibrous roots have been removed, the rhizomes are dried in the sun and cut into slices. The herb can be used either raw or carbonized.

Properties & Taste: Bitter and slightly cold
Meridians: Liver and spleen

134

Functions: 1. To kill parasites; 2. To clear heat and release toxins; 3. To stop bleeding

Indications & Combinations:

1. Parasites in the intestines: a) hookworm—Basket fern (Guanzhong) is used with Torrya seed (Feizi) and Areca seed (Binglang); b) tapeworm—Basket fern (Guanzhong) is used with Omphalia (Leiwan) and Areca seed (Binglang); c) pinworm—Basket fern (Guanzhong) is used with Chinaberry bark (Kulianpi) and Carpesium fruit (Heshi).

2. Wind-heat common cold, warm-heat maculopapule and acute parotitis. Basket fern (Guanzhong) is used with Honeysuckle flower (Jinyinhua), Forsythia fruit (Lianqiao), Isatis leaf (Daqingye) and Isatis root (Banlangen).

3. Extravasation of blood by heat manifested as vomiting of blood, epistaxis, bloody stool and functional uterine bleeding. Basket fern (Guanzhong) is used with Biota tops (Cebaiye), Agrimony (Xianhecao) and Carbonized petiole of windmill palm (Zonglütan).

Dosage: 10-15 g

Cautions & Contraindications: The carbonized herb is used to stop bleeding.

XI. Herbs That Stop Bleeding

Herbs that stop bleeding, or hemorrhaging, are used to treat cases of vomiting blood, epistaxis, cough with blood, bloody stool, bloody urine, uterine bleeding or traumatic bleeding.

The herbs stop bleeding by different methods, including cooling the blood, astringing, resolving blood stasis and warming the channels. Based on the cause of bleeding and its accompanying manifestations, the appropriate herb should be selected in combination with other herbs. For example, if bleeding is due to extravasation of blood by heat, herbs that clear heat and cool the blood are used in combination. If bleeding is due to deficiency of *yin* with hyperactivity of *yang*, herbs that tonify *yin* and subside *yang* should be chosen. If bleeding is due to deficiency and cold, herbs that warm *yang*, promote *qi* and strengthen the spleen should be combined. In cases of great loss of blood leading to collapse of *qi*, herbs must be added to tonify the source *qi*, so as to prevent further collapse.

It is important to remember that blood stagnation can be a factor in bleeding. In such cases, herbs that invigorate the blood and remove stasis should be added.

163. Japanese thistle (Daji)

Pharmaceutical Name: Herba seu Radix Cirsii japonici
Botanical Name: Cirsium japonicum DC.
Common Name: Japanese thistle
Source of Earliest Record: Mingyi Bielu
Part Used & Method for Pharmaceutical Preparations: The aerial parts of the plant are gathered in summer or autumn when the thistle is flowering. The root can be dug in late autumn. Both are dried in the sun and cut into pieces.
Properties & Taste: Sweet, bitter and cool
Meridians: Heart and liver
Functions: 1. To cool blood and stop bleeding; 2. To reduce swelling and resolve stagnation
Indications & Combinations:

1. Hemorrhages due to extravasation of blood by heat manifested as cough with blood, epistaxis, uterine bleeding, and hematuria. Japanese thistle (Daji) is used with Small thistle (Xiaoji) and Biota tops (Cebaiye).

2. Boils, carbuncles and swelling. Japanese thistle (Daji) is used both externally and internally.
Dosage: 10-15 g (60 g for fresh herb)

164. Small thistle (Xiaoji)

Pharmaceutical Name: Herba Cirsii segeti
Botanical Name: Cirsium segetum Bge.
Common Name: Small thistle
Source of Earliest Record: Mingyi Bielu
Part Used & Method for Pharmaceutical Preparations: The aerial parts of the plant and its rhizome are harvested in summer when the thistle is flowering. Then they are cleaned, dried in the sun and cut into pieces.
Properties & Taste: Sweet and cool
Meridians: Heart and liver
Functions: 1. To cool blood and stop bleeding; 2. To promote urination
Indications & Combinations:

1. Hemorrhages due to extravasation of blood by heat. Small thistle (Xiaoji) is used with Imperata rhizome (Baimaogen), Cattail pollen (Puhuang) and Biota tops (Cebaiye).

2. Bloody urine, painful urination. Small thistle (Xiaoji) is used with Lotus node (Oujie), Talc (Huashi) and Clematis stem (Mutong) in the formula Xiaoji Yinzi.

Dosage: 10-15 g (30-60 g for fresh herb)

165. Burnet root (Diyu)

Pharmaceutical Name: Radix Sanguisorbae
Botanical Name: Sanguisorba officinalis L.
Common Name: Sanguisorba root, Burnet root
Source of Earliest Record: Shennong Bencao Jing
Part Used & Method for Pharmaceutical Preparations: The roots are dug in spring or autumn. After the fibrous roots have been removed, the roots are then cleaned, dried in the sun and cut into slices.
Properties & Taste: Bitter, sour and slightly cold
Meridians: Liver, stomach and large intestine
Functions: 1. To cool blood and stop bleeding; 2. To dispel toxins and promote healing of ulcers
Indications & Combinations:

1. Hemorrhages due to extravasation of blood by heat: a) uterine bleeding—Burnet root (Diyu) is used with fried Cattail pollen (Puhuang), Scutellaria root (Huangqin) and Fresh rehmannia root (Shengdihuang); b) hemorrhages, bleeding and dysentery—Burnet root (Diyu) is used with Sophora flower (Huaihua), Coptis root (Huanglian) and Costus root (Muxiang).

2. Burns, eczema, ulcers of the skin. Burnet root (Diyu) is used with Coptis root (Huanglian) for external use.

Dosage: 10-15 g

Cautions & Contraindications: This herb is contraindicated for large burns. The ointment made from the herb may cause a toxic infection after absorption by the body.

166. Imperata rhizome (Baimaogen)

Pharmaceutical Name: Rhizoma Imperatae
Botanical Name: Imperata cylindrical Beauv. var. major (Nees.) C. E. Hubb.

Common Name: Imperata rhizome, Woody grass
Source of Earliest Record: Shennong Bencao Jing
Part Used & Method for Pharmaceutical Preparations: The rhizomes are dug in spring or autumn, cleaned, dried in the sun and cut into small pieces.
Properties & Taste: Sweet and cold
Meridians: Lung, stomach and urinary bladder
Functions: 1. To cool blood and stop bleeding; 2. To clear heat and promote urination
Indications & Combinations:

1. Hemorrhages due to extravasation of blood by heat. Imperata rhizome (Baimaogen) is used with Biota tops (Cebaiye), Small thistle (Xiaoji) and Cattail pollen (Puhuang).

2. Hot urination, edema and damp-heat jaundice. Imperata rhizome (Baimaogen) is used with Plantain seed (Cheqianzi) and Lysimachia (Jinqiancao).

Dosage: 15-30 g (30-60 g, if fresh herb)

167. Sophora flower (Huaihua)

Pharmaceutical Name: Flos Sophorae
Botanical Name: Sophora japonica L.
Common Name: Sophora flower, Pagoda tree flower
Source of Earliest Record: Rihuazi Bencao
Part Used & Method for Pharmaceutical Preparations: The flower buds are gathered in June or July and dried in the sun.
Properties & Taste: Bitter and slightly cold
Meridians: Liver and large intestine
Functions: To cool blood and stop bleeding
Indications & Combinations: Hemorrhages due to extravasation of blood by heat: a) dysentery and bleeding due to hemorrhoids—Sophora flower (Huaihua) is used with Burnet root (Diyu); b) cough with blood and epistaxis—Sophora flower (Huaihua) is used with Biota tops (Cebaiye), Imperata rhizome (Baimaogen) and Agrimony (Xianhecao).
Dosage: 10-15 g

168. Biota tops (Cebaiye)

Pharmaceutical Name: Cacumen Biotae
Botanical Name: Biota orientalis (L.) Endl.

Common Name: Biota tops, Acborvitae tops
Source of Earliest Record: Mingyi Bielu
Part Used & Method for Pharmaceutical Preparations: The leafy twigs are gathered all year round. They are dried in a shady place and cut into pieces.
Properties & Taste: Bitter, astringent and slightly cold
Meridians: Lung, liver and large intestine
Functions: To cool blood and stop bleeding
Indications & Combinations:

1. Hemorrhages due to extravasation of blood by heat manifested as cough with blood, vomiting with blood, epistaxis, hematuria and uterine bleeding. Biota tops (Cebaiye) is used with Japanese thistle (Daji), Small thistle (Xiaoji) and Imperata rhizome (Baimaogen).

2. Hemorrhages due to deficiency and cold. Biota tops (Cebaiye) is used with Mugwort leaf (Aiye).
Dosage: 10-15 g

169. Agrimony (Xianhecao)

Pharmaceutical Name: Herba Agrimoniae
Botanical Name: Agrimonia pilosa Ledeb. Nakai
Common Name: Agrimony
Source of Earliest Record: Diannan Bencao
Part Used & Method for Pharmaceutical Preparations: The entire plant is gathered in summer or autumn. It is cleaned, dried in the sun and cut into pieces.
Properties & Taste: Bitter, astringent and neutral
Meridians: Lung, liver and spleen
Functions: 1. To stop bleeding; 2. To relieve dysentery; 3. To kill parasites
Indications & Combinations:

1. Hemorrhages due to extravasation of blood by heat manifested as cough with blood, vomiting with blood, epistaxis, hematuria, bloody stool and uterine bleeding. Agrimony (Xianhecao) is used with Fresh rehmannia root (Shengdihuang), Moutan bark (Mudanpi), Capejasmine (Zhizi) and Biota tops (Cebaiye).

2. Hemorrhages due to deficient *yang qi* leading to failure of the spleen to control blood, which results in bloody stool or uterine bleeding. Agrimony (Xianhecao) is used with Ginseng (Renshen), As-

tragalus root (Huangqi) and Prepared rehmannia root (Shudihuang).

3. Trichomonas vaginitis with itching; 120 g of the herb is prepared in decoction, a cotton ball soaked in the decoction is then put into the vagina for 3-4 hours. Treatment is given once daily for one week.

Dosage: 10-15 g

170. Bletilla tuber (Baiji)

Pharmaceutical Name: Rhizoma Bletillae
Botanical Name: Bletilla striata (Thunb.) Reichb. f.
Common Name: Bletilla tuber
Source of Earliest Record: Shennong Bencao Jing
Part Used & Method for Pharmaceutical Preparations: The rhizomes are dug in summer or autumn. After the fibrous roots have been removed, the rhizomes are cleaned, boiled in water, dried in the sun and cut into slices.
Properties & Taste: Bitter, sweet, astringent and slightly cold
Meridians: Liver, lung and stomach
Functions: 1. To stop bleeding; 2. To reduce swelling and promote healing
Indications & Combinations:

1. Hemorrhages: a) cough with blood due to deficient *yin* of the lungs—Bletilla tuber (Baiji) is used with Donkey hide gelatin (Ejiao), Lotus node (Oujie) and Loquat leaf (Pipaye); b) vomiting with blood —Bletilla tuber (Baiji) is used with Cuttlefish bone (Wuzeigu) in the formula Wu Ji San; c) hemorrhage due to external injuries. Bletilla tuber (Baiji) can be applied alone or with the powder of Calcine gypsum (Duanshigao) for external use.

2. Boils, carbuncles and swelling: a) affected areas with redness, swelling, hot sensation and pain—Bletilla tuber (Baiji) is used with Honeysuckle flower (Jinyinhua), Tendrilled fritillary bulb (Chuanbeimu), Trichosanthes root (Tianhuafen) and Honeylocust thorn (Zaojiaoci) in the formula Neixiao San; b) chronic non-healing ulcers—the powder of Bletilla tuber (Baiji) is applied directly to wounds.

3. Chapped skin or cracked hands or feet. The powder of Bletilla tuber (Baiji) is mixed with sesame oil for external use.

Dosage: 3-10 g

Cautions & Contraindications: This herb counteracts Sichuan aconite root (Wutou).

171. Carbonized petiole of windmill palm (Zonglütan)

Pharmaceutical Name: Petiolus Trachycarpi carbonisatus
Botanical Name: Trachycarpus fortunei H. wendl.
Common Name: Carbonized palm fiber, Carbonized petiole of windmill palm
Source of Earliest Record: Bencao Shiyi
Part Used & Method for Pharmaceutical Preparations: The palm fiber is gathered in the period of the Winter Solstice (twenty-second solar term), and then it is carbonized.
Properties & Taste: Bitter, astringent and neutral
Meridians: Lung, liver and large intestine
Functions: To stop bleeding
Indications & Combinations:

1. Hemorrhages due to extravasation of blood by heat manifested as cough with blood, vomiting with blood, epistaxis, bloody stool and uterine bleeding. Carbonized petiole of windmill palm (Zonglütan) is used with Imperata rhizome (Baimaogen), Japanese thistle (Daji), Small thistle (Xiaoji) and Capejasmine (Zhizi) in the formula Shihui San.

2. Hemorrhages due to deficiency of *yang qi* leading to failure of the spleen to control blood manifested as uterine bleeding or bloody stool. Carbonized petiole of windmill palm (Zonglütan) is used with Astragalus root (Huangqi), Ginseng (Renshen) and White atractylodes (Baizhu).
Dosage: 3-10 g

172. Carbonized human hair (Xueyutan)

Pharmaceutical Name: Crinis carbonisatus
Common Name: Carbonized human hair
Source of Earliest Record: Mingyi Bielu
Part Used & Method for Pharmaceutical Preparations: Human hairs are carbonized.
Properties & Taste: Bitter and neutral
Meridians: Liver and stomach
Functions: To stop bleeding and release blood stagnation
Indications & Combinations: Hemorrhages: a) bleeding occurring in the upper part of the body—Carbonized human hair (Xueyutan) is used with the juice of Lotus node (Oujie); b) bleeding occurring in the lower part of the body—Carbonized human hair (Xueyutan) is used

with Carbonized petiole of windmill palm (Zonglütan).

Dosage: 6-10 g

173a. Notoginseng (Sanqi)

Pharmaceutical Name: Radix Notoginseng
Botanical Name: Panax notoginseng (Burk.) F. H. Chen
Common Name: Pseudoginseng, Notoginseng
Source of Earliest Record: Bencao Gangmu
Part Used & Method for Pharmaceutical Preparations: The roots are dug in spring or winter. The spring roots have a stronger pharmacological effect than winter roots. After cleaning, the roots are dried in the sun.
Properties & Taste: Sweet, bitter and warm
Meridians: Liver and stomach
Functions: 1. To stop bleeding and release stagnation; 2. To invigorate blood circulation and stop pain
Indications & Combinations:

1. Hemorrhage in the interior or at the surface of the body. The powder of Notoginseng (Sanqi) is taken alone, or it may be used with Ophicalcite (Huaruishi) and Carbonized human hair (Xueyutan) in the formula Huaxue Dan.

2. Hemorrhages and swelling due to external injuries. Powdered Notoginseng (Sanqi) is used alone externally.

Dosage: 3-10 g; 1-1.5 g for powder.

173b. Gynurasegetum (Juyesanqi)

The root and leaves of Gynurasegetum (Juyesanqi) are sweet, slightly bitter and neutral in properties, and enter the meridians of the liver and stomach. It stops bleeding and dispels toxins. The herb is used for epistaxis, carbuncles and mastitis. The recommended dosage is 6-10 g.

173c. Sedum (Jingtiansanqi)

The entire plant or root of Sedum Aizoon L. is sweet, slightly sour and neutral in properties and stops bleeding and releases stagnation to nourish the blood and calm the mind. The entire plant is used for epistaxis, cough with blood, vomiting with blood, insomnia, irritability, etc. The root stops bleeding, reduces swelling and relieves pain. It is used for epistaxis and traumatic hemorrhage. The recommended dosage is 15-30 g for the plant, 6-10 g for the root.

174. Rubia root (Qiancao)

Pharmceutical Name: Radix Rubiae
Botanical Name: Rubia cordifolia L.
Common Name: Madder root, Rubia root
Source of Earliest Record: Shennong Bencao Jing
Part Used & Method for Pharmaceutical Preparations: The roots are dug in spring or autumn, and cleaned and dried in the sun.
Properties & Taste: Bitter and cold
Meridian: Liver
Functions: 1. To cool blood and stop bleeding; 2. To invigorate blood circulation and release stagnation
Indications & Combinations:

1. Hemorrhages due to extravasation of blood by heat. Rubia root (Qiancao) is used with Japanese thistle (Daji), Small thistle (Xiaoji) and Biota tops (Cebaiye).

2. Amenorrhea caused by blood stagnation. Rubia root (Qiancao) is used with Chinese angelica root (Danggui), Chuanxiong rhizome (Chuanxiong) and Cyperus tuber (Xiangfu).

3. Blood stasis and pain caused by external injuries. Rubia root (Qiancao) is used with Safflower (Honghua), Chinese angelica root (Danggui) and Red peony (Chishao).

4. Wind-damp obstruction syndrome (painful joints). Rubia root (Qiancao) is used with Spatholobus stem (Jixueteng) and Futokadsura stem (Haifengteng).
Dosage: 10-15 g

175. Cattail pollen (Puhuang)

Pharmaceutical Name: Pollen Typhae
Botanical Name: 1. Typha orientalis Presl; 2. Typha angustifolia L.
Common Name: Cattail pollen, Bullrush pollen
Source of Earliest Record: Shennong Bencao Jing
Part Used & Method for Pharmaceutical Preparations: The pollen is gathered in May or June.
Properties & Taste: Sweet and neutral
Meridians: Liver and pericardium

Functions: 1. To stop bleeding; 2. To release stagnation and stop pain
Indications & Combinations:

1. Hemorrhages manifested as cough with blood, vomiting with blood, hematuria, bloody stool and uterine bleeding. Cattail pollen (Puhuang) is used with Agrimony (Xianhecao), Eclipta (Mohanlian) and Biota tops (Cebaiye).

2. Hemorrhages caused by external injuries. Cattail pollen (Puhuang) can be used alone and dry for external use.

3. Blood stagnation manifested as cardiac pain, abdominal pain, dysmenorrhea or postpartum abdominal pain. Cattail pollen (Puhuang) is used with Trogopterus dung (Wulingzhi) in the formula Shixiao San.

Dosage: 3-10 g

Cautions & Contraindications: The carbonized herb is effective in stopping bleeding; the raw herb is used for releasing stagnation and stopping pain.

176. Ophicalcite (Huaruishi)

Pharmaceutical Name: Ophicalcitum
Mineral Name: Ophicalcite
Common Name: Ophicalcite
Source of Earliest Record: Jiayou Bencao
Part Used & Method for Pharmaceutical Preparations: The ophicalcite stone is burned and ground into powder.
Properties & Taste: Sour, astringent and neutral
Meridian: Liver
Functions: 1. To stop bleeding; 2. To release stagnation
Indications & Combinations:

1. Vomiting with blood and cough with blood accompanied by blood stagnation. Ophicalcite (Huaruishi) is used with Notoginseng (Sanqi), Rubia stem (Qiancaotan) and Carbonized human hair (Xueyutan).

2. Hemorrhages caused by external injuries. The powder of Ophicalcite (Huaruishi) can be applied directly, externally.

Dosage: 10-15 g

177. Mugwort leaf (Aiye)

Pharmaceutical Name: Folium Artemisiae Argyi
Botanical Name: Artemisia argyi Levl. et Vant.

Common Name: Mugwort leaf

Source of Earliest Record: Mingyi Bielu

Part Used & Method for Pharmaceutical Preparations: The leaves are gathered in spring or summer, when the mugwort is flowering. They are dried in a shady place.

Properties & Taste: Bitter, pungent and warm

Meridians: Liver, spleen and kidney

Functions: 1. To warm the channels and stop bleeding; 2. To dispel cold and stop pain

Indications & Combinations:

1. Hemorrhages due to deficiency and cold, especially uterine bleeding. Mugwort leaf (Aiye) is used with Donkey hide gelatin (Ejiao) in the formula Jiao Ai Tang.

2. Deficiency and cold in the lower *jiao* manifested as abdominal cold pain, irregular menstruation, amenorrhea and leukorrhagia. Mugwort leaf (Aiye) is used with Chinese angelica root (Danggui), Cyperus tuber (Xiangfu), Chuanxiong rhizome (Chuanxiong) and Lindera root (Wuyao).

Dosage: 3-10 g

Note: This herb is used for moxibustion and can be made into moxa sticks or used as moxa cones. It warms meridians and promotes the circulation of *qi* and blood.

178. Lotus node (Oujie)

Pharmaceutical Name: Nodus Nelumbinis Rhizomatis

Botanical Name: Nelumbo nucifera Gaertn.

Common Name: Lotus node

Source of Earliest Record: Yaoxing Lun

Part Used & Method for Pharmaceutical Preparations: The lotus rhizomes are dug in autumn or winter. The nodes of the rhizomes are removed, cleaned and dried in the sun.

Properties & Taste: Sweet, astringent and neutral

Meridians: Liver, lung and stomach

Functions: To promote healing and stop bleeding

Indications & Combinations: Hemorrhages, especially cough with blood and vomiting with blood. Lotus node (Oujie) is used with Bletilla tuber (Baiji), Biota tops (Cebaiye) and Imperata rhizome (Baimaogen).

Dosage: 10-15 g

XII. Herbs That Invigorate Blood and Resolve Blood Stagnation

These herbs harmonize blood, promote blood circulation, resolve blood stagnation, reduce swelling and stop pain. Blood stagnation has various causes, and herbs from other categories should be added to the formulas based upon these causes. If blood stagnation is due to contraction from cold and *qi* stagnation, herbs that warm the interior and dispel cold should be combined. If the blood stagnation is caused by damage to the *yin* and blood due to excessive heat, herbs that clear heat and cool blood should be added to the formula. If the stagnation is due to invasion by pathogenic wind-damp, herbs that dispel wind-damp should be added.

Qi and blood are closely related in the body; circulation of *qi* promotes circulation of blood, and stagnation of *qi* leads to stagnation of blood. In using herbs that invigorate blood and resolve blood stagnation, it is necessary to add herbs that promote *qi* circulation to enhance therapeutic effects.

These herbs should be used with caution during excessive menstrual flow or pregnancy.

179. Chuanxiong rhizome (Chuanxiong)

Pharmaceutical Name: Radix chuanxiong
Botanical Name: Ligusticum chuanxiong Hort.
Common Name: Chuanxiong rhizome, Szechuan lovage root
Source of Earliest Record: Shennong Bencao Jing
Part Used & Method for Pharmaceutical Preparations: The rhizomes are dug in late May. The fibrous roots are soaked and cut into slices.
Properties & Taste: Pungent and warm
Meridians: Liver, gall bladder and pericardium
Functions: 1. To invigorate blood and promote *qi* circulation; 2. To expel wind and stop pain
Indications & Combinations:

1. Blood and *qi* stagnation: a) irregular menstruation, dysmenorrhea and amenorrhea—Chuanxiong rhizome (Chuanxiong) is used with Chinese angelica root (Danggui), Red peony (Chishao), Cyperus tuber (Xiangfu) and Motherwort (Yimucao); b) difficult labor

—Chuanxiong rhizome (Chuanxiong) is used with Cyathula root (Niuxi) and Tortoise plastron (Guiban); c) postpartum abdominal pain—Chuanxiong rhizome (Chuanxiong) is used with Motherwort (Yimucao), Peach seed (Taoren) and Safflower (Honghua); d) hypochondric pain—Chuanxiong rhizome (Chuanxiong) is used with Bupleurum root (Chaihu), Cyperus tuber (Xiangfu) and Curcuma root (Yujin); e) numbness of the limbs—Chuanxiong rhizome (Chuanxiong) is used with Red peony (Chishao), Earthworm (Dilong) and Spatholobus stem (Jixueteng).

2. Headache: a) wind-cold headache—Chuanxiong rhizome (Chuanxiong) is used with Dahurian angelica root (Baizhi) and Asarum herb (Xixin) in the formula Chuanxiong Cha Tiao San; b) wind-heat headache—Chuanxiong rhizome (Chuanxiong) is used with Chrysanthemum flower (Juhua), Gypsum (Shigao) and White-stiff silkworm (Baijiangcan) in the formula Chuanxiong San; c) wind-damp headache —Chuanxiong rhizome (Chuanxiong) is used with Notopterygium root (Qianghuo), Ligusticum root (Gaoben) and Ledebouriella (Fangfeng) in the formula Qianghuo Shengshi Tang; d) headache due to blood stagnation—Chuanxiong rhizome (Chuanxiong) is used with Red peony (Chishao), Red sage root (Danshen) and Safflower (Honghua); e) headache due to deficient blood—Chuanxiong rhizome (Chuanxiong) is used with Chinese angelica root (Danggui) and White peony root (Baishao).

3. Wind-damp obstruction syndrome (painful joints). Chuanxiong rhizome (Chuanxiong) is used with Notopterygium root (Qianghuo), Pubescent angelica root (Duhuo), Ledebouriella (Fangfeng) and Mulberry twigs (Sangzhi).

Dosage: 3-10 g

Cautions & Contraindications: This herb is contraindicated during hemorrhagic diseases and during profuse menstrual flow.

180. Frankincense (Ruxiang)

Pharmaceutical Name: Resina oliani; Olibanum
Botanical Name: Boswellia carterii Birdw.
Common Name: Frankincense, Mastic
Source of Earliest Record: Mingyi Bielu
Part Used & Method for Pharmaceutical Preparations: The gum-resin is gathered in spring or summer, after the bark of the tree is cut. Then

the gum-resin is fried.

Properties & Taste: Pungent, bitter and warm

Meridians: Heart, liver and spleen

Functions: 1. To invigorate blood and stop pain; 2. To reduce swelling

Indications & Combinations:

1. Pains caused by blood stagnation: a) dysmenorrhea—Frankincense (Ruxiang) is used with Chinese angelica root (Danggui), Chuanxiong rhizome (Chuanxiong) and Cyperus tuber (Xiangfu); b) stomach pain—Frankincense (Ruxiang) is used with Sichuan chinaberry (Chuanlianzi) and Corydalis tuber (Yanhusuo); c) general pain or joint pain due to invasion of wind-cold-damp. Frankincense (Ruxiang) is used with Notopterygium root (Qianghuo), Futokadsura stem (Haifengteng), Large-leaf gentian root (Qinjiao), Chinese angelica root (Danggui) and Chuanxiong rhizome (Chuanxiong) in the formula Juanbi Tang; d) pains caused by external injuries—Frankincense (Ruxiang) is used with Myrrh (Moyao), Dragon's blood (Xuejie) and Safflower (Honghua) in the formula Qili San; e) pain from carbuncles and furuncles with swelling—Frankincense (Ruxiang) is used with Myrrh (Moyao), Red peony (Chishao) and Honeysuckle flower (Jinyinhua) in the formula Xianfang Huoming Yin.

2. Boils and ulcers. The powders of Frankincense (Ruxiang) and Myrrh (Moyao) are used externally. The combination is called Haifu San.

Dosage: 3-10 g

Cautions & Contraindications: This herb is contraindicated during pregnancy.

181. Myrrh (Moyao)

Pharmaceutical Name: Myrrha; Resina myrrhae

Botanical Name: Commiphora myrrha Engl.

Common Name: Myrrh

Source of Earliest Record: Kaibao Bencao

Part Used & Method for Pharmaceutical Preparations: After the stem is cut, the gum-resin is gathered and then carbonized.

Properties & Taste: Bitter and neutral

Meridians: Heart, liver and spleen

Functions: 1. To invigorate blood and stop pain; 2. To reduce swelling and promote healing

Indications & Combinations: The indications and combinations of Myrrh (Moyao) are the same as those for Frankincense (Ruxiang).

Dosage: 3-10 g

Cautions & Contraindications: This herb is contraindicated during pregnancy.

182. Corydalis tuber (Yanhusuo)

Pharmaceutical Name: Rhizoma corydalis Yanhusuo

Botanical Name: Corydalis turtschaninovii Bess. f. Yanhusuo, Y. H. Chow et C. C. Hsu

Common Name: Corydalis tuber

Source of Earliest Record: Kaibao Bencao

Part Used & Method for Pharmaceutical Preparations: The rhizomes are dug at the Beginning of Summer (seventh solar term). After the fibrous roots have been removed, the rhizomes are boiled for three minutes, dried in the sunshine and pounded into pieces.

Properties & Taste: Pungent, bitter and warm

Meridians: Heart, liver and spleen

Functions: 1. To invigorate blood and promote *qi* circulation; 2. To stop pain

Indications & Combinations: Pains due to *qi* and blood stagnation. Corydalis tuber (Yanhusuo) is used with Sichuan chinaberry (Chuanlianzi), Chinese angelica root (Danggui), Chuanxiong rhizome (Chuanxiong), Frankincense (Ruxiang) and Myrrh (Moyao).

Dosage: 5-10 g

Note: Frying with vinegar enhances this herb's ability to stop pain.

183. Curcuma root (Yujin)

Pharmaceutical Name: Radix Curcumae

Botanical Name: 1. Curcuma longa L.; 2. C. aromatica salisb.; 3. Curcuma zedoaria Rosc.; 4. Curcuma kwangsiensis S. Lee et C. F. Liang

Common Name: Curcuma root

Source of Earliest Record: Xinxiu Bencao

Part Used & Method for Pharmaceutical Preparations: The tuberous roots are dug in autumn or winter. After removing the fibrous roots, the roots are cleaned, boiled, dried in the sun and cut into slices.

Properties & Taste: Pungent, bitter and cold

Meridians: Heart, liver and gall bladder

Functions: 1. To invigorate blood and stop pain; 2. To promote *qi* circulation and release stagnation; 3. To cool blood and clear heat in the heart; 4. To relieve jaundice and facilitate gall bladder function

Indications & Combinations:

1. *Qi* and blood stagnation: a) pain in the chest, abdominal or hypochondriac regions—Curcuma root (Yujin) is used with Red sage root (Danshen), Cyperus tuber (Xiangfu), Bupleurum root (Chaihu) and Bitter orange (Zhiqiao); b) dysmenorrhea due to *qi* and blood stagnation. Curcuma root (Yujin) is used with Bupleurum root (Chaihu), Cyperus tuber (Xiangfu), White peony root (Baishao) and Chinese angelica root (Danggui).

2. Mental derangement due to interior damp-warm attacking. Curcuma root (Yujin) is used with Grass-leaved sweetflag (Shichangpu) in the formula Changpu Yujin Tang.

3. Jaundice due to interior accumulation of damp-heat. Curcuma root (Yujin) is used with Oriental wormwood (Yinchenhao) and Capejasmine (Zhizi).

Dosage: 6–12 g

Cautions & Contraindications: This herb should not be combined with Cloves (Dingxiang).

184. Turmeric (Jianghuang)

Pharmaceutical Name: Rhizoma Curcumae longae

Botanical Name: Curcuma longa L.

Common Name: Turmeric

Source of Earliest Record: Xinxiu Bencao

Part Used & Method for Pharmaceutical Preparations: The rhizomes are dug in autumn or winter. After the bark and fibrous roots have been removed, the rhizomes are cleaned, boiled, dried in the sun and cut into slices.

Properties & Taste: Pungent, bitter and warm

Meridians: Liver and spleen

Functions: 1. To invigorate blood and promote *qi* circulation; 2. To promote menstruation and stop pain

Indications & Combinations:

1. *Qi* and blood stagnation manifested as chest pain, hypochondriac

pain, amenorrhea and abdominal pain. Turmeric (Jianghuang) is used with Chinese angelica root (Danggui), Curcuma root (Yujin), Cyperus tuber (Xiangfu) and Corydalis tuber (Yanhusuo).

2. Wind-damp obstruction syndrome manifested as rigid neck, shoulder pain and motor impairment of the limbs. Turmeric (Jianghuang) is used with Notopterygium root (Qianghuo) and Chinese angelica root (Danggui) in the formula Shujing Tang.

Dosage: 5-10 g

185. Zedoary (Ezhu)

Pharmaceutical Name: Rhizoma Zedoariae

Botanical Name: 1. Curcuma zedoaria Rosc.; 2. Curcuma aromatica Salisb.; 3. Curcuma Kwangsiensis S. Lee et C. F. Liang

Common Name: Zedoary, Zedoaria

Source of Earliest Record: Yaoxing Lun

Part Used & Method for Pharmaceutical Preparations: The rhizomes are dug in autumn or winter. They are cleaned, boiled and dried. After the fibrous roots have been removed, the rhizomes are cut into slices.

Properties & Taste: Pungent and bitter

Meridians: Liver and spleen

Functions: 1. To invigorate blood and move stagnation; 2. To promote *qi* circulation and stop pain

Indications & Combinations:

1. *Qi* and blood stagnation manifested as abdominal pain, amenorrhea, abdominal or epigastric masses. Zedoary (Ezhu) is used with Burreed tuber (Sanleng) in the formula Ezhu Wan.

2. Dysfunction of the spleen in transforming and transporting manifested as retention of food, epigastric and abdominal distension, fullness and pain. Zedoary (Ezhu) is used with Burreed tuber (Sanleng), Hawthorn fruit (Shanzha), Costus root (Muxiang) and Immature bitter orange (Zhishi).

Dosage: 3-10 g

Cautions & Contraindications: This herb is contraindicated during pregnancy and during profuse menstrual flow.

186. Burreed tuber (Sanleng)

Pharmaceutical Name: Rhizoma Sparganii

Botanical Name: Sparganium stoloniferum Buch.-Ham.

Common Name: Burreed tuber, Sparganium, Scirpus

Source of Earliest Record: Bencao Shiyi

Part Used & Method for Pharmaceutical Preparations: The rhizomes are dug in winter or spring. After the fibrous roots have been removed, the rhizomes are dried in the sun.

Properties & Taste: Bitter and neutral

Meridians: Liver and spleen

Functions: 1. To invigorate blood and move stagnation; 2. To promote *qi* circulation and stop pain

Indications & Combinations:

1. *Qi* and blood stagnation manifested as amenorrhea, abdominal pain and epigastric or abdominal masses. Burreed tuber (Sanleng) is used with Zedoary (Ezhu) in the formula Ezhu Wan.

2. Retention of food and *qi* stagnation manifested as epigastric and abdominal distension and pain. Burreed tuber (Sanleng) is used with Zedoary (Ezhu), Green tangerine peel (Qingpi) and Germinated barley (Maiya).

Dosage: 3-10 g

Cautions & Contraindications: Prepared with vinegar can help the function of stopping pain. This herb is contraindicated during pregnancy and during profuse menstrual flow.

187. Red sage root (Danshen)

Pharmaceutical Name: Radix Salviae militiorrhizae

Botanical Name: Salvia miltiorrhiza Bge.

Common Name: Salvia root, Red sage root

Source of Earliest Record: Shennong Bencao Jing

Part Used & Method for Pharmaceutical Preparations: The roots are dug in autumn, and then cleaned, soaked, cut into slices and dried in the sun. They can also be fried with wine.

Properties & Taste: Bitter and slightly cold

Meridians: Heart, pericardium and liver

Functions: 1. To invigorate blood and move stagnation; 2. To cool blood and reduce carbuncles; 3. To clear heat in the heart and soothe irritability

Indications & Combinations:

1. Internal blood stagnation manifested as irregular menstruation, amenorrhea, abdominal pain or postpartum abdominal pain. Red sage

root (Danshen) is used with Motherwort (Yimucao), Peach seed (Tao-ren), Safflower (Honghua) and Chinese angelica root (Danggui).

2. *Qi* and blood stagnation manifested as cardiac pain, abdominal pain or epigastric pain. Red sage root (Danshen) is used with Amomum fruit (Sharen) and Sandalwood (Tanxiang) in the formula Danshen Yin.

3. Blood stagnation manifested as general pain or joint pain. Red sage root (Danshen) is used with Chinese angelica root (Danggui), Chuanxiong rhizome (Chuanxiong) and Safflower (Honghua).

4. Carbuncles, furuncles and swellings. Red sage root (Danshen) is used with Honeysuckle flower (Jinyinhua), Forsythia fruit (Lianqiao) and Frankincense (Ruxiang) in the formula Xiaoru Tang.

5. Febrile disease with pathogenic wind invading the nutritive level manifested as high fever, irritability, dull maculopapule and a red or deep red tongue proper with scanty coating. Red sage root (Danshen) is used with Fresh rehmannia root (Shengdihuang), Scrophularia (Xuanshen) and Bamboo leaf (Zhuye).

6. Deficiency of nutritive blood with internal heat manifested as palpitations, irritability and insomnia. Red sage root (Danshen) is used with Wild jujube seed (Suanzaoren) and Multiflower knotweed (Ye-jiaoteng).

Dosage: 5-15 g

Cautions & Contraindications: Blood invigoration is enhanced by frying with wine. Do not combine with the herb Black false bellebore (Lilu).

188. Motherwort (Yimucao)

Pharmaceutical Name: Herba Leonuri
Botanical Name: Leonurus heterophyllus Sweet
Common Name: Motherwort
Source of Earliest Record: Shennong Bencao Jing
Part Used & Method for Pharmaceutical Preparations: The entire plant is gathered in May or June, when it is flowering. It is then dried in the sun.
Properties & Taste: Pungent, bitter and slightly cold
Meridians: Heart, liver and urinary bladder
Functions: 1. To invigorate blood and move stagnation; 2. To promote urination and reduce edema
Indications & Combinations:

1. Blood stagnation manifested as irregular menstruation, dysmenorrhea, amenorrhea, postpartum abdominal pain and swelling and pain due to external injuries. Motherwort (Yimucao) is used with Chinese angelica root (Danggui), Chuanxiong rhizome (Chuanxiong) and Red peony (Chishao). Motherwort (Yimucao) may also be used alone.

2. Dysuria or edema. Motherwort (Yimucao) is used with fresh Imperata rhizome (Baimaogen).

Dosage: 10-15 g

189. Spatholobus stem (Jixueteng)

Pharmaceutical Name: Caulis Millettiae; Caulis spatholobi
Botanical Name: 1. Spatholobus suberectus Dunn; 2. Millettia dielsiana Harms ex Diels
Common Name: Milletia, Spatholobus stem
Source of Earliest Record: Bencao Gangmu Shiyi
Part Used & Method for Pharmaceutical Preparations: The stems are gathered in autumn, dried in sun, soaked in water and cut into slices.
Properties & Taste: Bitter, slightly sweet and warm
Meridian: Liver
Functions: 1. To invigorate the blood; 2. To nourish the blood; 3. To relax and activate the tendons
Indications & Combinations:

1. Blood deficiency and blood stagnation manifested as irregular menstruation, dysmenorrhea or menorrhea. Spatholobus stem (Jixueteng) is used with Chinese angelica root (Danggui), White peony root (Baishao) and Chuanxiong rhizome (Chuanxiong).

2. Soreness and painful joints caused by invasion of wind-cold-damp manifested as numbness of the limbs, or paralysis caused by poor nourishment of tendons and muscles due to deficient blood. Spatholobus stem (Jixueteng) is used with Chinese angelica root (Danggui), Chuanxiong rhizome (Chuanxiong), Chaenomeles fruit (Mugua) and Mulberry mistletoe (Sangjisheng).

Dosage: 10-15 g

190. Peach seed (Taoren)

Pharmaceutical Name: Semen Persicae
Botanical Name: 1. Prunus persica (L.) Batch; 2. Prunus davidiana

(Carr.) Franch.

Common Name: Persica seed, Peach seed

Source of Earliest Record: Shennong Bencao Jing

Part Used & Method for Pharmaceutical Preparations: Ripe peaches are gathered in July or September. The seeds are removed and their shells broken. After the seeds are dried in the sun, the skin of the seeds is rubbed off.

Properties & Taste: Bitter and neutral

Meridians: Heart, liver, lung and large intestine

Functions: 1. To invigorate blood and remove stagnation; 2. To lubricate the intestines and move feces downward

Indications & Combinations:

1. Blood stagnation manifested as amenorrhea, dysmenorrhea, postpartum abdominal pain and pain and swelling due to external injuries. Peach seed (Taoren) is used with Red peony (Chishao), Safflower (Honghua), Chinese angelica root (Danggui) and Chuanxiong rhizome (Chuanxiong) in the formula Tao Hong Siwu Tang.

2. Constipation due to dryness in the intestines. Peach seed (Taoren) is used with Chinese angelica root (Danggui), Arborvitae seed (Baiziren), Hemp seed (Huomaren) and Apricot seed (Xingren).

Dosage: 6-10 g

Cautions & Contraindications: This herb is pounded into pieces before decoction. It is contraindicated during pregnancy.

191a. Safflower (Honghua)

Pharmaceutical Name: Flos Carthami

Botanical Name: Carthamus tinctorius L.

Common Name: Carthamus, Safflower

Source of Earliest Record: Kaibao Bencao

Part Used & Method for Pharmaceutical Preparations: The flowers are gathered in summer, when they turn bright red. They are then dried in the shade.

Properties & Taste: Pungent and warm

Meridians: Heart and liver

Functions: 1. To invigorate blood and release stagnation; 2. To promote menstruation

Indications & Combinations: Blood stagnation manifested as amenorrhea, dysmenorrhea, postpartum abdominal pain and pain and swelling due to external injuries. Safflower (Honghua) is used with Peach seed (Taoren), Chinese angelica root (Danggui), Chuanxiong rhizome (Chuanxiong) and Red peony (Chishao) in the formula Tao Hong Siwu Tang.

Dosage: 3-10 g

Cautions & Contraindications: This herb is contraindicated during pregnancy.

191b. Saffron (Fanhonghua)

The dried stigmas and the top of the style of the Saffron Crocus are used in place of Safflower (Honghua), but they have a stronger action. Saffron (Fanhonghua) has as its properties and taste sweet and cold. It enters the heart and liver channels and invigorates the blood, removes stagnation and clears channels, and also cools the blood and releases toxins. Saffron (Fanhonghua) is used to treat cases with indications such as high fever, maculopapule and febrile disease in which pathogenic heat has entered the blood. The recommended dosage is 1.5-3 g.

192. Cyathula root (Niuxi)

Pharmaceutical Name: Radix Achyranthis bidentatae; Radix Cyathulae

Botanical Name: 1. Achyranthes bidentata Bl.; 2. Cyathula Officinalis Kuan

Common Name: Achyranthes root, Cyathula root

Source of Earliest Record: Shennong Bencao Jing

Part Used & Method for Pharmaceutical Preparations: The roots are dug in winter, dried and cut into slices.

Properties & Taste: Bitter, sour and neutral

Meridians: Liver and kidney

Functions: 1. To invigorate blood, release stagnation and promote menstruation; 2. To tonify liver and kidneys, and strengthen the tendons and muscles; 3. To promote urination and relieve urinary disorders; 4. To conduct blood flow downward

Indications & Combinations:

1. Blood stagnation manifested as amenorrhea, dysmenorrhea, irregular menstruation and pains due to external injuries. Cyathula root (Niuxi) is used with Peach seed (Taoren), Safflower (Honghua), Chinese angelica root (Danggui) and Corydalis tuber (Yanhusuo).

156

2. Deficiency of the liver and kidneys manifested as soreness and weakness in the lumbar region and legs. Cyathula root (Niuxi) is used with Mulberry mistletoe (Sangjisheng), Eucommia bark (Duzhong) and Cibot rhizome (Gouji).

3. Extravasation of blood by heat manifested as vomiting with blood and epistaxis. Cyathula root (Niuxi) is used with Small thistle (Xiaoji), Biota tops (Cebaiye) and Imperata rhizome (Baimaogen).

4. Deficient *yin* with hyperactive *yang* leading to internal liver wind going upward manifested as headache, dizziness and vertigo. Cyathula root (Niuxi) is used with Red ochre (Daizheshi), Oyster shell (Muli) and Dragon's bone (Longgu) in the formula Zhengan Xifeng Tang.

5. Deficient *yin* and excessive fire manifested as ulceration of the mouth and gum swelling. Cyathula root (Niuxi) is used with Fresh rehmannia root (Shengdihuang) and Anemarrhena rhizome (Zhimu).

6. Urinary tract disorders manifested as painful urination, hematuria and dysuria. Cyathula root (Niuxi) is used with Ricepaper pith (Tongcao), Talc (Huashi) and Pink (Qumai) in the formula Niuxi Tang.

Dosage: 6-15 g

Cautions & Contraindications: This herb is contraindicated during pregnancy, or with profuse menstrual flow.

193. Pangolin scales (Chuanshanjia)

Pharmaceutical Name: Squama Manitis
Zoological Name: Manis pentadactyla L.
Common Name: Anteater scales, Pangolin scales
Source of Earliest Record: Shennong Bencao Jing
Part Used & Method for Pharmaceutical Preparations: The anteater scales are removed, cleaned and dried in the sun.
Properties & Taste: Salty and slightly cold
Meridians: Liver and stomach
Functions: 1. To invigorate blood and promote menstruation; 2. To promote lactation; 3. To reduce swelling and dispel pus
Indications & Combinations:

1. Amenorrhea caused by blood stagnation. Pangolin scales (Chuanshanjia) is used with Chinese angelica root (Danggui), Chuanxiong rhizome (Chuanxiong) and Safflower (Honghua).

2. Postpartum insufficient lactation. Pangolin scales (Chuanshanjia)

is used with Vaccaria seed (Wangbuliuxing), Ricepaper pith (Tongcao) and Chinese angelica root (Danggui).

3. Wind-damp obstruction syndrome manifested as joint pain and motor impairment. Pangolin scales (Chuanshanjia) is used with Chuanxiong rhizome (Chuanxiong), Notopterygium root (Qianghuo), Pubescent angelica root (Duhuo) and Ledebouriella (Fangfeng).

4. Beginning of carbuncles and swelling manifested as red, hot, painful swollen skin. Pangolin scales (Chuanshanjia) is used with Honeylocust thorn (Zaojiaoci), Tendrilled fritillary bulb (Chuanbeimu), Frankincense (Ruxiang), Myrrh (Moyao), Red peony (Chishao) and Honeysuckle flower (Jinyinhua).

Dosage: 3-10 g

Cautions & Contraindications: Pangolin scales (Chuanshanjia) should be used cautiously in sores that have already ulcerated. This substance is contraindicated during pregnancy.

194. Cockroach (Chechong)

Pharmaceutical Name: Eupolyphaga

Zoological Name: 1. Eupolyphaga sinensis walk.; 2. Steleophaga plancyi (Bol.)

Common Name: Cockroach

Source of Earliest Record: Shennong Bencao Jing

Part Used & Method for Pharmaceutical Preparations: The cockroach is caught in summer, killed by boiling in water and then dried in the sun.

Properties & Taste: Salty, cold and slightly toxic

Meridian: Liver

Functions: To invigorate blood and remove stagnation

Indications & Combinations:

1. Amenorrhea or postpartum abdominal pain due to blood stagnation. Cockroach (Chechong) is used with Rhubarb (Dahuang) and Peach seed (Taoren) in the formula Xia Yuxue Tang.

2. Abdominal or epigastric masses. Cockroach (Chechong) is used with Turtle shell (Biejia), Rhubarb (Dahuang), Moutan bark (Mudanpi) and Peach seed (Taoren) in the formula Biejia Jian Wan.

3. Pains caused by external injuries or lumbar pain due to sprain. Cockroach (Chechong) is used with Peach seed (Taoren), Frankincense (Ruxiang) and Myrrh (Moyao). Cockroach (Chechong) may also be taken

alone.

Dosage: 3-10 g; 1-1.5 g for powder

Cautions & Contraindications: This substance is contraindicated during pregnancy.

195. Leech (Shuizhi)

Pharmaceutical Name: Hirudo seu whitmaniae

Zoological Name: 1. Whitmania pigra (Whitman); 2. Hirudo nipponica Whitman; 3. Whitmania acranulata (Whitman)

Common Name: Leech

Source of Earliest Record: Shennong Bencao Jing

Part Used & Method for Pharmaceutical Preparations: The leeches are caught from May to June or in autumn. They are killed and dried in the sun, and then pounded into powder or carbonized.

Properties & Taste: Salty, bitter, neutral and slightly toxic

Meridian: Liver

Functions: 1. To invigorate blood and remove stagnation; 2. To promote menstruation

Indications & Combinations:

1. Amenorrhea or abdominal and epigastric masses caused by blood stagnation. Leech (Shuizhi) is used with Peach seed (Taoren), Burreed tuber (Sanleng) and Chinese angelica root (Danggui).

2. Chest pain, abdominal pain and constipation caused by blood stagnation due to external injury. Leech (Shuizhi) is used with Pharbitis seed (Qianniuzi) and Rhubarb (Dahuang) in the formula Duoming Dan.

Dosage: 3-6 g; 0.3-0.5 g for baked powder

Cautions & Contraindications: This substance is contraindicated during pregnancy.

196. Gadfly (Mengchong)

Pharmaceutical Name: Tabanus

Zoological Name: Tabanus bivittatus Mats.

Common Name: Gadfly

Source of Earliest Record: Shennong Bencao Jing

Part Used & Method for Pharmaceutical Preparations: The female gadfly is caught in May or June. It is boiled or steamed, and then dried in the sun.

Properties & Taste: Bitter, slightly cold and slightly toxic

Meridian: Liver

Functions: To invigorate blood and remove stagnation

Indications & Combinations:

1. Amenorrhea or abdominal and epigastric masses caused by blood stagnation. Gadfly (Mengchong) is used with Leech (Shuizhi), Cockroach (Chechong), Peach seed (Taoren) and Rhubarb (Dahuang) in the formula Dahuang Zhechong Wan.

2. Pain due to external injury. Gadfly (Mengchong) is used with Frankincense (Ruxiang), Myrrh (Moyao) and Peach seed (Taoren).

Dosage: 1-1.5 g; 0.3 g for baked powder

Cautions & Contraindications: This substance is contraindicated during pregnancy.

197. Dalbergia wood (Jiangxiang)

Pharmaceutical Name: Lignum Dalbergiae Odoriferae

Botanical Name: Dalbergia odorifera T. Chen

Common Name: Dalbergia wood

Source of Earliest Record: Haiyao Bencao

Part Used & Method for Pharmaceutical Preparations: The heart wood of dalbergia odorifera is sawed into small pieces, then dried in the shade.

Properties & Taste: Pungent and warm

Meridians: Heart and liver

Functions: 1. To invigorate blood and remove stagnation; 2. To stop bleeding and pain; 3. To conduct *qi* downward and resolve turbid dampness

Indications & Combinations:

1. *Qi* and blood stagnation manifested as stifling sensation in the chest and hypochondriac pain. Dalbergia wood (Jiangxiang) is used with Curcuma root (Yujin), Pilose asiabell root (Dangshen), Peach seed (Taoren) and Vegetable sponge (Sigualuo).

2. Swellings and pains due to external injuries. Dalbergia wood (Jiangxiang) is used with Frankincense (Ruxiang) and Myrrh (Moyao).

3. Interior turbid dampness with vomiting and abdominal pain. Dalbergia wood (Jiangxiang) is used with Agastache (Huoxiang) and Costus root (Muxiang).

4. Hemorrhage and pain due to external injuries. Dalbergia wood (Jiangxiang) can be used alone, externally.

Dosage: 3-6 g; 1-2 g for powder

198. Bugleweed (Zelan)

Pharmaceutical Name: Herba Lycopi
Botanical Name: Lycopus lucidus Turcz. var. hirtus Regel
Common Name: Bugleweed
Source of Earliest Record: Shennong Bencao Jing
Part Used & Method for Pharmaceutical Preparations: The aerial part of the entire plant is gathered in summer, dried in the sun and cut into pieces.
Properties & Taste: Bitter, pungent and slightly warm
Meridians: Liver and spleen
Functions: 1. To invigorate blood and remove stagnation; 2. To promote urination and reduce edema
Indications & Combinations:

1. Blood stagnation manifested as amenorrhea, dysmenorrhea, irregular menstruation or postpartum abdominal pain. Bugleweed (Zelan) is used with Chinese angelica root (Danggui), Red sage root (Danshen) and Red peony (Chishao).

2. Chest pain or hypochondriac pain caused by external injuries. Bugleweed (Zelan) is used with Curcuma root (Yujin) and Red sage root (Danshen).

3. Carbuncles, furuncles, swellings. Bugleweed (Zelan) is used with Honeysuckle flower (Jinyinhua), Chinese angelica root (Danggui) and Licorice root (Gancao).

Dosage: 10-15 g

199. Chinese rose flower (Yuejihua)

Pharmaceutical Name: Flos Rosae chinensis
Botanical Name: Rosa chinensis Jacq.
Common Name: Chinese rose flower
Source of Earliest Record: Bencao Gangmu
Part Used & Method for Pharmaceutical Preparations: The flower buds are gathered in June or July in fair weather. Then the buds are opened and dried in the shade.
Properties & Taste: Sweet and warm
Meridian: Liver
Functions: 1. To invigorate blood and regulate menstruation; 2. To

reduce swelling

Indications & Combinations:

1. *Qi* and blood stagnation in the liver manifested as irregular menstruation, dysmenorrhea or amenorrhea. Chinese rose flower (Yuejihua) is used with Chinese angelica root (Danggui), Red sage root (Danshen) and Cyperus tuber (Xiangfu).

2. Scrofula and swellings. Chinese rose flower (Yuejihua) is used with Prunella spike (Xiakucao), Tendrilled fritillary bulb (Chuanbeimu) and Oyster shell (Muli).

Dosage: 3-6 g

Cautions & Contraindications: Excessive use of this herb may cause diarrhea. It should be used with caution in cases with weakness of the spleen and stomach. It is also contraindicated during pregnancy.

200. Campsis flower (Lingxiaohua)

Pharmaceutical Name: Flos Campsis

Botanical Name: Campsis grandiflora (Thunb.) K. Schum.

Common Name: Campsis flower

Source of Earliest Record: Shennong Bencao Jing

Part Used & Method for Pharmaceutical Preparations: The flowers are gathered in full bloom. They are then dried in the shade.

Properties & Taste: Pungent and slightly cold

Meridians: Liver and pericardium

Functions: 1. To release stagnation and clear the meridians; 2. To cool the blood and dispel wind

Indications & Combinations:

1. Amenorrhea caused by blood stagnation. Campsis flower (Lingxiaohua) is used with Chinese angelica root (Danggui), Safflower (Honghua), Red peony (Chishao) and Siphonostegia (Liujinu).

2. General itching due to endogenous wind caused by excessive heat in the blood. Campsis flower (Lingxiaohua) is used with Moutan bark (Mudanpi), Fresh rehmannia root (Shengdihuang), Tribulus fruit (Baijili) and Cicada slough (Chantui).

Dosage: 3-10 g

Cautions & Contraindications: This herb is contraindicated during pregnancy.

201. Vaccaria seed (Wangbuliuxing)

Pharmaceutical Name: Semen Vaccariae
Botanical Name: Vaccaria segetalis (Neck.) Garcke
Common Name: Vacarria seed, Cow soapwort seed
Source of Earliest Record: Shennong Bencao Jing
Part Used & Method for Pharmaceutical Preparations: The whole plant is harvested in June or July. After it has been dried in the sun, the seeds are removed from their shells. They are then dried again.
Properties & Taste: Bitter and neutral
Meridians: Liver and stomach
Functions: 1. To invigorate blood and promote menstruation; 2. To promote lactation
Indications & Combinations:

1. Dysmenorrhea by retardation of blood circulation or amenorrhea caused by blood stagnation. Vaccaria seed (Wangbuliuxing) is used with Chinese angelica root (Danggui), Chuanxiong rhizome (Chuanxiong), Safflower (Honghua) and Motherwort (Yimucao).

2. Postpartum insufficient lactation. Vaccaria seed (Wangbuliuxing) is used with Pangolin scales (Chuanshanjia) and Rice paper pith (Tongcao). If there is deficiency of *qi* and blood, Astragalus root (Huangqi) and Chinese angelica root (Danggui) are added.

3. Mastitis with pain and swollen breasts. Vaccaria seed (Wangbuliuxing) is used with Dandelion herb (Pugongying), Honeysuckle flower (Jinyinhua) and Trichosanthes fruit (Gualou).

Dosage: 6-10 g
Cautions & Contraindications: This herb should be used with caution during pregnancy.

202. Siphonostegia (Liujinu)

Pharmaceutical Name: Herba siphonostegiae; Herba Artemisiae anomalae
Botanical Name: 1. Artemsia anomala S. Moore; 2. Siphonostegia chinensis Benth.
Common Name: Siphonostegia
Source of Earliest Record: Xinxiu Bencao
Part Used & Method for Pharmaceutical Preparations: The whole plant is gathered in August or September and dried in the sun.
Properties & Taste: Bitter and warm

Meridians: Heart and spleen

Functions: 1. To invigorate blood and open the channels; 2. To stop pain

Indications & Combinations:

1. Blood stagnation manifested as dysmenorrhea, amenorrhea, post-partum abdominal pain or swelling and pain due to external injuries. Siphonostegia (Liujinu) is used with Chinese angelica root (Danggui), Corydalis tuber (Yanhusuo) and Chuanxiong rhizome (Chuanxiong).

2. Hemorrhages and pain due to external injuries. The powder of Siphonostegia (Liujinu) is used alone, externally.

Dosage: 3-10 g

Cautions & Contraindications: This herb is contraindicated during pregnancy.

203. Sappan wood (Sumu)

Pharmaceutical Name: Lignum Sappan

Botanical Name: Caesalpinia sappan L.

Common Name: Sappan wood

Source of Earliest Record: Xinxiu Bencao

Part Used & Method for Pharmaceutical Preparations: The heart wood is sawn into pieces or steamed and cut into slices.

Properties & Taste: Sweet, salty, slightly pungent and neutral

Meridians: Heart, liver and spleen

Functions: 1. To invigorate blood and promote menstruation; 2. To stop pain and reduce swelling

Indications & Combinations:

1. Blood stagnation manifested as dysmenorrhea, amenorrhea and postpartum abdominal pain. Sappan wood (Sumu) is used with Chinese angelica root (Danggui), Red peony (Chishao) and Safflower (Hong-hua).

2. Swellings and pains caused by external injuries. Sappan wood (Sumu) is used with Frankincense (Ruxiang) and Myrrh (Moyao).

Dosage: 3-10 g

Cautions & Contraindications: This herb is contraindicated during pregnancy.

204. Dragon's blood (Xuejie)

Pharmaceutical Name: Sanguis Draconis

Botanical Name: Daemonorops draco Bl.

Common Name: Calamus gum, Dragon's blood

Source of Earliest Record: Xinxiu Bencao

Part Used & Method for Pharmaceutical Preparations: The red resinous secretion from the fruit and stem is collected during the summer. It is heated or steamed into a solid resin, then pounded into powder.

Properties & Taste: Sweet, salty and neutral

Meridians: Heart and liver

Functions: 1. To stop bleeding and promote the healing of wounds; 2. To invigorate blood and remove stagnation; 3. To stop pain

Indications & Combinations:

1. Hemorrhages due to external injuries. Dragon's blood (Xuejie) can be taken alone for external use, or it can be combined with Cattail pollen (Puhuang).

2. Chronic ulcers. Dragon's blood (Xuejie) is used with Frankincense (Ruxiang) and Myrrh (Moyao) for external use.

3. Swelling and pain due to blood stagnation caused by external injuries. Dragon's blood (Xuejie) is used with Frankincense (Ruxiang) and Myrrh (Moyao) in the formula Qili San.

Dosage: 1-1.5 g in pill form

Cautions & Contraindications: This herb is contraindicated in the absence of signs of blood stagnation.

XIII. Herbs That Resolve Phlegm and Stop Cough and Asthma

Herbs that resolve phlegm and stop cough and asthma are used in cases with profuse sputum; thick, sticky phlegm; asthma; or symptoms related to phlegm, such as scrofula, goiter, epilepsy, convulsions and *yin* carbuncles.

The selection of herbs depends upon the cause and manifestations. For example, if phlegm is accompanied by an exterior syndrome, herbs that release the exterior are added. If phlegm is complicated with heat signs, herbs that clear heat are put into the formula. If an interior cold syndrome exists, herbs that warm the interior and dispel cold are added to the formula. If there are signs of cough and asthma with fatigue or weakness, herbs that nourish and tonify are added. For epilepsy and convulsions, herbs that pacify the liver, subdue endogenous wind and tranquilize the mind are added. For goiter and scrofula, herbs that soften hardness are added. For *yin* carbuncles, herbs that dispel cold and remove stagnation are added.

205. Pinellia tuber (Banxia)

Pharmaceutical Name: Rhizoma Pinelliae
Botanical Name: Pinellia ternata (Thunb.) Breit.
Common Name: Pinellia tuber
Source of Earliest Record: Shennong Bencao Jing
Part Used & Method for Pharmaceutical Preparations: The tuberous rhizomes are dug in the period between summer and autumn. After the bark and fibrous roots have been removed, the rhizomes are dried in the sun.
Properties & Taste: Pungent, warm and toxic
Meridians: Spleen, stomach and lung
Functions: 1. To dry dampness and resolve phlegm; 2. To conduct rebellious *qi* downward and stop vomiting; 3. To reduce distension and disperse nodules
Indications & Combinations:

1. Phlegm-damp cough due to deficient spleen manifested as cough with profuse, dilute and white sputum. Pinellia tuber (Banxia) is used with Tangerine peel (Chenpi) and Poria (Fuling) in the formula Erchen Tang.

2. Nausea and vomiting due to rebellious stomach *qi*: a) stomach cold type—Pinellia tuber (Banxia) is used with Fresh ginger (Shengjiang) in the formula Xiao Banxia Tang; b) stomach heat type —Pinellia tuber (Banxia) is used with Bamboo shavings (Zhuru) and Loquat leaf (Pipaye); c) pregnancy type—Pinellia tuber (Banxia) is used with Perilla stem (Sugeng) and Amomum fruit (Sharen); d) stomach weakness type—Pinellia tuber (Banxia) is used with Ginseng (Renshen) and Jujube (Dazao).

3. Globus hystericus due to *qi* stagnation and accumulation of phlegm-damp manifested as a feeling of having a foreign body in the throat, fullness and distension in the chest and epigastric region and nausea. Pinellia tuber (Banxia) is used with Magnolia bark (Houpo), Perilla leaf (Zisuye) and Poria (Fuling) in the formula Banxia Houpo Tang.

4. Goiter, scrofula and subcutaneous nodule. Pinellia tuber (Banxia) is used with Laminaria (Kunbu), Seaweed (Haizao) and Tendrilled fritillary bulb (Chuanbeimu).

Dosage: 5-10 g

Cautions & Contraindications: This herb is contraindicated in cases with dry cough due to deficient *yin,* or cough due to phlegm-heat. Also, it cannot be used together with the herb Sichuan aconite root (Wutou).

206a. Arisaema tuber (Tiannanxing)

Pharmaceutical Name: Rhizoma Arisaematis

Botanical Name: 1. Arisaema consanguineum Schott.; 2. Arisaema amurense Maxim.; 3. Arisaema heterophyllum Bl.

Common Name: Arisaema tuber

Source of Earliest Record: Shennong Bencao Jing

Part Used & Method for Pharmaceutical Preparations: The tuberous rhizomes are dug in autumn or winter. After the fibrous roots and bark have been removed, the rhizomes are dried in the sun and cut into slices.

Properties & Taste: Bitter, pungent and warm

Meridians: Lung, liver and spleen

Functions: 1. To dry dampness and resolve phlegm; 2. To dispel wind and stop spasms

Indications & Combinations:

1. Phlegm-damp cough manifested as profuse, dilute and white sputum and stifling sensation in the chest. Arisaema tuber (Tiannanxing) is used with Pinellia tuber (Banxia), Tangerine peel (Chenpi) and Immature bitter orange (Zhishi) in the formula Daotan Tang.

2. Phlegm-heat in the lungs manifested as cough with profuse, yellow and thick sputum and stifling sensation in the chest. Arisaema tuber with bile (Dannanxing) is used with Scutellaria root (Huangqin) and Trichosanthes fruit (Gualou).

3. Wind-phlegm manifested as dizziness, vertigo, rattling sound in the windpipe, facial paralysis, epilepsy and convulsions in tetanus. Arisaema tuber (Tiannanxing) is used with Pinellia tuber (Banxia), Gastrodia tuber (Tianma) and Typhonium tuber (Baifuzi).

Dosage: 5-10 g

Cautions & Contraindications: This herb is contraindicated during pregnancy. In general, the raw herb is not used for internal use.

206b. Arisaema tuber with bile (Dannanxing)

When arisaema tuber is powdered and mixed with ox bile, it is called Arisaema tuber with bile (Dannanxing). The combination is bitter and cool. It clears heat and resolves phlegm, dispels wind and stops convulsions. It is used to treat convulsions, windstroke and epilepsy. The recommended dosage is 2-5 g.

207. Typhonium tuber (Baifuzi)

Pharmaceutical Name: Rhizoma Typhonii gigantei seu Radix Aconiti coreani

Botanical Name: 1. Typhonium giganteum Engl.; 2. Aconitum coreanum (Lévl.) Raip.

Common Name: Typhonus, Typhonium tuber

Source of Earliest Record: Zhongyao Zhi

Part Used & Method for Pharmaceutical Preparations: The tuberous rhizomes are dug in autumn. After the fibrous roots and bark have been removed, the rhizomes are steamed with sulphur once or twice. Then they are dried in the sun and cut into slices.

Properties & Taste: Pungent, sweet, warm and toxic

Meridians: Spleen and stomach

Functions: 1. To dry dampness and resolve phlegm; 2. To dispel wind and stop spasms; 3. To release toxins and disperse nodules

Indications & Combinations:

1. Excessive wind-phlegm manifested as spasms, convulsions and facial paralysis. Typhonium tuber (Baifuzi) is used with Arisaema tuber (Tiannanxing), Pinellia tuber (Banxia), Gastrodia tuber (Tianma) and Scorpion (Quanxie).

2. Convulsions and spasms in tetanus. Typhonium tuber (Baifuzi) is used with Arisaema tuber (Tiannanxing), Gastrodia tuber (Tianma) and Ledebouriella (Fangfeng).

3. One-sided headache (migraine). Typhonium tuber (Baifuzi) is used with Chuanxiong rhizome (Chuanxiong) and Dahurian Angelica root (Baizhi).

Dosage: 3-5 g

Cautions & Contraindications: This herb is contraindicated during pregnancy. In general, the raw herb is not taken internally.

208. White mustard seed (Baijiezi)

Pharmaceutical Name: Semen Sinapsis seu Brassicae

Botanical Name: 1. Sinapis alba (L.) Boiss.; 2. Brassica Juncea (L.) Czern. et Coss.

Common Name: Brassica seed, White mustard seed

Source of Earliest Record: Mingyi Bielu

Part Used & Method for Pharmaceutical Preparations: After the white mustard ripens in summer or autumn, the seeds are gathered and dried in the sun.

Properties & Taste: Pungent and warm

Meridian: Lung

Functions: 1. To warm the lungs and resolve phlegm; 2. To invigorate *qi* circulation and disperse nodules; 3. To open the channels and stop pain

Indications & Combinations:

1. Lungs blocked by cold-phlegm manifested as cough with profuse, dilute and white sputum and stifling sensation in the chest. White mustard seed (Baijiezi) is used with Perilla seed (Suzi) and Radish seed (Laifuzi) in the formula Sanzi Yangqing Tang.

2. Retention of phlegm-damp in the chest and diaphragm manifested as distension and pain in the chest and hypochondriac region. White mustard seed (Baijiezi) is used with Kansui root (Gansui) and Peking spurge root (Daji).

3. Channels and collaterals obstructed by phlegm-damp manifested as joint pain and numbness of the limbs. White mustard seed (Baijiezi) is used with Myrrh (Moyao) and Costus root (Muxiang).

4. *Yin* carbuncles and swellings without discoloration of the skin. White mustard seed (Baijiezi) is used with Antler glue (Lujiaojiao), Cinnamon bark (Rougui) and Prepared rehmannia root (Shudihuang) in the formula Yanghe Tang.

Dosage: 3-10 g

Cautions & Contraindications: This herb is contraindicated in cases with skin allergies.

209. Platycodon root (Jiegeng)

Pharmaceutical Name: Radix Platycodi

Botanical Name: Platycodon grandiflorum (Jacq.) A. DC.

Common Name: Platycodon root, Balloonflower root

Source of Earliest Record: Shennong Bencao Jing

Part Used & Method for Pharmaceutical Preparations: The Platycodon roots are dug in either spring or autumn, but the autumn roots are better quality. After the root bark has been removed, the roots are dried in the sun and cut into slices.

Properties & Taste: Bitter, pungent and neutral

Meridian: Lung

Functions: 1. To promote the dispersing function of the lungs; 2. To resolve phlegm; 3. To expel pus

Indications & Combinations:

1. Failure of lung *qi* to disperse due to invasion of exogenous pathogenic factors manifested as cough with profuse sputum or sputum that is difficult to expectorate, fullness and distension in the chest and hypochondriac region, sore throat and hoarse voice. Platycodon root (Jiegeng) is used with Apricot seed (Xingren), Perilla leaf (Zisuye) and Tangerine peel (Chenpi) for wind-cold cough. Platycodon root (Jiegeng) is used with Mulberry leaf (Sangye), Apricot seed (Xingren) and Trichosanthes fruit (Gualou) for wind-heat cough. Platycodon root (Jiegeng) is used with Scrophularia (Xuanshen), Licorice root (Gancao) and Arctium fruit (Niubangzi) for sore throat and hoarse voice.

2. Toxic heat accumulated in the lungs (lung abscess) manifested as cough with blood or pus, yellow and offensive smelling sputum and chest pain. Platycodon root (Jiegeng) is used with Houttuynia (Yuxingcao), Benincasa seed (Dongguaren) and Trichosanthes fruit (Gualou).

Dosage: 3-10 g

210. Inula flower (Xuanfuhua)

Pharmaceutical Name: Flos Inulae

Botanical Name: 1. Inula britannica L.; 2. Inula japonica Thunb.

Common Name: Inula flower

Source of Earliest Record: Shennong Bencao Jing

Part Used & Method for Pharmaceutical Preparations: The flower is gathered in summer and autumn, when it is blooming, and is dried in the sun.

Properties & Taste: Bitter, pungent, salty and slightly warm

Meridians: Lung, spleen, stomach and large intestine

Functions: 1. To resolve phlegm and promote water metabolism; 2.

To conduct *qi* downward and stop vomiting

Indications & Combinations:

1. Phlegm fluid blocking the lungs manifested as asthma and cough with profuse sputum. Inula flower (Xuanfuhua) is used with Pinellia tuber (Banxia) and Asarum herb (Xixin).

2. Phlegm fluid blocking the stomach leading to rebellious *qi* manifested as eructation, vomiting and epigastric full sensation. Inula flower (Xuanfuhua) is used with Red ochre (Daizheshi), in the formula Xuanfu Daizhe Tang.

Dosage: 3-10 g

Cautions & Contraindictions: When decocting this herb should be wrapped in cloth.

211. Swallowwort rhizome (Baiqian)

Pharmaceutical Name: Radix et Rhizome Stauntoni

Botanical Name: 1. Cynanchum stauntoni (Decne.) Schltr. ex Lévl.; 2. Dynanchum glaucescens Hand.-Mazz.

Common Name: Cynanchum root, Swallowwort rhizome

Source of Earliest Record: Mingyi Bielu

Part Used & Method for Pharmaceutical Preparations: The roots are dug in autumn, cleaned and dried in the sun and cut into pieces.

Properties & Taste: Pungent, sweet and neutral

Meridian: Lung

Functions: 1. To resolve phlegm and stop cough; 2. To conduct *qi* downward

Indications & Combinations:

1. Cough due to invasion by exogenous pathogenic factors. Swallowwort rhizome (Baiqian) is used with Schizonepeta (Jingjie) and Platycodon root (Jiegeng) in the formula Zhisuo San.

2. Turbid phlegm blocking the lungs: a) cold-phlegm cough—Swallowwort rhizome (Baiqian) is used with Pinellia tuber (Banxia) and Perilla seed (Suzi); b) phlegm-heat cough—Swallowwort rhizome (Baiqian) is used with Trichosanthes fruit (Gualou).

3. Cough, asthma, edema and rattling sound in the throat. Swallowwort rhizome (Baiqian) is used with Aster root (Ziwan) and Peking spurge root (Daji) in the formula Baiqian Tang.

Dosage: 3-10 g

212. Peucedanum root (Qianhu)

Pharmaceutical Name: Radix Peucedani
Botanical Name: 1. Peucedanum praeruptorum Dunn.; 2. Peucedanum decursivum Maxim.
Common Name: Peucedanum root, Hogfennel root
Source of Earliest Record: Mingyi Bielu
Part Used & Method for Pharmaceutical Preparations: The roots are dug in winter or spring, and cleaned and dried in the sun. After the root bark has been removed, the roots are soaked in warm water and cut into slices.
Properties & Taste: Bitter, pungent and slightly cold
Meridian: Lung
Functions: 1. To promote dispersing function of the lungs and clear heat; 2. To resolve phlegm and stop cough
Indications & Combinations:

1. Phlegm-heat accumulating in the lungs manifested as cough with yellow and thick sputum. Peucedanum root (Qianhu) is used with Mulberry bark (Sangbaipi), Trichosanthes fruit (Gualou) and Tendrilled fritillary bulb (Chuanbeimu) in the formula Qianhu San.

2. Cough due to invasion by exogenous pathogenic wind and heat. Peucedanum root (Qianhu) is used with Mentha (Bohe), Arctium fruit (Niubangzi) and Platycodon root (Jiegeng).
Dosage: 6-10 g

213. Trichosanthes fruit (Gualou)

Pharmaceutical Name: Fructus Trichosanthes
Botanical Name: 1. Trichosanthes kirilowii Maxim.; 2. Trichosanthes rosthornii Harms.
Common Name: Trichosanthes fruit, Snakeground fruit
Source of Earliest Record: Mingyi Bielu
Part Used & Method for Pharmaceutical Preparations: The fruit is gathered in autumn and dried in the shade.
Properties & Taste: Sweet and cold
Meridians: Lung, stomach and large intestine
Functions: 1. To clear heat and resolve phlegm; 2. To moisten dryness and move feces; 3. To regulate *qi* in the chest and release nodules
Indications & Combinations:

1. Phlegm-heat cough manifested as cough with yellow and thick sputum, stifling sensation in the chest and constipation. Trichosanthes fruit (Gualou) is used with Arisaema tuber with bile (Dannanxing) and Scutellaria root (Huangqin) in the formula Qingqi Huatan Wan.

2. Phlegm, dampness and stagnated blood blocking the chest manifested as stifling sensation and pain in the chest, and chest pain referring to the back of the body. Trichosanthes fruit (Gualou) is used with Macrostem onion (Xiebai) and Pinellia tuber (Banxia) in the formula Gualou Xiebai Banxia Tang.

3. Phlegm and heat accumulating in the chest and epigastric region manifested as fullness and stifling sensation in the chest and epigastric region. Trichosanthes fruit (Gualou) is used with Coptis root (Huanglian) and Pinellia tuber (Banxia) in the formula Xiao Xianxiong Tang.

4. Constipation. Trichosanthes fruit (Gualou) is used with Hemp seed (Huomaren), Bush-cherry seed (Yuliren) and Bitter orange (Zhiqiao).

5. Mastitis (swollen and painful breasts). Trichosanthes fruit (Gualou) is used with Dandelion herb (Pugongying), Frankincense (Ruxiang) and Myrrh (Moyao).

Dosage: 10-20 g

Cautions & Contraindications: This herb cannot be used with Sichuan aconite root (Wutou), as they counteract each other.

214. Tendrilled fritillary bulb (Chuanbeimu)

Pharmaceutical Name: Bulbus fritillariae cirrhosae

Botanical Name: 1. Fritillaria cirrhosa D. Don; 2. Fritillaria unibracteata Hsiao et K. C. Hsia; 3. Fritillaria Przewalskii Maxim; 4. Fritillaria Delavayi Franch.

Common Name: Tendrilled fritillary bulb

Source of Earliest Record: Shennong Bencao Jing

Part Used & Method for Pharmaceutical Preparations: The bulbs are dug in summer and dried in the sun. The bulb bark is removed.

Properties & Taste: Bitter, sweet and slightly cold

Meridians: Lung and heart

Functions: 1. To moisten the lungs and resolve phlegm; 2. To stop cough; 3. To clear heat and release nodules

Indications & Combinations:

1. Cough: a) chronic cough due to lung deficiency manifested as

dry cough and dry throat—Tendrilled fritillary bulb (Chuanbeimu) is used with Ophiopogon root (Maidong) and Glehnia root (Shashen); b) phlegm-heat cough manifested as yellow and thick sputum—Tendrilled fritillary bulb (Chuanbeimu) is used with Anemarrhena rhizome (Zhimu), Scutellaria root (Huangqin) and Trichosanthes fruit (Gualou); c) wind-heat cough—Tendrilled fritillary bulb (Chuanbeimu) is used with Mulberry leaf (Sangye), Peucedanum root (Qianhu) and Apricot seed (Xingren).

2. Scrofula, mastitis and lung abscess: a) scrofula—Tendrilled fritillary bulb (Chuanbeimu) is used with Scrophularia (Xuanshen) and Oyster shell (Muli); b) mastitis—Tendrilled fritillary bulb (Chuanbeimu) is used with Dandelion herb (Pugongying) and Forsythia fruit (Lianqiao); c) lung abscess—Tendrilled fritillary bulb (Chuanbeimu) is used with Houttuynia (Yuxingcao) and Coix seed (Yiyiren).

Dosage: 3-10 g

Cautions & Contraindications: This herb cannot be used with Sichuan aconite root (Wutou), as they counteract each other.

215. Bamboo shavings (Zhuru)

Pharmaceutical Name: Caulis bambusae in taenis
Botanical Name: Phyliostachys nigra var. henonis Stapf
Common Name: Bamboo shavings
Source of Earliest Record: Mingyi Bielu
Part Used & Method for Pharmaceutical Preparations: After the outside green skin has been removed, shavings are taken from the outer part of the bamboo. This can be done all year round.

Properties & Taste: Sweet and slightly cold
Meridians: Lung, stomach and gall bladder
Functions: 1. To clear heat and resolve phlegm; 2. To relieve irritability and stop vomiting
Indications & Combinations:

1. Cough due to heat in the lungs manifested as cough with yellow thick sputum. Bamboo shavings (Zhuru) is used with Scutellaria root (Huangqin) and Trichosanthes fruit (Gualou).

2. Mind disturbed by phlegm-heat manifested as irritability, insomnia, palpitations, stifling sensation in the chest and cough with yellow sputum. Bamboo shavings (Zhuru) is used with Immature bitter orange (Zhishi), Tangerine peel (Chenpi) and Poria (Fuling) in the formula

Wendan Tang.

3. Nausea and vomiting caused by heat in the stomach. Bamboo shavings (Zhuru) is used with Coptis root (Huanglian), Tangerine peel (Chenpi), Pinellia tuber (Banxia) and Fresh ginger (Shengjiang).

Dosage: 6-10 g

216. Bamboo juice (Zhuli)

Pharmaceutical Name: Saccus Bambusae in Taeniam

Botanical Name: 1. Phyllostachys nigra var. henonis Stapf; 2. Bambusa tuldoides Munro; 3. Sinocalamus breecheyanus (Munro) McClure var. pubescens P. F. Li

Common Name: Bamboo juice

Source of Earliest Record: Mingyi Bielu

Part Used & Method for Pharmaceutical Preparations: The bamboo juice is collected after the green bamboo has been burned.

Properties & Taste: Sweet and cold

Meridians: Lung and stomach

Functions: To clear heat and resolve phlegm

Indications & Combinations:

1. Phlegm-heat cough manifested as cough with thick, yellow sputum and chest pain. Bamboo juice (Zhuli) is used with Loquat leaf (Pipaye) and Trichosanthes fruit (Gualou).

2. Windstroke due to heart misted by phlegm, epilepsy or manic psychosis. Bamboo juice (Zhuli) is used with Ginger juice (Jiangzhi).

Dosage: 30-50 g

Cautions & Contraindications: This herb is contraindicated for cough caused by cold and in cases with diarrhea caused by spleen deficiency.

217. Costazia bone (Haifushi)

Pharmaceutical Name: Pumice; Pumex

Zoological Name: Costazia aculeata Canu et Bassler

Common Name: Pumice, Costazia bone

Source of Earliest Record: Rihuazi Bencao

Part Used & Method for Pharmaceutical Preparations: The dried bone is collected from Costazia Sp.

Properties & Taste: Salty and cold

Meridian: Lung

Functions: 1. To clear heat in the lungs and resolve phlegm; 2. To soften hardness and release nodules

Indications & Combinations:

1. Phlegm-heat cough manifested as cough with yellow, sticky and thick sputum or sputum difficult to expectorate. Costazia bone (Haifushi) is used with Sea clam shell (Haigeqiao), Trichosanthes fruit (Gualou), Capejasmine (Zhizi) and Natural indigo (Qingdai).

2. Scrofula and goiter caused by phlegm and *qi* accumulation. Costazia bone (Haifushi) is used with Oyster shell (Muli), Tendrilled fritillary bulb (Chuanbeimu), Scrophularia (Xuanshen) and Laminaria (Kunbu).

Dosage: 6-10 g

218. Sea clam shell (Haigeqiao)

Pharmaceutical Name: Concha Meretricis seu Cyclinae
Zoological Name: 1. Cyclina sinensis Gmelin; 2. Meretrix meretrix L.
Common Name: Clam shell
Source of Earliest Record: Shennong Bencao Jing
Part Used & Method for Pharmaceutical Preparations: The clam shells are collected from the seashore and pounded into powder.
Properties & Taste: Bitter, salty and cold
Meridians: Lung and stomach
Functions: 1. To clear heat in the lungs and resolve phlegm; 2. To soften hardness and release nodules

Indications & Combinations:

1. Phlegm-heat cough manifested as cough with thick yellow sputum, asthma, chest pain and hypochondriac pain. Sea clam shell (Haigeqiao) is used with Costazia bone (Haifushi), Swallowwort rhizome (Baiqian), Mulberry bark (Sangbaipi), Capejasmine (Zhizi) and Trichosanthes fruit (Gualou).

2. Scrofula and goiter. Sea clam shell (Haigeqiao) is used with Laminaria (Kunbu), Seaweed (Haizao) and Ark shell (Walengzi) in the formula Hanhua Wan.

Dosage: 10-15 g

Cautions & Contraindications: This substance is normally used in powdered form and should be placed in a cloth bag for decoction or removed from the decoction with a strainer.

219. Seaweed (Haizao)

Pharmaceutical Name: Sargassum
Botanical Name: 1. Sargassum pallidum (Turn.) G. Ag.; 2. Sargassum fusiforme (Harv.) Setch.
Common Name: Sargassum, seaweed
Source of Earliest Record: Shennong Bencao Jing
Part Used & Method for Pharmaceutical Preparations: Entire plant. It is collected in summer, cleaned, cut into pieces and dried in the shade.
Properties & Taste: Salty and cold
Meridians: Liver, stomach and kidney
Functions: 1. To resolve phlegm and soften hardness; 2. To promote water metabolism
Indications & Combinations:

1. Goiter. Seaweed (Haizao) is used with Laminaria (Kunbu) in the formula Haizao Yuhu Tang.

2. Scrofula. Seaweed (Haizao) is used with Prunella spike (Xiakucao), Scrophularia (Xuanshen) and Tendrilled fritillary bulb (Chuanbeimu) in the formula Neixiao Lei Li Wan.

3. Edema of the foot or general edema. Seaweed (Haizao) is used with Poria (Fuling) and Alismatis rhizome (Zexie).

Dosage: 10-15 g
Cautions & Contraindications: This herb should not be combined with Licorice root (Gancao), as they counteract each other.

220. Laminaria (Kunbu)

Pharmaceutical Name: Thallus Laminariae seu Eckloniae
Botanical Name: 1. Laminaria japonica Aresch.; 2. Ecklonia kurome Okam.
Common Name: Laminaria, Kelp, Kunbu sea cress
Source of Earliest Record: Mingyi Bielu
Part Used & Method for Pharmaceutical Preparations: The laminaria thallus is collected from the sea in summer or autumn. It is cleaned, cut into pieces and dried in the shade.
Properties & Taste: Salty and cold
Meridians: Liver, stomach and kidney
Functions: 1. To resolve phlegm and soften hardness; 2. To promote water metabolism
Indications & Combinations:

1. Goiter manifested as enlarged neck and stifling sensation in the throat. Laminaria (Kunbu) is used with Seaweed (Haizao) and Sea clam shell (Haigeqiao) in the formula Kunbu Wan.

2. Edema of the foot or general edema. Laminaria (Kunbu) is used with Poria (Fuling) and Alismatis rhizome (Zexie).

Dosage: 10-15 g

221. Boat sterculia seed (Pangdahai)

Pharmaceutical Name: Semen Sterculiae lychnopherae
Botanical Name: Sterculia lychnophera Hance
Common Name: Boat sterculia seed
Source of Earliest Record: Bencao Gangmu Shiyi
Part Used & Method for Pharmaceutical Preparations: The seeds are collected from April to June after the fruit ripens, and then they are dried in the sun.

Properties & Taste: Sweet and cold
Meridians: Lung and large intestine
Functions: 1. To clear heat in the lungs and promote the dispersing function of *qi* in the lungs; 2. To moisten the intestines and move feces

Indications & Combinations:

1. Failure of lung *qi* to disperse, resulting in accumulation of heat in the lungs manifested as sore throat, coarse voice, cough with yellow, thick and sticky sputum and sputum difficult to expectorate. Boat sterculia seed (Pangdahai) is used with Platycodon root (Jiegeng), Cicada slough (Chantui), Mentha (Bohe) and Licorice root (Gancao). The herb can also be used alone in boiled water as tea.

2. Constipation due to accumulation of heat. Boat sterculia seed (Pangdahai) is used alone in boiled water as tea, or it is combined with other herbs that move stool.

Dosage: 3-5 g (The dosage for powder form should be halved.)

222. Dichroa root (Changshan)

Pharmaceutical Name: Radix Dichroae
Botanical Name: Dichroa fibrifuga Lour.
Common Name: Dichroa root
Source of Earliest Record: Shennong Bencao Jing
Part Used & Method for Pharmaceutical Preparations: The roots are dug in autumn. After the fibrous roots have been removed, the roots

are dried in the sun and cut into slices. They can also be fried with wine.

Properties & Taste: Bitter, pungent, cold and toxic

Meridians: Lung, heart and liver

Functions: To expel phlegm and relieve malaria

Indications & Combinations: Malaria. Dichroa root (Changshan) is used with Tsaoko (Caoguo), Anemarrhena rhizome (Zhimu) and Areca seed (Binglang).

Dosage: 5-10 g

Cautions & Contraindications: This herb may cause vomiting and nausea; it should be used with caution, especially with weak patients.

223. Ark shell (Walengzi)

Pharmaceutical Name: Concha Arcae

Zoological Name: 1. Arca granosa L.; 2. Arca subcrenata Lischke; 3. Arca inflata Reeve

Common Name: Ark shell

Source of Earliest Record: Mingyi Bielu

Part Used & Method for Pharmaceutical Preparations: The shells are collected from the sea when the tide is out. After the flesh is removed, the shell is dried and ground into powder.

Properties & Taste: Salty and neutral

Meridians: Lung, stomach and liver

Functions: 1. To resolve phlegm and stagnation; 2. To soften hardness and disperse nodules

Indications & Combinations:

1. Scrofula and goiter. Ark shell (Walengzi) is used with Seaweed (Haizao) and Laminaria (Kunbu).

2. Stomach pain and acid regurgitation. Ark shell (Walengzi) is used with Cuttlefish bone (Wuzeigu).

3. Subcutaneous nodules. Ark shell (Walengzi) is used with Burreed tuber (Sanleng), Zedoary (Ezhu) and Turtle shell (Biejia).

Dosage: 10-30 g

Cautions & Contraindications: The raw substance is used for nodules; the baked substance is better for treating acid regurgitation and pain.

224a. Apricot seed (Xingren)

Pharmaceutical Name: Semen Armeniacae

Botanical Name: 1. Prunus armeniaca L. var. ansu maxim.; 2. Prunus mandshurica (Maxim.) Koehne; 3. Prunus sibirica L.

Common Name: Apricot seed, Bitter apricot seed or kernel

Source of Earliest Record: Shennong Bencao Jing

Part Used & Method for Pharmaceutical Preparations: The seeds are collected after the apricot ripens in summer. They are then dried in the sun and pounded into pieces.

Properties & Taste: Bitter, slightly warm and slightly toxic

Meridians: Lung and large intestine

Functions: 1. To stop cough and relieve asthma; 2. To moisten the intestines and move stool

Indications & Combinations:

1. Cough and asthma: a) cough due to invasion by exogenous pathogenic wind and heat—Apricot seed (Xingren) is used with Mulberry leaf (Sangye) and Chrysanthemum flower (Juhua) in the formula Sang Ju Yin; b) cough due to dysfunction of the lungs caused by dryness and heat—Apricot seed (Xingren) is used with Mulberry leaf (Sangye), Tendrilled fritillary bulb (Chuanbeimu) and Glehnia root (Shashen) in the formula Sang Xing Tang; c) cough and asthma due to accumulated heat in the lungs—Apricot seed (Xingren) is used with Gypsum (Shigao) and Ephedra (Mahuang) in the formula Ma Xing Shi Gan Tang.

2. Constipation due to dryness in the intestines. Apricot seed (Xingren) is used with Hemp seed (Huomaren) and Chinese angelica root (Danggui) in the formula Runchang Wan.

Dosage: 3-10 g

Cautions & Contraindications: This herb is slightly toxic, so overdosing should be avoided. It should be used with caution in infants.

224b. Sweet apricot seed (Tianxingren)

The apricot seed comes from the cultivated prunus armeniaca. Its properties and taste are sweet and neutral. Its functions are quite similar to those of bitter apricot seed, but it is more effective for moistening. Sweet apricot seed (Tianxingren) is indicated in cough and asthma caused by weakness of the body and fatigue. The recommended dosage is 3-10 g.

225. Stemona root (Baibu)

Pharmaceutical Name: Radix Stemonae

Botanical Name: 1. Stemona sessilifolia Miq.; 2. Stemona japonica (Bl.) Miq.; 3. Stemona tuberosa Lour.

Common Name: Stemona root

Source of Earliest Record: Mingyi Bielu

Part Used & Method for Pharmaceutical Preparations: The roots are dug in spring or autumn. After the fibrous roots have been removed, the roots are cleaned and put into boiling water. Then they are dried in the sun and cut into pieces.

Properties & Taste: Sweet, bitter and neutral

Meridian: Lung

Functions: 1. To moisten the lungs and stop cough; 2. To kill lice and parasites

Indications & Combinations:

1. Cough in common cold. Stemona root (Baibu) is used with Schizonepeta (Jingjie), Platycodon root (Jiegeng) and Aster root (Ziwan).

2. Whooping cough. Stemona root (Baibu) is used with Glehnia root (Beishashen), Tendrilled fritillary bulb (Chuanbeimu) and Swallowwort rhizome (Baiqian).

3. Cough due to tuberculosis. Stemona root (Baibu) is used with Ophiopogon root (Maidong) and Fresh rehmannia root (Shengdihuang).

4. Lice of the head or body. The herb is made into a 20% tincture, or a 50% decoction used as an external wash.

5. Pinworm. The 30-ml 100% decoction as an enema before sleep, daily for five days.

Dosage: 5-10 g

226. Aster root (Ziwan)

Pharmaceutical Name: Radix Asteris

Botanical Name: Aster tataricus L. f.

Common Name: Aster root, Purple aster root

Source of Earliest Record: Shennong Bencao Jing

Part Used & Method for Pharmaceutical Preparations: The roots, or rhizomes, are dug in spring or autumn. Then they are cleaned, dried in the sun and cut into pieces.

Properties & Taste: Bitter, sweet and slightly warm

Meridian: Lung

Functions: To resolve phlegm and stop cough

Indications & Combinations: Cough: a) cough due to invasion by exogenous pathogenic factors manifested as cough with profuse sputum—Aster root (Ziwan) is used with Schizonepeta (Jingjie) and Swallowwort rhizome (Baiqian); b) cough due to deficiency of the lungs manifested as cough with scanty sputum or with bloody sputum. Aster root (Ziwan) is used with Anemarrhena rhizome (Zhimu), Tendrilled fritillary bulb (Chuanbeimu) and Donkey hide gelatin (Ejiao) in the formula Ziwan Tang.

Dosage: 5-10 g

227. Coltsfoot flower (Kuandonghua)

Pharmaceutical Name: Flos Farfarae
Botanical Name: Tussilago farfara L.
Common Name: Coltsfoot flower, Tussilago
Source of Earliest Record: Shennong Bencao Jing
Part Used & Method for Pharmaceutical Preparations: After the plant begins to flower before winter, the flower buds are gathered and dried in the shade.
Properties & Taste: Pungent and warm
Meridian: Lung
Functions: 1. To moisten the lungs and resolve phlegm; 2. To stop cough

Indications & Combinations: Cough. Coltsfoot flower (Kuandonghua) is used with Aster root (Ziwan). It is more powerful than Aster root (Ziwan) in stopping cough and resolving phlegm.

Dosage: 5-10 g

228. Perilla seed (Suzi)

Pharmaceutical Name: Fructus Perillae
Botanical Name: Perilla frutescens (L.) Britt.
Common Name: Purple perilla fruit, Perilla seed
Source of Earliest Record: Mingyi Bielu
Part Used & Method for Pharmaceutical Preparations: The fruit is gathered in autumn, when it ripens. Then it is dried in the sun and pounded into pieces.
Properties & Taste: Pungent and warm
Meridians: Lung and large intestine

Functions: 1. To stop cough and soothe asthma; 2. To moisten the intestines and move feces

Indications & Combinations:

1. Upward perversion of lung *qi* caused by excessive phlegm fluid manifested as cough with white profuse sputum, or asthma and fullness and stifling sensation in the chest and hypochondriac region. Perilla seed (Suzi) is used with White mustard seed (Baijiezi) and Radish seed (Laifuzi) in the formula Sanzi Yangqing Tang.

2. Constipation due to dryness in the intestines. Perilla seed (Suzi) is used with Hemp seed (Huomaren), Trichosanthes seed (Gualouren) and Apricot seed (Xingren).

Dosage: 5-10 g

229. Mulberry bark (Sangbaipi)

Pharmaceutical Name: Cortex Mori
Botanical Name: Morus alba L.
Common Name: Mulberry bark, Morus bark
Source of Earliest Record: Shennong Bencao Jing
Part Used & Method for Pharmaceutical Preparations: The bark of the root is collected in winter. It is cleaned, cut into pieces and dried in the sun.
Properties & Taste: Sweet and cold
Meridian: Lung
Functions: 1. To reduce heat from the lungs and soothe asthma; 2. To promote urination and reduce edema
Indications & Combinations:

1. Heat in the lungs manifested as cough with excessive sputum and asthma. Mulberry bark (Sangbaipi) is used with Wolfberry bark (Digupi) and Licorice root (Gancao) in the formula Xiebai San.

2. Dysuria or edema. Mulberry bark (Sangbaipi) is used with Areca nut shell (Dafupi) and Poria peel (Fulingpi) in the formula Wupi Yin.

Dosage: 10-15 g

230. Lepidium seed (Tinglizi)

Pharmaceutical Name: Semen Lepiddi seu Descurainiae
Botanical Name: 1. Lepidium apetalum Willd.; 2. Descurainia sophia (L.) Webb et prantl
Common Name: Lepidium seed, Descurainia seed

Source of Earliest Record: Shennong Bencao Jing

Part Used & Method for Pharmaceutical Preparations: The whole plant is harvested in the period of the Beginning of Summer (seventh solar term) and dried in the sun. Then the seeds are collected.

Properties & Taste: Bitter, pungent and very cold

Meridians: Lung and urinary bladder

Functions: 1. To reduce phlegm in the lungs and soothe asthma; 2. To promote urination and reduce edema

Indications & Combinations:

1. Retention of phlegm fluid in the lungs manifested as cough with profuse sputum, asthma, fullness and distension in the chest and hypochondriac region, asthma in which patient cannot lie flat and edema of the face. Lepidium seed (Tinglizi) is used with Jujube (Dazao) in the formula Tingli Dazao Xiefei Tang.

2. Edema or dysuria. Lepidium seed (Tinglizi) is used with Tetrandra root (Fangji) and Rhubarb (Dahuang) in the formula Ji Jiao Li Huang Wan.

Dosage: 3-10 g

231. Datura flower (Yangjinhua)

Pharmaceutical Name: Flos Daturae

Botanical Name: Datura metel L.

Common Name: Datura flower, Jimson weed

Source of Earliest Record: Bencao Gangmu

Part Used & Method for Pharmaceutical Preparations: The flowers are gathered in the period from April to November, and then they are dried in the sun.

Properties & Taste: Pungent, warm and toxic

Meridians: Heart, lung and spleen

Functions: To stop asthma

Indications & Combinations:

1. Asthma manifested as cough with no sputum and stifling sensation in the chest. Datura flower (Yangjinhua) is used to roll a "cigarette" which is lighted and which the patient sniffs.

2. Epigastric and abdominal pain, wind-damp obstruction pain and pain due to external injuries. Datura flower (Yangjinhua) is used alone or with Chuanxiong rhizome (Chuanxiong) and Tetrandra root (Fangji).

Dosage: 0.3-0.6 g

Cautions & Contraindications: This herb is toxic. It is contraindicated during glaucoma and should be used with caution in cases of weakness of the body and hypertension, and in children and pregnant women.

232. Loquat leaf (Pipaye)

Pharmaceutical Name: Folium Eriobotryae
Botanical Name: Eriobotrya japonica (Thunb.) Lindl.
Common Name: Eriobotrya leaf, Loquat leaf
Source of Earliest Record: Mingyi Bielu
Part Used & Method for Pharmaceutical Preparations: The leaves are gathered in late spring or early summer and dried in the sun. Then the down of the leaves is brushed off and the leaves are cut into pieces.
Properties & Taste: Bitter and neutral
Meridians: Lung and stomach
Functions: 1. To resolve phlegm and stop cough; 2. To conduct rebellious *qi* downward and stop vomiting
Indications & Combinations:

1. Heat in the lungs manifested as cough and asthma. Loquat leaf (Pipaye) is used with Mulberry bark (Sangbaipi), Swallowwort rhizome .(Baiqian) and Platycodon root (Jiegeng).

2. Heat in the stomach manifested as nausea and vomiting. Loquat leaf (Pipaye) is used with Bamboo shavings (Zhuru) and Reed root (Lugen).
Dosage: 10-15 g

233. Birthwort fruit (Madouling)

Pharmaceutical Name: Fructus Aristlochiae
Botanical Name: 1. Aristolochia contorta Bge.; 2. Aristolochia debilis Sieb. et Zucc.
Common Name: Aristolochia fruit, Birthwort fruit
Source of Earliest Record: Yaoxing Lun
Part Used & Method for Pharmaceutical Preparations: The ripe fruit is gathered in autumn and dried in the sun.
Properties & Taste: Bitter, slightly pungent and cold
Meridians: Lung and large intestine
Functions: 1. To clear the lungs and resolve phlegm; 2. To stop cough and soothe asthma
Indications & Combinations:

1. Heat in the lungs manifested as cough with profuse yellow

sputum and asthma. Birthwort fruit (Madouling) is used with Loquat leaf (Pipaye), Peucedanum root (Qianhu), Mulberry bark (Sangbaipi) and Scutellaria root (Huangqin).

2. Deficiency of the lungs manifested as cough with scanty sputum or with bloody sputum and shortness of breath. Birthwort fruit (Madouling) is used with Glehnia root (Shashen), Ophiopogon root (Maidong), Aster root (Ziwan) and Donkey hide gelatin (Ejiao).

Dosage: 3-10 g

Cautions & Contraindications: Overdosage of the herb may cause nausea and vomiting.

234. Ginkgo seed (Baiguo)

Pharmaceutical Name: Semen Ginkgo
Botanical Name: Ginkgo biloba L.
Common Name: Ginkgo seed
Source of Earliest Record: Bencao Gangmu
Part Used & Method for Pharmaceutical Preparations: The ripe seeds are gathered in autumn, cleaned and dried in the sun. After the shells of the seeds have been broken, the seeds are removed and pounded into pieces.
Properties & Taste: Sweet, bitter, astringent, neutral and slightly toxic
Meridian: Lung
Functions: 1. To strengthen lung *qi* and soothe asthma; 2. To relieve leukorrhea
Indications & Combinations:

1. Asthma: a) asthma with stifling sensation in the chest and cough with profuse, dilute sputum—Ginkgo seed (Baiguo) is used with Ephedra (Mahuang) and Licorice root (Gancao); b) asthma with stifling sensation in the chest and cough with thick yellow sputum—Ginkgo seed (Baiguo) is used with Scutellaria root (Huangqin) and Mulberry bark (Sangbaipi) in the formula Dingchuan Tang.

2. Leukorrhea: a) downward flowing of damp-heat manifested as yellow, odorous leukorrhea—Ginkgo seed (Baiguo) is used with Phellodendron bark (Huangbai) and Plantain seed (Cheqianzi) in the formula Yihuang Tang; b) deficiency of kidney *yang* manifested as whitish, odorless leukorrhea—Ginkgo seed (Baiguo) is used with Cinnamon bark (Rougui), Astragalus root (Huangqi) and Dogwood fruit (Shanzhuyu).

Dosage: 6-10 g
Cautions & Contraindications: Overdosage of the herb is toxic.

XIV. Herbs That Tranquilize the Mind

Herbs that tranquilize the mind are used for deficient *qi* of the heart, deficient blood in the heart or flaring up of fire in the heart, which are manifested as restlessness, palpitations, anxiety, insomnia, dream-disturbed sleep, convulsions, epilepsy and manic psychotic disorders. The selection of herbs should follow the pathological condition. For example, when accompanied by deficient *yin* and blood, herbs that replenish blood and nourish *yin* are added to the combination. If the condition is due to hyperactivity of liver *yang*, herbs that pacify the liver and subdue *yang* are added to the combination. If there are complications of flaring up of heart fire, herbs that clear heart fire are added. In cases of epilepsy and convulsions, herbs that resolve phlegm and open the orifices, or pacify the liver and subdue endogenous wind, are selected as the main herbs. Tranquilizing herbs, in these cases, are added as supplemental herbs.

235. Dragon's bone (Longgu)

Pharmaceutical Name: Os draconis
Zoological Name: 1. Stegodon orientalis; 2. Rhinocerus senensia
Common Name: Dragon's bone, Fossilized bone
Source of Earliest Record: Shennong Bencao Jing
Part Used & Method for Pharmaceutical Preparations: The fossilized vertebrae and other bones of ancient large mammals, such as Rhinocerus or Rechistaric reptiles, are collected and broken into pieces.
Properties & Taste: Sweet, astringent and slightly cold
Meridians: Heart and liver
Functions: 1. To pacify the liver and subdue the *yang*; 2. To calm the heart and soothe the mind; 3. To relieve leukorrhea and arrest seminal emissions or sweating
Indications & Combinations:

1. Deficient *yin* of the liver and kidneys with hyperactive *yang* of the liver manifested as dizziness, vertigo, blurred vision or irritability. Dragon's bone (Longgu) is used with Oyster shell (Muli), Red ochre

(Daizheshi) and White peony root (Baishao) in the formula Zhengan Xifeng Tang.

2. Seminal emissions due to deficient kidneys. Dragon's bone (Longgu) is used with Oyster shell (Muli), Flattened milkvetch seed (Shayuanzi) and Euryale seed (Qianshi).

3. Palpitations and insomnia. Dragon's bone (Longgu) is used with Oyster shell (Muli), Polygala root (Yuanzhi) and Wild jujube seed (Suanzaoren).

4. Leukorrhea due to deficient kidneys. Dragon's bone (Longgu) is used with Oyster shell (Muli), Dioscorea (Shanyao) and Cuttlefish bone (Wuzeigu).

5. Spontaneous sweating and night sweating. Dragon's bone (Longgu) is used with Oyster shell (Muli) and Schisandra fruit (Wuweizi).

Dosage: 15-30 g

Cautions & Contraindications: This herb should be cooked before adding other herbs.

236. Amber (Hupo)

Pharmaceutical Name: Succinus
Botanical Name: Pinus spp.
Common Name: Amber, Succinus
Source of Earliest Record: Mingyi Bielu
Part Used & Method for Pharmaceutical Preparations: The brownish fossil resin is taken from a pine tree which has been buried underground for a long time. It is then ground into powder.
Properties & Taste: Sweet and neutral
Meridians: Heart, liver and urinary bladder
Functions: 1. To calm and tranquilize the mind; 2. To invigorate the blood and release stagnation; 3. To promote urination
Indications & Combinations:

1. Infantile convulsions and epilepsy. Amber (Hupo) is used with Centipede (Wugong) and Scorpion (Quanxie).

2. Palpitations, insomnia and dream-disturbed sleep. Amber (Hupo) is used with Wild jujube seed (Suanzaoren) and Multiflower knotweed (Yejiaoteng).

3. Dysmenorrhea or amenorrhea due to blood stagnation. Amber (Hupo) is used with Chinese angelica root (Danggui), Zedoary (Ezhu) and Lindera root (Wuyao) in the formula Hupo San.

4. Urinary tract disorders manifested as frequent urination, painful urination, bloody urine or calculus formation in the urinary tract. Amber (Hupo) is used with Lysimachia (Jinqiancao), Clematis stem (Mutong) and Imperata rhizome (Baimaogen).

Dosage: 1.5-3 g (powder form)

Cautions & Contraindications: This substance is used in powder and pills, not in decoctions.

237. Wild jujube seed (Suanzaoren)

Pharmaceutical Name: Semen Zizyphi spinosae
Botanical Name: Zizyphus spinosa Hu
Common Name: Wild jujube seed, Zizyphus seed
Source of Earliest Record: Shennong Bencao Jing
Part Used & Method for Pharmaceutical Preparations: After the wild jujube ripens in late autumn or early winter, the seeds are collected and dried.

Properties & Taste: Sweet and neutral
Meridians: Heart and liver
Functions: 1. To nourish the blood and tranquilize the mind; 2. To stop sweating

Indications & Combinations:

1. Deficient blood in the heart and liver manifested as irritability, insomnia, palpitations and forgetfulness. Wild jujube seed (Suanzaoren) is used with Chinese angelica root (Danggui), Polygala root (Yuanzhi), White peony root (Baishao), Fleeceflower root (Heshouwu) and Long-an aril (Longyanrou).

2. Spontaneous sweating and night sweating due to weakness of the body. Wild jujube seed (Suanzaoren) is used with Schisandra fruit (Wuweizi) and Ginseng (Renshen).

Dosage: 10-18 g

238. Arborvitae seed (Baiziren)

Pharmaceutical Name: Semen Biotae
Botanical Name: Biota orientalis (L.) Endl.
Common Name: Biota seed, Arborvitae seed
Source of Earliest Record: Shennong Bencao Jing
Part Used & Method for Pharmaceutical Preparations: The fruit is gathered in autumn. After being shelled and dried in the shade, the

seeds are broken into pieces.

Properties & Taste: Sweet and neutral

Meridians: Heart, kidney and large intestine

Functions: 1. To nourish the blood and tranquilize the mind; 2. To moisten the intestines and move feces

Indications & Combinations:

1. Deficient blood of the heart manifested as irritability, insomnia, palpitations and anxiety. Arborvitae seed (Baiziren) is used with Wild jujube seed (Suanzaoren) and Schisandra fruit (Wuweizi).

2. Night sweating due to *yin* deficiency. Arborvitae seed (Baiziren) is used with Ginseng (Renshen), Oyster shell (Muli) and Schisandra fruit (Wuweizi).

3. Constipation due to dryness in the intestines. Arborvitae seed (Baiziren) is used with Apricot seed (Xingren), Bush-cherry seed (Yuliren) and Peach seed (Taoren) in the formula Wuren Wan.

Dosage: 10-18 g

Cautions & Contraindications: This herb is contraindicated in cases with loose stool or excessive phlegm.

239. Polygala root (Yuanzhi)

Pharmaceutical Name: Radix Polygalae

Botanical Name: 1. Polygala tenuifolia Willd.; 2. Polygala Sibirica L.

Common Name: Polygala root

Source of Earliest Record: Shennong Bencao Jing

Part Used & Method for Pharmaceutical Preparations: The roots are dug in spring or autumn. After the fibrous roots have been removed, the roots are cleaned in water and dried in the sun.

Properties & Taste: Pungent, bitter and slightly warm

Meridians: Lung and heart

Functions: 1. To calm the heart and soothe the mind; 2. To resolve phlegm and clear the orifices (sense organs)

Indications & Combinations:

1. Insomnia and forgetfulness. Polygala root (Yuanzhi) is used with Ginseng (Renshen) and Grass-leaved sweetflag (Shichangpu) in the formula Buwang San.

2. Palpitations and restlessness. Polygala root (Yuanzhi) is used with Wild jujube seed (Suanzaoren) and Dragon's bone (Longgu).

3. Turbid phlegm disturbing the heart manifested as mental disor-

ders and unconsciousness. Polygala root (Yuanzhi) is used with Grass-leaved sweetflag (Shichangpu) and Curcuma root (Yujin).

4. Cough with excessive thick sputum or sputum that is difficult to expectorate. Polygala root (Yuanzhi) is used with Apricot seed (Xingren), Platycodon root (Jiegeng) and Licorice root (Gancao).

Dosage: 3-10 g

Cautions & Contraindications: This herb should be used with caution in cases with gastric ulcer or gastritis.

240. Albizia bark (Hehuanpi)

Pharmaceutical Name: Cortax Albiziae
Botanical Name: Albizia julibrissin Durazz.
Common Name: Albizia bark, Mimosa tree bark
Source of Earliest Record: Shennong Bencao Jing
Part Used & Method for Pharmaceutical Preparations: The bark is collected in summer or autumn, and then cut into pieces.
Properties & Taste: Sweet and neutral
Meridians: Heart and liver
Functions: 1. To tranquilize the mind and relieve depression; 2. To invigorate the blood and reduce swelling
Indications & Combinations:

1. Insomnia, forgetfulness and irritability due to depression or anger. Albizia bark (Hehuanpi) is used with Arborvitae seed (Baiziren) and Multiflower knotweed (Yejiaoteng).

2. Swelling and pain due to external injury. Albizia bark (Hehuanpi) is used with Chinese angelica root (Danggui) and Chuanxiong rhizome (Chuanxiong).

3. Carbuncles and furuncles. Albizia bark (Hehuanpi) is used with Wild chrysanthemum flower (Yejuhua), Dandelion herb (Pugongying) and Forsythia fruit (Lianqiao).

Dosage: 10-15 g

XV. Herbs That Pacify the Liver and Subdue Endogenous Wind

Herbs that pacify the liver and subdue endogenous wind stop tremors and subdue the *yang*. They are mainly indicated in tremors, convulsions and spasms caused by the stirring of liver wind, and in dizziness or vertigo due to hyperactivity of liver *yang*. As endogenous wind can arise from extreme heat, hyperactivity of the liver *yang* or deficient *yin* and blood, corresponding herbs should be used in the prescriptions. For example, if endogenous wind is due to extreme heat, herbs that clear heat should be added with those that subdue wind.

241. Antelope's horn (Lingyangjiao)

Pharmaceutical Name: Cornus Saigae Tataricae
Zoological Name: Saiga tatarica L.
Common Name: Antelope's horn
Source of Earliest Record: Shennong Bencao Jing
Part Used & Method for Pharmaceutical Preparations: The antelope's horn is sawn off in autumn and ground into powder or cut into very thin slices.
Properties & Taste: Salty and cold
Meridians: Liver and heart
Functions: 1. To pacify the liver and subdue endogenous wind; 2. To clear liver fire and brighten the eyes; 3. To clear heat and release toxins

Indications & Combinations:

1. Endogenous wind due to extreme heat manifested as high fever, spasms and convulsions. Antelope's horn (Lingyangjiao) is used with Uncaria stem (Gouteng), Chrysanthemum flower (Juhua) and Fresh rehmannia root (Shengdihuang) in the formula Lingjiao Gouteng Tang.

2. Hyperactivity of liver *yang* manifested as dizziness, distending sensation in the head and blurred vision. Antelope's horn (Lingyangjiao) is used with Sea-ear shell (Shijueming), Prunella spike (Xiakucao) and Chrysanthemum flower (Juhua).

3. Flaring up of liver fire manifested as red eyes, painful and swollen eyes and headache. Antelope's horn (Lingyangjiao) is used with Capejasmine (Zhizi), Chinese gentian (Longdancao) and Cassia seed (Juemingzi) in the formula Lingyangjiao San.

4. High fever, loss of consciousness, delirium and mania. Antelope's horn (Lingyangjiao) is used with Gypsum (Shigao) and Rhinoceros horn (Xijiao) in the formula Zixue Dan.

Dosage: 1-3 g; 0.3-0.5 g for powder

242. Sea-ear shell (Shijueming)

Pharmaceutical Name: Concha Haliotidis
Zoological Name: 1. Haliotis diversicolor Reeve; 2. Haliotis discus hannai lno; 3. Haliotis ovina Gmelin; 4. Haliotis ruber (Leach); 5. Haliotis asinina L.; 6. Haliotis laevigata (Donovan)
Common Name: Abalone shell, Sea-ear shell, Haliotis shell
Source of Earliest Record: Mingyi Bielu
Part Used & Method for Pharmaceutical Preparations: The shells are collected from the ocean in summer or autumn. They are dried in the sun and broken into pieces.
Properties & Taste: Salty and cold
Meridian: Liver
Functions: 1. To pacify the liver and subdue *yang*; 2. To clear the fire in the liver and brighten the eyes
Indications & Combinations:

1. Deficient *yin* of the liver and kidneys and hyperactivity of liver *yang*: a) dizziness, vertigo and blurred vision manifestations—Sea-ear shell (Shijueming) is used with Oyster shell (Muli), White peony root (Baishao) and Tortoise plastron (Guiban) to nourish *yin* and subdue *yang*; b) distending sensation of the head and eyes, headache, eye pain and red face manifestations—Sea-ear shell (Shijueming) is used with Uncaria stem (Gouteng), Chrysanthemum flower (Juhua) and Prunella spike (Xiakucao) to pacify the liver and clear heat.

2. Flaring up of liver fire manifested as red, swollen and painful eyes and blurred vision. Sea-ear shell (Shijueming) is used with Chrysanthemum flower (Juhua) and Cassia seed (Juemingzi).

3. Deficiency of liver blood manifested as chronic blurred vision and dryness of the eyes. Sea-ear shell (Shijueming) is used with Prepared rehmannia root (Shudihuang) in the formula Shijueming Wan.
Dosage: 15-30 g

243. Oyster shell (Muli)

Pharmaceutical Name: Concha Ostreae
Zoological Name: 1. Ostrea gigas Thunb.; 2. Ostrea talienwhanensis Cross; 3. Ostrea rivularia Gould
Common Name: Oyster shell
Source of Earliest Record: Shennong Bencao Jing
Part Used & Method for Pharmaceutical Preparations: Oyster shells

are collected from the ocean in winter or spring. They are cleaned and dried in the sun, then pounded into powder.

Properties & Taste: Salty and slightly cold

Meridians: Liver and kidney

Functions: 1. To pacify the liver and subdue the *yang*; 2. To soften hardness and release nodules; 3. To stop perspiration, nocturnal emissions and leukorrhagia by astringents

Indications & Combinations:

1. Deficient *yin* of the liver and kidneys and upward flaring of *yang* manifested as dizziness, vertigo, blurred vision, tinnitus, palpitations, irritability and insomnia. Oyster shell (Muli) is used with Dragon's bone (Longgu), Tortoise plastron (Guiban) and White peony root (Baishao).

2. Late stage of febrile disease with exhaustion of *yin* and body fluids which leads to malnutrition of tendons and muscles manifested as spasms, or convulsions. Oyster shell (Muli) is used with Tortoise plastron (Guiban), Donkey hide gelatin (Ejiao), White peony root (Baishao) and Turtle shell (Biejia) in the formula Sanjia Fumai Tang.

3. Scrofula due to phlegm and fire. Oyster shell (Muli) is used with Thunberg fritillary bulb (Zhebeimu) and Scrophularia (Xuanshen) in the formula Xiaolei Wan.

4. Spontaneous sweating and night sweating due to weakness of the body. Oyster shell (Muli) is used with Astragalus root (Huangqi), Ephedra root (Mahuanggen) and Light wheat (Fuxiaomai) in the formula Muli San.

5. Nocturnal emissions due to kidney deficiency. Oyster shell (Muli) is used with Flattened milkvetch seed (Shayuanzi), Euryale seed (Qianshi) and Lotus stamen (Lianxu) in the formula Jinsuo Gujing Wan.

6. Uterine bleeding and leukorrhagia due to deficient Chong and Ren meridians. Oyster shell (Muli) is used with Dragon's bone (Longgu), Dioscorea (Shanyao) and Schisandra fruit (Wuweizi).

Dosage: 15-30 g

244. Mother-of-pearl (Zhenzhumu)

Pharmaceutical Name: Margarita

Zoological Name: 1. Pteria martensii (Dunker); 2. Hyriopsis cumingii (Lea); 3. Cristaria plicata (Leach)

Common Name: Mother-of-pearl, pearl

Source of Earliest Record: Haiyao Bencao

Part Used & Method for Pharmaceutical Preparations: The pearl shells are collected and ground into powder.

Properties & Taste: Salty and cold

Meridians: Heart and liver

Functions: 1. To pacify the liver and subdue the *yang*; 2. To clear heat in the liver and brighten the eyes

Indications & Combinations:

1. Deficient *yin* of the liver and kidneys and hyperactivity of liver *yang* manifested as headache, dizziness, vertigo, tinnitus, irritability and insomnia. Mother-of-pearl (Zhenzhumu) is used with White peony root (Baishao), Fresh rehmannia root (Shengdihuang), Sea-ear shell (Shijueming) and Dragon's bone (Longgu).

2. Deficient blood in the liver manifested as blurred vision and night blindness. Mother-of-pearl (Zhenzhumu) is used with Atractylodes rhizome (Cangzhu), Pig liver (Zhugan) and Chicken's liver (Jigan) or Rabbit's liver (Tugan).

3. Wind and heat in the liver meridian manifested as red, swollen and painful eyes and photophobia. Mother-of-pearl (Zhenzhumu) is used with Chrysanthemum flower (Juhua) and Plantain seed (Cheqianzi).

Dosage: 15-30 g; 0.3-1 g (for pills)

245. Purple cowrie shell (Zibeichi)

Pharmaceutical Name: Concha Mauritiae

Zoological Name: Mauritia arabica (L)

Common Name: Purple cowrie shell

Source of Earliest Record: Xinxiu Bencao

Part Used & Method for Pharmaceutical Preparations: The shells are collected in summer, then cleaned, dried in the sun and broken into pieces.

Properties & Taste: Salty and neutral

Meridian: Liver

Functions: 1. To calm the heart and tranquilize the mind; 2. To clear heat in the liver and brighten eyes

Indications & Combinations:

1. Palpitations, irritability, insomnia, dream-disturbed sleep or infantile convulsions due to high fever. Purple cowrie shell (Zibeichi) is used with Coptis root (Huanglian), Mother-of-pearl (Zhenzhumu) and Ante-

195

lope's horn (Lingyangjiao).

2. Wind and heat in the liver meridian manifested as red, swollen and painful eyes or visual obstruction; or hyperactivity of liver *yang* manifested as dizziness, vertigo and headache. Purple cowrie shell (Zibeichi) is used with Chrysanthemum flower (Juhua), Mulberry leaf (Sangye) and Uncaria stem (Gouteng).

Dosage: 10-15 g

Cautions & Contraindications: The substance is cooked before the other herbs.

246. Red ochre (Daizheshi)

Pharmaceutical Name: Hematitum
Mineral Name: Hematite
Common Name: Hematite, Red ochre
Source of Earliest Record: Shennong Bencao Jing
Part Used & Method for Pharmaceutical Preparations: The hematite mineral is dug and smashed into small pieces or ground into powder.
Properties & Taste: Bitter and cold
Meridians: Liver and heart
Functions: 1. To pacify the liver and subdue the *yang*; 2. To conduct rebellious *qi* downward and stop vomiting; 3. To stop bleeding
Indications & Combinations:

1. Deficient *yin* of the liver and kidneys and hyperactivity of liver *yang* manifested as distension and pain in the head and eyes, dizziness and vertigo. Red ochre (Daizheshi) is used with Dragon's bone (Longgu), Oyster shell (Muli), White peony root (Baishao), Tortoise plastron (Guiban) and Cyathula root (Niuxi) in the formula Zhengan Xifeng Tang.

2. Rebellious stomach *qi* manifested as vomiting and belching. Red ochre (Daizheshi) is used with Inula flower (Xuanfuhua), Fresh ginger (Shengjiang) and Pinellia tuber (Banxia) in the formula Xuanfu Daizhe Tang.

3. Asthma due to deficiency of the lung and kidneys. Red ochre (Daizheshi) is used with Ginseng (Renshen) and Dogwood fruit (Shanzhuyu).

4. Extravasation of blood by heat manifested as vomiting with blood and epistaxis. Red ochre (Daizheshi) is used with White peony

root (Baishao), Bamboo shavings (Zhuru) and Arctium fruit (Niubang-zi) in the formula Hanjiang Tang.

5. Chronic uterine bleeding manifested as dizziness and blurred vision due to deficient blood. Red ochre (Daizheshi) is used with Limonite (Yuyuliang), Red halloysite (Chishizhi), Frankincense (Ru-xiang) and Myrrh (Moyao) in the formula Zhenling Dan.

Dosage: 10-30 g

Cautions & Contraindications: This substance should be used with caution during pregnancy.

247. Uncaria stem (Gouteng)

Pharmaceutical Name: Ramulus Uncariae cum Uncis

Botanical Name: 1. Uncaria rhynchophylla (Miq.) Jacks.; 2. Uncaria hirsuta Havil.; 3. Uncaria sinensis (Oliv.) Havil; 4. Uncaria sessilifructus Roxb.

Common Name: Uncaria stem with hooks

Source of Earliest Record: Mingyi Bielu

Part Used & Method for Pharmaceutical Preparations: The uncaria stems with hooks are gathered in spring or autumn, dried in the sun and cut into pieces.

Properties & Taste: Sweet and slightly cold

Meridians: Liver and pericardium

Functions: 1. To eliminate endogenous wind and stop spasms; 2. To clear heat and pacify the liver

Indications & Combinations:

1. Stirring up of the liver wind by excessive heat manifested as high fever, spasms and convulsions. Uncaria stem (Gouteng) is used with Antelope's horn (Lingyangjiao), Chrysanthemum flower (Juhua) and Gypsum (Shigao).

2. Deficient *yin* of the liver and kidneys and hyperactivity of liver *yang* or excessive heat in the liver meridian manifested as dizziness, vertigo, blurred vision and headache. Uncaria stem (Gouteng) is used with Prunella spike (Xiakucao), Scutellaria root (Huangqin), Sea-ear shell (Shijueming) and Chrysanthemum flower (Juhua).

Dosage: 10-15 g

Cautions & Contraindications: This herb should not be cooked for a long time.

248. Gastrodia tuber (Tianma)

Pharmaceutical Name: Rhizoma Gastrodiae
Botanical Name: Gastrodia elata Bl.
Common Name: Gastrodia tuber
Source of Earliest Record: Shennong Bencao Jing
Part Used & Method for Pharmaceutical Preparations: The rhizomes are dug in winter or spring. After the bark has been removed, the rhizomes are cleaned, boiled or steamed and baked. They are then soaked again and cut into slices.
Properties & Taste: Sweet and neutral
Meridian: Liver
Functions: 1. To eliminate endogenous wind and stop spasms; 2. To pacify the liver and subdue the *yang*
Indications & Combinations:

1. Internal stirring up of liver wind manifested as spasms and convulsions. Gastrodia tuber (Tianma) is used with Uncaria stem (Gouteng) and Scorpion (Quanxie).

2. Spasms or convulsions in tetanus. Gastrodia tuber (Tianma) is used with Ledebouriella (Fangfeng), Arisaema tuber (Tiannanxing) and Typhonium tuber (Baifuzi) in the formula Yuzhen San.

3. Headache and dizziness due to hyperactivity of liver *yang*. Gastrodia tuber (Tianma) is used with Uncaria stem (Gouteng), Scutellaria root (Huangqin) and Cyathula root (Niuxi) in the formula Tianma Gouteng Yin.

4. Vertigo and dizziness caused by upward attack of wind-phlegm due to deficiency of the spleen and stagnation of *qi* in the liver. Gastrodia tuber (Tianma) is used with Pinellia tuber (Banxia), White atractylodes (Baizhu) and Poria (Fuling) in the formula Banxia Baizhu Tianma Tang.

5. Unilateral headache (migraine) and frontal headache. Gastrodia tuber (Tianma) is used with Chuanxiong rhizome (Chuanxiong) in the formula Tianma Wan.

6. Pain due to wind-damp obstruction (joint pain). Gastrodia tuber (Tianma) is used with Frankincense (Ruxiang) and Scorpion (Quanxie).

7. Numbness of limbs due to deficient blood in the channels. Gastrodia tuber (Tianma) is used with Chinese angelica root (Danggui) and Cyathula root (Niuxi).

Dosage: 3-10 g; 1-1.5 g for powder

249. Tribulus fruit (Baijili)

Pharmaceutical Name: Fructus Tribuli
Botanical Name: Tribulus terestris L.
Common Name: Tribulus fruit, Puncture-vine fruit
Source of Earliest Record: Shennong Bencao Jing
Part Used & Method for Pharmaceutical Preparations: The ripe fruit is gathered in autumn, dried in the sun and baked until the fruit turns yellow.
Properties & Taste: Bitter, pungent and neutral
Meridian: Liver
Functions: 1. To pacify the liver and subdue the *yang*; 2. To promote the free flow of *qi* in the liver and release stagnation; 3. To expel wind and stop itching; 4. To brighten the eyes
Indications & Combinations:

1. Hyperactivity of liver *yang* manifested as dizziness, vertigo, distension and pain in the head. Tribulus fruit (Baijili) is used with Uncaria stem (Gouteng), Chrysanthemum flower (Juhua) and White peony root (Baishao).

2. *Qi* stagnation of the liver manifested as distension in the breasts, uncomfortable feeling in the chest and hypochondriac regions and obstructed lactation. Tribulus fruit (Baijili) is used with Bupleurum root (Chaihu), Tangerine leaf (Juye), Green tangerine peel (Qingpi) and Cyperus tuber (Xiangfu).

3. Wind and heat in the liver meridian manifested as red eyes and profuse lacrimation. Tribulus fruit (Baijili) is used with Chrysanthemum flower (Juhua), Chastetree fruit (Manjingzi) and Cassia seed (Jueming-zi).

4. Wind and heat in the blood manifested as rubella and itching. Tribulus fruit (Baijili) is used with Schizonepeta (Jingjie) and Cicada slough (Chantui).
Dosage: 6-10 g

250. Cassia seed (Juemingzi)

Pharmaceutical Name: Semen Sennae
Botanical Name: 1. Cassia angustifolia Vahl; 2. Cassia acutifolia Delile
Common Name: Foetid Cassia seed
Source of Earliest Record: Shennong Bencao Jing
Part Used & Method for Pharmaceutical Preparations: The seeds are

gathered in autumn and dried in the sun.

Properties & Taste: Sweet, bitter and slightly cold

Meridians: Liver and large intestine

Functions: 1. To clear heat in the liver and brighten the eyes; 2. To dispel wind and clear heat; 3. To moisten the intestines and move feces

Indications & Combinations:

1. Upward disturbance of liver fire or invasion of exogenous wind and heat manifested as red, swollen and painful eyes and photophobia. Cassia seed (Juemingzi) is used with Chrysanthemum flower (Juhua), Mulberry leaf (Sangye), Capejasmine (Zhizi) and Prunella spike (Xia-kucao).

2. Constipation due to dryness in the intestines. Cassia seed (Jue-mingzi) can be used alone.

3. Hyperactivity of liver *yang* manifested as dizziness, vertigo and blurred vision. Cassia seed (Juemingzi) is used with Uncaria stem (Gouteng) and raw Oyster shell (Muli).

4. Deficient *yin* of the liver and kidneys manifested as blurred vision and cataracts. Cassia seed (Juemingzi) is used with Flattened milkvetch seed (Shayuanzi), Tribulus fruit (Baijili), Grossy privet fruit (Nüzhenzi) and Wolfberry fruit (Gouqizi).

Dosage: 10-15 g

251. Scorpion (Quanxie)

Pharmaceutical Name: Scorpio

Zoological Name: Buthus martensi Karsch

Common Name: Scorpion

Source of Earliest Record: Kaibao Bencao

Part Used & Method for Pharmaceutical Preparations: The scorpion is caught in spring or autumn and then boiled and dried in the sun.

Properties & Taste: Pungent, neutral and toxic

Meridian: Liver

Functions: 1. To subdue endogenous wind and stop spasms; 2. To dispel toxins; 3. To dispel wind and stop pain

Indications & Combinations:

1. Convulsions due to high fever or epileptic spasms. Scorpion (Quanxie) is used with Centipede (Wugong) in the formula Zijing San.

2. Facial paralysis manifested as deviation of the eye and mouth and incomplete closing of the eyelids. Scorpion (Quanxie) is used with

Typhonium tuber (Baifuzi) and White-stiff silkworm (Baijiangcan) in the formula Qianzhen San.

3. Tetanus manifested as spasms of the limbs and opisthotonos. Scorpion (Quanxie) is used with Arisaema tuber (Tiannanxing) and Cicada slough (Chantui) in the formula Wuhu Zhuifeng San.

4. Chronic convulsions caused by chronic diarrhea due to deficiency of the spleen manifested as spasms of the hands and feet. Scorpion (Quanxie) is used with Pilose asiabell root (Dangshen), White atractylodes (Baizhu) and Gastrodia tuber (Tianma).

5. Stubborn headache and rheumatic pain. Scorpion (Quanxie) is used with Centipede (Wugong) and White-stiff silkworm (Baijiangcan).

Dosage: 2-5 g; 0.6-1 g for powder

Cautions & Contraindications: This substance is toxic and overdosing should be avoided. Use with caution for a person with endogenous wind caused by deficient blood. This substance is contraindicated during pregnancy.

252. Centipede (Wugong)

Pharmaceutical Name: Scolopendra
Zoological Name: Scolopendra subspinipes mutilams L. Koch
Common Name: Centipede
Source of Earliest Record: Shennong Bencao Jing
Part Used & Method for Pharmaceutical Preparations: The centipede is caught in spring, and then it is boiled, dried and pounded into powder, or fixed to bamboo slats to dry.
Properties & Taste: Pungent, warm and toxic
Meridian: Liver
Functions: 1. To subdue endogenous wind and stop spasms; 2. To dispel toxins; 3. To clear collaterals and stop pain
Indications & Combinations:

1. Acute and chronic convulsions or tetany manifested as spasms, convulsions of the limbs and ophisthotonos. Centipede (Wugong) is used with Scorpion (Quanxie), White-stiff silkworm (Baijiangcan) and Uncaria stem (Gouteng).

2. Stubborn headache and rheumatic pain. Centipede (Wugong) is used with Scorpion (Quanxie), Gastrodia tuber (Tianma), White-stiff silkworm (Baijiangcan) and Chuanxiong rhizome (Chuanxiong).

Dosage: 1-3 g; 0.6-1 g for powder

Cautions & Contraindications: This substance is toxic. Overdosing should be avoided. This substance is contraindicated during pregnancy.

253. White-stiff silkworm (Baijiangcan)

Pharmaceutical Name: Bombyx Batryticatus
Zoological Name: Bombyx mori L.
Common Name: White-stiff silkworm
Source of Earliest Record: Shennong Bencao Jing
Part Used & Method for Pharmaceutical Preparations: The silkworm, dead and stiffened due to the infection of beavveria bassiana, is dried in the sun.
Properties & Taste: Salty, pungent and neutral
Meridians: Liver and lung
Functions: 1. To subdue endogenous wind and stop spasms; 2. To expel wind and stop pain; 3. To dispel toxins and disperse nodules
Indications & Combinations:

1. Convulsions due to high fever and epileptic spasms. White-stiff silkworm (Baijiangcan) is used with Gastrodia tuber (Tianma), Arisaema tuber with bile (Dannanxing) and Ox gallstone (Niuhuang) in the formula Qianjin San.

2. Chronic convulsions with prolonged diarrhea due to deficiency of the spleen. White-stiff silkworm (Baijiangcan) is used with Pilose asiabell root (Dangshen), White atractylodes (Baizhu) and Gastrodia tuber (Tianma).

3. Windstroke manifested as deviation of eyes and mouth or facial spasms. White-stiff silkworm (Baijiangcan) is used with Scorpion (Quanxie) and Typhonium tuber (Baifuzi) in the formula Qianzhen San.

4. Wind-heat headache and lacrimation from exposure to wind. White-stiff silkworm (Baijiangcan) is used with Schizonepeta (Jingjie), Mulberry leaf (Sangye) and Shave grass (Muzei) in the formula Baijiangcan San.

5. Wind-heat sore throat. White-stiff silkworm (Baijiangcan) is used with Platycodon root (Jiegeng), Ledebouriella (Fangfeng) and Licorice root (Gancao).

6. Rubella and itching. White-stiff silkworm (Baijiangcan) is used with Cicada slough (Chantui) and Mentha (Bohe).

7. Scrofula. White-stiff silkworm (Baijiangcan) is used with Ten-

drilled fritillary bulb (Chuanbeimu) and Prunella spike (Xiakucao).

Dosage: 3-10 g

Cautions & Contraindications: The raw substance is used for wind-heat syndrome, the fried substance for other applications.

254. Earthworm (Dilong)

Pharmaceutical Name: Lumbricus

Zoological Name: 1. Pheretima aspergilum (Perrier); 2. Allolobo-phora caliginosa (Savigny) trapezoides (Ant. Duges)

Common Name: Earthworm

Source of Earliest Record: Shennong Bencao Jing

Part Used & Method for Pharmaceutical Preparations: The earth-worm is caught in summer or autumn. It is cleaned in warm water, and then dried in the sun.

Properties & Taste: Salty and cold

Meridians: Liver, spleen and urinary bladder

Functions: 1. To clear heat and subdue endogenous wind; 2. To soothe asthma; 3. To promote urination; 4. To clear the collaterals

Indications & Combinations:

1. Convulsions and spasms due to high fever. Earthworm (Dilong) is used with Uncaria stem (Gouteng), White-stiff silkworm (Bai-jiangcan) and Scorpion (Quanxie).

2. Damp-heat obstruction syndrome manifested as red, swollen, painful joints and motor impairment. Earthworm (Dilong) is used with Mulberry twigs (Sangzhi), Honeysuckle stem (Rendongteng) and Red peony (Chishao).

3. Wind-cold-damp obstruction syndrome manifested as cold, pain-ful joints with motor impairment. Earthworm (Dilong) is used with Wild aconite root (Caowu) and Arisaema tuber (Tiannanxing) in the formula Xiao Huolu Dan.

4. Hemiplegia due to obstruction of meridians by *qi* deficiency and blood stagnation. Earthworm (Dilong) is used with Chinese angelica root (Danggui), Chuanxiong rhizome (Chuanxiong) and Astragalus root (Huangqi) in the formula Buyang Huanwu Tang.

5. Heat accumulated in the urinary bladder manifested as dysuria. Earthworm (Dilong) is used with Plantain seed (Cheqianzi) and Clema-tis stem (Mutong).

6. Asthma. Earthworm (Dilong) is used with Ephedra (Mahuang)

and Apricot seed (Xingren).
Dosage: 5-15 g (10-20 g if fresh)

255. Dogbane (Luobuma)

Pharmaceutical Name: Folium Apocyni veneti
Botanical Name: Apocynum venetum L.
Common Name: Dogbane leaf
Source of Earliest Record: Shennong Bencao Jing
Part Used & Method for Pharmaceutical Preparations: The leaves or whole plant are gathered in summer, dried in the sun and then cut into pieces.
Properties & Taste: Tasteless, astringent and slightly cold
Meridian: Liver
Functions: 1. To pacify the liver and clear heat; 2. To promote urination
Indications & Combinations:

1. Hyperactivity of liver *yang* manifested as headache, vertigo, dizziness, irritability and insomnia. Dogbane (Luobuma) is used with Prunella spike (Xiakucao), Uncaria stem (Gouteng) and Chrysanthemum flower (Juhua). Also, Dogbane (Luobuma) can be used alone to make tea.

2. Dysuria and edema. Dogbane (Luobuma) can be used alone or with other herbs to promote urination.
Dosage: 3-10 g

XVI. Herbs That Open the Orifices

Herbs that open the orifices are aromatic substances that open the sense organs (orifices) and restore consciousness. They are used when heat attacks the pericardium or turbid phlegm mists the heart. Manifestations include loss of consciousness, delirium, epilepsy and convulsions or coma from windstroke.

Comas are ranked according to their severity into two types: tense syndrome and flaccid syndrome. The tense syndrome is an excess syndrome manifested as mouth agape, clenched fists and forceful pulse. The flaccid syndrome is a deficiency syndrome manifested as cold sweating, cold limbs and fading pulse. The tense syndrome may be

204

divided into a cold-tense syndrome and a heat-tense syndrome. The cold-tense syndrome is manifested in such symptoms as green complexion, cold body, white tongue coating and slow pulse, the heat-tense syndrome in red face, hot body, yellow tongue coating and rapid pulse. To treat flaccid syndrome, use herbs that recapture *yang* so as to prevent collapse, as well as those that tonify *qi*. When treating flaccid syndrome, herbs that open the orifices are not allowed. Herbs that open the orifices can be added to other combinations in treating tense syndrome. In cold-tense syndrome, herbs that dispel cold and promote *qi* are added. In heat-tense syndrome, herbs that clear heat and release toxins are added.

Aromatic herbs that open the orifices are used for first-aid treatment. Since they may consume primary *qi*, they should be used only for short periods of time.

256. Musk (Shexiang)

Pharmaceutical Name: Moschus
Zoological Name: 1. Moschus berezovskii Flerov; 2. Moschus sifanicus Przewalski; 3. Moschus moschiferus L.
Common Name: Musk
Source of Earliest Record: Shennong Bencao Jing
Part Used & Method for Pharmaceutical Preparations: The secretion is obtained from the naval musk gland of male musk deers. It is dried in the shade in winter or spring.
Properties & Taste: Pungent and warm
Meridians: Heart and spleen
Functions: 1. To open the orifices and clear the mind; 2. To invigorate the blood and disperse nodules; 3. To stop pain; 4. To expel placenta labor
Indications & Combinations:

1. Unconsciousness due to high fever. Musk (Shexiang) is used with Ox gallstone (Niuhuang) and Rhinoceros horn (Xijiao) in the formula Zhibao Dan.

2. Unconsciousness due to windstroke. Musk (Shexiang) is used with Storax (Suhexiang) and Cloves (Dingxiang) in the formula Suhexiang Wan.

3. Carbuncles, furuncles and swellings. Musk (Shexiang) is used with Frankincense (Ruxiang), Myrrh (Moyao) and Realgar (Xiong-

huang) in the formula Xingxiao Wan.

4. Sudden severe pain in the chest and abdominal region. Musk (Shexiang) is used with Costus root (Muxiang), Peach seed (Taoren) and herbs that invigorate the blood in a formula such as Shexiang Tang.

5. Swelling and pain caused by external injuries. Musk (Shexiang) is used with Sappan wood (Sumu), Myrrh (Moyao) and Safflower (Honghua) in the formula Bali San.

6. Dead fetus or placenta failing to be expelled. Musk (Shexiang) is used with Cinnamon bark (Rougui) in the formula Xiang Gui San.

Dosage: 0.06-0.1 g (in pill form)

Cautions & Contraindications: The substance must not be cooked. It is contraindicated during pregnancy.

257. Borneol (Bingpian)

Pharmaceutical Name: Borneolum Syntheticum

Mineral Name: 1. Dryobalanops aromatica Gaertn. f.; 2. Blumea balsamifera DC.

Common Name: Borneol

Source of Earliest Record: Xinxiu Bencao

Part Used & Method for Pharmaceutical Preparations: The stems of dryobalanops aromatica are steamed and then cooled into crystals.

Properties & Taste: Pungent, bitter and slightly cold

Meridians: Heart, spleen and lung

Functions: 1. To open the orifices and clear the mind; 2. To clear heat and stop pain

Indications & Combinations:

1. Unconsciousness due to high fever. Borneol (Bingpian) is used with Musk (Shexiang) in the formula Angong Niuhuang Wan.

2. Red, swollen and painful eyes. Borneol (Bingpian) can be used alone as eye drops.

3. Sore throat or ulceration of the mouth. Borneol (Bingpian) is used with Sodium borate (Pengsha) and the compound of Licorice root (Gancao) and Glauber's salt (Mangxiao), also called Xuanming Fen, in the formula Bing Peng San.

Dosage: 0.03-0.1 g (in pill form)

Cautions & Contraindications: This substance should be used with caution during pregnancy.

258. Storax (Suhexiang)

Pharmaceutical Name: Styrax
Botanical Name: Liquidambar orientalis Mill.
Common Name: Storax
Source of Earliest Record: Mingyi Bielu
Part Used & Method for Pharmaceutical Preparations: The resin, or balsam, from the trunk or bark is collected in autumn.
Properties & Taste: Pungent and warm
Meridians: Heart and spleen
Functions: 1. To open the orifices and clear the mind; 2. To stop pain
Indications & Combinations:

1. Sudden coma caused by *qi* stagnation or unconsciousness due to windstroke. Storax (Suhexiang) is used with Musk (Shexiang), Cloves (Dingxiang) and Benzoin (Anxixiang) in the formula Suhexiang Wan.

2. Stifling sensation and pain in the chest. Storax (Suhexiang) is used with Borneol (Bingpian), Sandalwood (Tanxiang) and Cloves (Dingxiang) in formulas such as Guanxin Suhexiang Wan and Su Bing Diwan.

Dosage: 0.3-1 g (in pill form)

259. Grass-leaved sweetflag (Shichangpu)

Pharmaceutical Name: Rhizome Acori graminei
Botanical Name: Acorus gramineus Soland.
Common Name: Grass-leaved sweetflag rhizome
Source of Earliest Record: Shennong Bencao Jing
Part Used & Method for Pharmaceutical Preparations: The rhizomes are dug in early spring and cleaned and dried in the sun. When the fresh rhizome is used for medical purposes, it should be dug in late summer.
Properties & Taste: Pungent and warm
Meridians: Heart and stomach
Functions: 1. To open the orifices; 2. To transform dampness and harmonize the stomach; 3. To tranquilize the mind
Indications & Combinations:

1. Unconsciousness due to blockage of the pericardium by turbid phlegm or accumulation of dampness and heat. Grass-leaved sweetflag (Shichangpu) is used with fresh Bamboo juice (Zhuli) and Curcuma

root (Yujin) in the formula Changpu Yujin Tang.

2. Dampness blocking the middle *jiao* (spleen and stomach) manifested as stifling sensation, distension and pain in the chest and abdominal region. Grass-leaved sweetflag (Shichangpu) is used with Tangerine peel (Chenpi) and Magnolia bark (Houpo).

3. Damp-heat blocking the middle *jiao* manifested as dysentery and vomiting after meals. Grass-leaved sweetflag (Shichangpu) is used with Coptis root (Huanglian).

4. Insomnia, forgetfulness, tinnitus and deafness. Grass-leaved sweetflag (Shichangpu) is used with Polygala root (Yuanzhi) and Poria (Fuling) in the formula Anshen Dingzhi Wan.

Dosage: 5-8 g (double dosage for the fresh herb)

XVII. Herbs That Tonify Deficiencies

Herbs that tonify deficiencies strengthen or supplement the body's resistance against disease. These herbs are usually subdivided into herbs which tonify either *qi, yang*, blood or *yin*. As *qi*, blood, *yin* and *yang* are interdependent in the body, a deficient condition in any one of them will affect the others. Therefore, practitioners must be flexible when using these herbs. It is very important that tonifying herbs are only applied in cases with weakness of anti-pathogenic factors, and not during excess pathogenic factors.

a) Herbs That Tonify *Qi*

Herbs that tonify *qi* are used for deficient *qi* syndrome, which is often seen as deficient *qi* in the spleen or deficient *qi* in the lungs. Deficient *qi* of the spleen is manifested as poor appetite, loose stool, abdominal distension, lassitude, edema or prolapsed anus. The symptoms of deficient *qi* in the lungs are shortness of breath, dysphasia and spontaneous sweating.

When *qi* deficiency is accompanied by *yin* deficiency or *yang* deficiency, herbs that tonify *yin* or *yang* should be added to the combination. Because *qi* is responsible for the generation and circulation of blood, these herbs are also used in the acute phase of severe blood loss to prevent collapse and to stop bleeding.

In general, overdosing of these herbs is not recommended, as it may cause stifling sensation in the chest, abdominal distension or poor appetite.

260. Ginseng (Renshen)

Pharmaceutical Name: Radix Ginseng
Botanical Name: Panax ginseng C. A. Mey.
Common Name: Ginseng
Source of Earliest Record: Shennong Bencao Jing
Part Used & Method for Pharmaceutical Preparations: There are many types of ginseng, including wild and cultivated. Cultivated ginseng from Jilin Province in China is the best quality. The ginseng roots are dug in autumn after being cultivated for six to seven years, and then they are cleaned, dried in the sun, steamed or baked and cut into slices.
Properties & Taste: Sweet, slightly warm
Meridians: Spleen and lung
Functions: 1. To replenish *qi*, prevent collapse and strengthen *yang*; 2. To tonify the spleen and lungs; 3. To promote body fluids and relieve thirst; 4. To calm the heart and soothe the mind
Indications & Combinations:

1. Collapsing syndrome due to severe deficiency of primary *qi*, severe loss of blood, severe vomiting or severe diarrhea manifested as sweating, cold limbs, shortness of breath and weak and fading pulse. Ginseng (Renshen) can be used alone or with Prepared aconite root (Fuzi) in the formula Shen Fu Tang.

2. Weakness of the spleen and stomach manifested as poor appetite, lassitude, fullness in the epigastric and abdominal regions and loose stool. Ginseng (Renshen) is used with White atractylodes (Baizhu), Poria (Fuling) and Licorice root (Gancao) in the formula Sijunzi Tang.

3. Deficient *qi* of the lungs manifested as shortness of breath, spontaneous sweating and lassitude. Ginseng (Renshen) is used with Gecko (Gejie) in the formula Renshen Gejie San.

4. Diabetes or exhaustion of *qi* and body fluids by febrile disease manifested as thirst, sweating, irritability, shortness of breath and weak pulse. Ginseng (Renshen) is used with Ophiopogon root (Maidong) and Schisandra fruit (Wuweizi) in the formula Shengmai San. If the above-mentioned manifestations are accompanied by fever, Ginseng (Renshen) can be taken with Gypsum (Shigao) and Anemarrhena rhizome (Zhimu) in the formula Baihu Jia Renshen Tang.

5. Mental restlessness manifested as palpitations, anxiety, insomnia, dream-disturbed sleep and forgetfulness. Ginseng (Renshen) is used with Wild jujube seed (Suanzaoren) and Chinese angelica root (Danggui) in the formula Guipi Tang.

6. Impotence and premature ejaculation in men or frigidity in women. Ginseng (Renshen) can be used alone or with Pilose antler (Lurong) and Human placenta (Ziheche).

Dosage: 5-10 g (for decoction), 1-2 g (for powder), 15-30 g (decoction for severe collapsing)

Cautions & Contraindications: This herb is contraindicated for a person with heat signs or excessive syndromes without deficiency of anti-pathogenic factor. It should not be mixed with Black false bellebore (Lilu), Trogopterus dung (Wulingzhi) and Chinese honey locust (Zaojia). When taking Ginseng (Renshen), do not drink tea or eat turnips.

261. American ginseng (Xiyangshen)

Pharmaceutical Name: 1. Radix Panacis quinquefolii; 2. Radix ginseng americane

Botanical Name: Panax quinquefolium L.

Common Name: American ginseng

Source of Earliest Record: Shennong Bencao Jing

Part Used & Method for Pharmaceutical Preparations: The three to six year old root is dug in autumn, dried in the sun and cut into slices.

Properties & Taste: Bitter, slightly sweet and cold

Meridians: Heart, lung and kidney

Functions: 1. To replenish *qi* and promote body fluids; 2. To nourish *yin* and clear heat

Indications & Combinations:

1. Deficient *yin* in the lungs and excessive fire manifested as asthma and cough with bloody sputum. American ginseng (Xiyangshen) is used with Ophiopogon root (Maidong), Donkey hide gelatin (Ejiao), Anemarrhena rhizome (Zhimu) and Tendrilled fritillary bulb (Chuanbeimu).

2. Exhaustion of *qi* and *yin* from febrile disease manifested as thirst, irritability, shortness of breath and deficient pulse. American ginseng (Xiyangshen) is used with Fresh rehmannia root (Shengdihuang), fresh Dendrobium (Shihu) and Ophiopogon root (Maidong).

Dosage: 3-6 g

Cautions & Contraindications: This herb should be cooked separately, then added into the decoction of other herbs. It is contraindicated for a person with cold and dampness in the stomach. It counteracts the herb Black false bellebore (Lilu). When frying or decocting, pots made from iron should not be used.

262. Pilose asiabell root (Dangshen)

Pharmaceutical Name: Radix Codonopsis pilosulae
Botanical Name: Codonopsis pilosula (Franch.) Nannf.
Common Name: Pilose asiabell root, Codonopsis
Source of Earliest Record: Bencao Congxin
Part Used & Method for Pharmaceutical Preparations: The roots are dug in spring or autumn, but autumn herbs are of better quality. They are dried in the sun and cut into pieces.
Properties & Taste: Sweet and neutral
Meridians: Spleen and lung
Functions: To replenish *qi*
Indications & Combinations:

1. Deficient *qi* in the middle *jiao* (spleen and stomach) manifested as tired limbs. Pilose asiabell root (Dangshen) is used with White atractylodes (Baizhu) and Poria (Fuling).

2. Deficient *qi* in the lungs manifested as shortness of breath, cough, asthma, lassitude, dysphasia, low voice, shallow breathing and deficient, forceless pulse. Pilose asiabell root (Dangshen) is used with Astragalus root (Huangqi) and Schisandra fruit (Wuweizi).

Dosage: 10-30 g

Cautions & Contraindications: This herb counteracts the herb Black false bellebore (Lilu).

263. Pseudostellaria root (Taizishen)

Pharmaceutical Name: Radix Pseudostellariae
Botanical Name: Pseudostellaria heterophylla (Miq.) Pax ex Pax et Hoffm.
Common Name: Pseudostellaria root
Source of Earliest Record: Zhongguo Yaoyong Zhiwu Zhi
Part Used & Method for Pharmaceutical Preparations: The tuberous roots of the cultivated pseudostellaris are dug in the period around the

211

Great Heat (twelfth solar term). After the fibrous roots are removed, the roots are dried in the sun.

Properties & Taste: Sweet, slightly bitter and neutral

Meridians: Spleen and lung

Functions: To replenish *qi* and promote body fluids

Indications & Combinations:

1. Deficiency of the spleen manifested as poor appetite and lassitude. Pseudostellaria root (Taizishen) is used with Dioscorea (Shanyao), Hyacinth bean (Biandou), Germinated millet (Guya) and Germinated barley (Maiya).

2. Deficient *yin* of the lungs manifested as dry cough or cough with scanty sputum. Pseudostellaria root (Taizishen) is used with Glehnia root (Shashen) and Ophiopogon root (Maidong).

3. Deficient *yin* of the stomach manifested as thirst. Pseudostellaria root (Taizishen) is used with Dendrobium (Shihu) and Trichosanthes root (Tianhuafen).

4. Deficiency of the spleen leading to deficiency of both *qi* and blood manifested as palpitations, insomnia and sweating. Pseudostellaria root (Taizishen) is used with Wild jujube seed (Suanzaoren) and Schisandra fruit (Wuweizi).

Dosage: 10-30 g

264. Astragalus root (Huangqi)

Pharmaceutical Name: Radix Astragali

Botanical Name: 1. Astragalus membranaceus (Fisch.) Bge.; 2. Astragalus membranaceus Bge. var. mongolicus (Bge.) Hsiao

Common Name: Astragalus root

Source of Earliest Record: Shennong Bencao Jing

Part Used & Method for Pharmaceutical Preparations: The four year old roots are dug in spring or autumn, but autumn ones are of better quality. After the fibrous roots are removed, the roots are dried in the sun, soaked again in water and cut into slices.

Properties & Taste: Sweet and slightly warm

Meridians: Spleen and lung

Functions: 1. To replenish *qi* and cause *yang* to ascend; 2. To benefit *qi* and stabilize the exterior; 3. To release toxins and promote healing; 4. To promote water metabolism and reduce edema

Indications & Combinations:

212

1. Deficient *qi* of the spleen and lungs manifested as poor appetite, loose stool, shortness of breath and lassitude. Astragalus root (Huangqi) is used with Ginseng (Renshen) and White atractylodes (Baizhu).

2. Deficient *qi* and weakened *yang* manifested as chills and sweating. Astragalus root (Huangqi) is used with Prepared aconite root (Fuzi).

3. *Qi* sinking in the middle *jiao* due to weakness of the spleen and stomach manifested as prolapsed anus, prolapsed uterus and gastroptosis. Astragalus root (Huangqi) is used with Ginseng (Renshen), White atractylodes (Baizhu) and Cimicifuga rhizome (Shengma) in the formula Buzhong Yiqi Tang.

4. Failure of deficient *qi* of the spleen in controlling blood manifested as blood in the stool and uterine bleeding. Astragalus root (Huangqi) is used with Ginseng (Renshen) and Chinese angelica root (Danggui) in the formula Guipi Tang.

5. Deficiency of *qi* and blood manifested as palpitations, anxiety, insomnia and forgetfulness. Astragalus root (Huangqi) is used with Longan aril (Longyanrou), Wild jujube seed (Suanzaoren) and Polygala root (Yuanzhi) in the formula Guipi Tang.

6. Spontaneous sweating due to exterior deficiency. Astragalus root (Huangqi) is used with Oyster shell (Muli), Light wheat (Fuxiaomai) and Ephedra root (Mahuanggen) in the formula Muli San.

7. Night sweating due to *yin* deficiency and excessive fire. Astragalus root (Huangqi) is used with Fresh rehmannia root (Shengdihuang) and Phellodendron bark (Huangbai) in the formula Danggui Liuhuang Tang.

8. Deficiency of the spleen leading to dysfunction in transportation and transformation of water manifested as edema and scanty urine. Astragalus root (Huangqi) is used with Tetrandra root (Fangji) and White atractylodes (Baizhu) in the formula Fangji Huangqi Tang.

9. Boils and ulcers due to *qi* and blood deficiency manifested as sores that have formed pus but have not drained or healed well. Astragalus root (Huangqi) is used with Cinnamon bark (Rougui), Chinese angelica root (Danggui) and Ginseng (Renshen).

10. Retardation of circulation of the blood due to deficiency of *qi* and blood manifested as hemiplegia. Astragalus root (Huangqi) is used with Chinese angelica root (Danggui), Chuanxiong rhizome (Chuanxiong) and Earthworm (Dilong) in the formula Buyang Huanwu Tang.

Dosage: 10-15 g (The maximum dosage can be 30-60 g.)

Cautions & Contraindications: This herb is contraindicated during *yin* deficiency and hyperactivity of *yang, qi* stagnation and accumulation of dampness, retention of food, exterior excess syndrome, and the early stage of carbuncles and furuncles.

265. White atractylodes (Baizhu)

Pharmaceutical Name: Rhizoma Atractylodis macrocephalae
Botanical Name: Atractylodes macrocephala Koidz.
Common Name: White atractylodes rhizome
Source of Earliest Record: Shennong Bencao Jing
Part Used & Method for Pharmaceutical Preparations: The rhizomes are dug in October, cleaned and dried in the sun or baked. They are then soaked in water and cut into slices.
Properties & Taste: Bitter, sweet and warm
Meridians: Spleen and stomach
Functions: 1. To replenish *qi* and strengthen the spleen; 2. To resolve dampness and promote water metabolism; 3. To stop sweating and calm the fetus
Indications & Combinations:

1. Weakness of the spleen in transportation and transformation of water manifested as poor appetite, loose stool, lassitude and epigastric and abdominal distension and fullness. White atractylodes (Baizhu) is used with Ginseng (Renshen) and Poria (Fuling) in the formula Sijunzi Tang.

2. Deficiency and cold in the spleen and stomach manifested as cold sensation and pain in the epigastric and abdominal regions, diarrhea and vomiting. White atractylodes (Baizhu) is used with Dried ginger (Ganjiang) and Ginseng (Renshen) in the formula Lizhong Wan.

3. *Qi* stagnation due to weakness of the spleen and stomach manifested as epigastric and abdominal fullness. White atractylodes (Baizhu) is used with Immature bitter orange (Zhishi) in the formula Zhi Zhu Wan.

4. Internal accumulation of water and dampness due to dysfunction of the spleen and stomach accompanied by edema or phlegm-fluid syndrome: a) for edema and ascites, White atractylodes (Baizhu) is used with Areca nut shell (Dafupi) and Poria (Fuling); b) for phlegm-damp syndrome manifested as palpitation, asthma, cough with excessive sputum and stifling sensation in the chest, White atractylodes (Baizhu)

is used with Cinnamon twigs (Guizhi) and Poria (Fuling) in the formula Ling Gui Zhu Gan Tang.

5. Spontaneous sweating due to *qi* deficiency. White atractylodes (Baizhu) is used with Astragalus root (Huangqi) and Ledebouriella (Fangfeng) in the formula Yupingfeng San.

6. Restlessness of fetus due to weakness of *qi* of the spleen during pregnancy: a) if accompanying manifestations include vaginal bleeding and pain in the lower abdomen, White atractylodes (Baizhu) is used with Ginseng (Renshen) and Poria (Fuling); b) if accompanying manifestations include dizziness, vertigo and palpitations, White atractylodes (Baizhu) is used with Prepared rehmannia root (Shudihuang), Chinese angelica root (Danggui), White peony root (Baishao) and Donkey hide gelatin (Ejiao); c) if accompanying manifestations include soreness and pain of the lumbar region due to deficiency of the kidneys, White atractylodes (Baizhu) is used with Eucommia bark (Duzhong), Teasel root (Xuduan) and Mulberry mistletoe (Sangjisheng); d) if accompanying manifestations include distention and fullness in the chest and abdominal region due to *qi* stagnation, White atractylodes (Baizhu) is used with Perilla stem (Sugeng) and Amomum fruit (Sharen); e) if accompanying manifestations include red tongue proper with yellow coating and rapid pulse due to internal heat, White atractylodes (Baizhu) is used with Scutellaria root (Huangqin).

Dosage: 5-15 g

Cautions & Contraindications: The raw herb is used for resolving dampness and promoting water metabolism. The fried herb is used for replenishing *qi* and strengthening the spleen. The carbonized herb is used for tonifying the spleen and stopping diarrhea. White atractylodes (Baizhu) is contraindicated in cases with thirst accompanied by exhaustion of body fluids.

266. Dioscorea (Shanyao)

Pharmaceutical Name: Rhizoma Dioscoreae
Botanical Name: Dioscorea opposita Thunb.
Common Name: Chinese yam, Dioscorea
Source of Earliest Record: Shennong Bencao Jing
Part Used & Method for Pharmaceutical Preparations: The rhizomes are dug in the period of Frost's Descent (eighteenth solar term). After the rough bark has been removed, the rhizomes are cleaned and dried

in either the sun or the shade. Then, they are soaked again and cut into slices.

Properties & Taste: Sweet and neutral

Meridians: Spleen, lung and kidney

Functions: 1. To strengthen the spleen and stomach; 2. To tonify the lungs and kidneys

Indications & Combinations:

1. Weakness of the spleen and stomach manifested as poor appetite, diarrhea and lassitude. Dioscorea (Shanyao) is used with Ginseng (Renshen), White atractylodes (Baizhu) and Poria (Fuling) in the formula Shen Ling Baizhu San.

2. Excessive dampness due to deficiency of the spleen manifested as whitish and dilute leukorrhagia and lassitude. Dioscorea (Shanyao) is used with White atractylodes (Baizhu), Poria (Fuling) and Euryale seed (Qianshi).

3. Excessive dampness transforming into heat manifested as yellow leukorrhea. Dioscorea (Shanyao) is used with Phellodendron bark (Huangbai) and Plantain seed (Cheqianzi) in the formula Yihuang Tang.

4. Leukorrhagia due to deficient kidneys manifested as leukorrhagia and lower back pain. Dioscorea (Shanyao) is used with Dogwood fruit (Shanzhuyu) and Dadder seed (Tusizi).

5. Diabetes manifested as extreme thirst, excessive drinking, excessive food intake, profuse urination and lassitude. Dioscorea (Shanyao) is used with Astragalus root (Huangqi), Trichosanthes root (Tianhuafen), Fresh rehmannia root (Shengdihuang) and Pueraria root (Gegen) in the formula Yuye Tang.

6. Nocturnal emissions due to deficient kidneys. Dioscorea (Shanyao) is used with Dogwood fruit (Shanzhuyu) and Prepared rehmannia root (Shudihuang) in the formula Liuwei Dihuang Wan.

7. Frequent urination due to kidney deficiency. Dioscorea (Shanyao) is used with Bitter cardamom (Yizhiren) and Mantis egg case (Sangpiaoxiao).

8. Chronic cough due to deficient lungs. Dioscorea (Shanyao) is used with Glehnia root (Shashen), Ophiopogon root (Maidong) and Schisandra fruit (Wuweizi).

Dosage: 10-30 g; 6-10 g (for powder)

Cautions & Contraindications: This herb is contraindicated during food retention.

267. Hyacinth bean (Biandou)

Pharmaceutical Name: Semen Dolichoris
Botanical Name: Dolichos lablab L.
Common Name: Dolichos seed, Hyacinth bean, Egyptian kidney bean
Source of Earliest Record: Mingyi Bielu
Part Used & Method for Pharmaceutical Preparations: The ripe seeds are gathered in autumn and then dried in the sun.
Properties & Taste: Sweet and slightly warm
Meridians: Spleen and stomach
Functions: To strengthen the spleen and transform dampness
Indications & Combinations:

1. Deficient spleen not transforming and transporting water manifested as lassitude, poor appetite, loose stool or diarrhea, or leukorrhea due to downward flowing of turbid dampness. Hyacinth bean (Biandou) is used with Ginseng (Renshen), White atractylodes (Baizhu) and Poria (Fuling) in the formula Shen Ling Baizhu San.

2. Disharmony of the spleen and stomach due to invasion from exogenous pathogenic summer-damp-heat manifested as vomiting and diarrhea. Hyacinth bean (Biandou) is used with Elsholtzia (Xiangru) and Magnolia bark (Houpo) in the formula Xiangru San.

Dosage: 10-20 g
Cautions & Contraindications: The raw herb is used for relieving summer-heat, the fried herb for strengthening the spleen and stopping diarrhea.

268. Licorice root (Gancao)

Pharmaceutical Name: Radix Glycyrrhizae
Botanical Name: 1. Glycyrrhiza uralensis Fisch.; 2. Glycyrrhiza inflata Bat.; 3. Glycyrrhiza glabra L.
Common Name: Licorice root
Source of Earliest Record: Shennong Bencao Jing
Part Used & Method for Pharmaceutical Preparations: The rhizomes are dug in spring or autumn. After the fibrous roots and bark have been removed, the rhizomes are cut into slices and dried in the sun.
Properties & Taste: Sweet and neutral

Meridians: Heart, lung, spleen and stomach

Functions: 1. To tonify the spleen and replenish *qi*; 2. To moisten the lungs and stop coughs; 3. To relax spasms and stop pain; 4. To moderate the action of herbs; 5. To reduce fire and release toxins

Indications & Combinations:

1. Deficient *qi* of the spleen and stomach manifested as poor appetite, loose stool and lassitude. Licorice root (Gancao) is used with White atractylodes (Baizhu), Poria (Fuling) and Ginseng (Renshen) in the formula Sijunzi Tang.

2. Cough and asthma. Licorice root (Gancao) is used with Apricot seed (Xingren) and Ephedra (Mahuang) in the formula Sanniu Tang.

3. Carbuncles, furuncles, sore throat and swelling due to toxic heat. Licorice root (Gancao) is used with Platycodon root (Jiegeng), Scrophu-laria (Xuanshen) and Arctium fruit (Niubangzi) for sore throat; Licorice root (Gancao) can also be used with Honeysuckle flower (Jinyinhua) and Forsythia fruit (Lianqiao) for carbuncles, furuncles and swellings.

4. Abdominal pain due to spasms of the stomach or intestines. Licorice root (Gancao) is used with White peony root (Baishao).

5. Moderating the action of other herbs. For example, Licorice root (Gancao) with Prepared aconite root (Fuzi) and Dried ginger (Ganjiang) can weaken the heating properties and lessen the side effects of some herbs. This combination is called Sini Tang.

Dosage: 2-10 g

Cautions & Contraindications: This herb is contraindicated during cases of excess dampness causing distension and fullness in the chest and abdominal region, or vomiting. It counteracts Peking spurge root (Daji), Genkwa flower (Yuanhua), Kansui root (Gansui) and Seaweed (Haizao). Prolonged overdosing of the herb may cause edema.

269. Jujube (Dazao)

Pharmaceutical Name: Fructus Jujubae

Botanical Name: Ziziphus jujuba Mill.

Common Name: Jujube, Chinese date

Source of Earliest Record: Shennong Bencao Jing

Part Used & Method for Pharmaceutical Preparations: The ripe fruit is gathered at the beginning of autumn and dried in the sun.

Properties & Taste: Sweet and warm

Meridians: Spleen and stomach

Functions: 1. To replenish *qi* in the middle *jiao* (spleen and stomach); 2. To nourish the blood and soothe the mind; 3. To moderate the action of herbs

Indications & Combinations:

1. Weakness of the spleen and stomach manifested as lassitude, poor appetite and loose stool. Jujube (Dazao) is used with Ginseng (Renshen) and White atractylodes (Baizhu).

2. Hysteria manifested as grief, weeping and sighing. Jujube (Dazao) is used with Licorice root (Gancao) and Light wheat (Fuxiaomai) in the formula Gan Mai Dazao Tang.

3. Moderating the action of other herbs. Jujube (Dazao) is used with Peking spurge root (Daji), Kansui root (Gansui) and Genkwa flower (Yuanhua) in the formula Shizao Tang.

Dosage: 3-12 g, or 10-30 g

Cautions & Contraindications: This herb is contraindicated in conditions of excessive dampness, epigastric and abdominal distension and fullness, retention of food, intestinal parasites, pain of decayed teeth and cough due to phlegm-heat.

b) Herbs That Tonify *Yang*

Herbs that tonify *yang* are used to treat deficient *yang* syndrome, mainly deficient *yang* of the kidneys. Deficient *yang* syndrome is manifested as aversion to cold, cold extremities, soreness and weakness or cold pain in the lower back and knees, impotence, spermatorrhea, sterility, watery leukorrhea, enuresis, white tongue coating, deep pulse, wheezing and diarrhea.

In general, herbs that tonify *yang* are warm and dry in nature. They can injure *yin* and give rise to fire, so they are contraindicated for a person with deficient *yin* and excessive fire syndrome.

270a. Pilose antler (Lurong)

Pharmaceutical Name: Cornu Cervi Pantotrichum
Zoological Name: 1. Cervus nippon Temminck; 2. Cervus elaphus L.
Common Name: Pilose antler, Pilose deer-horn
Source of Earliest Record: Shennong Bencao Jing
Part Used & Method for Pharmaceutical Preparations: The horn is sawn off in summer or autumn. It is boiled and dried in the shade, then boiled and dried again. Next it is put in a container in a cool, dry place.

Finally, the hairs on the horn are burned off and the horn is soaked in white wine. Later, it is cut into slices.

Properties & Taste: Sweet, salty and warm

Meridians: Liver and kidney

Functions: 1. To replenish blood and essence; 2. To tonify kidney *yang*; 3. To strengthen the bones and tendons

Indications & Combinations:

1. Deficient kidney *yang* manifested as weakness of the body, aversion to cold, cold extremities, impotence in men, frigidity in women, infertility, frequent urination, soreness and pain in the lower back and knees, dizziness, tinnitus, gradual loss of hearing and listlessness. Pilose antler (Lurong) is used with Ginseng (Renshen), Prepared rehmannia root (Shudihuang) and Dadder seed (Tusizi).

2. Deficiency of blood and essence manifested as soreness and weakness of bones and tendons and infantile maldevelopment. Pilose antler (Lurong) is used with Prepared rehmannia root (Shudihuang), Dioscorea (Shanyao) and Dogwood fruit (Shanzhuyu).

3. Deficiency and cold in the Chong and Ren meridians manifested as white and dilute leukorrhea or uterine bleeding. Pilose antler (Lurong) is used with Donkey hide gelatin (Ejiao), Chinese angelica root (Danggui), Dogwood fruit (Shanzhuyu) and Cuttlefish bone (Wuzeigu).

4. Chronic ulcers. Pilose antler (Lurong) is used with Prepared rehmannia root (Shudihuang), Cinnamon bark (Rougui) and Astragalus root (Huangqi).

Dosage: 1-3 g (for powder)

Cautions & Contraindications: Overdosing of this herb can cause dizziness or red eyes, and may consume *yin*. It is contraindicated in cases with deficient *yin* with hyperactive *yang*, heat in the blood, excessive fire in the stomach, phlegm-heat in the lungs and febrile disease due to exogenous pathogenic heat.

270b. Antler (Lujiao), Antler glue (Lujiaojiao) and Deglued antler powder (Lujiaoshuang)

Antler (Lujiao) is the ossified horn of a deer. Its taste is salty, its property warm. It enters the liver and kidney meridians. It tonifies the kidneys and strengthens *yang*. Although a weaker substitute for Pilose antler (Lurong), Antler (Lujiao) does invigorate the blood and reduce swelling. It is indicated for boils, ulcers, swelling, mastitis, pain due to blood stagnation and pain of tendons, bones and lower back. The recommended dosage is 5-10 g. Antler (Lujiao) is contraindicated during *yin* deficiency with excessive fire.

Antler glue (Lujiaojiao) is made from mature deer antlers. It is sweet, salty and warm, and enters the liver and kidney meridians, replenishing blood and essence and stopping bleeding. Antler glue (Lujiaojiao) is indicated for weakness of the body, vomiting, epistaxis, uterine bleeding, blood in the urine and *yin* boils. The recommended dosage is 5-10 g.

Deglued antler powder (Lujiaoshuang) is the residue from the process of preparing soft extract by cooking the deer horn for a long time. The astringent action of this substance is similar to that of Antler (Lujiao) but is less effective. Clinically, it is used mainly in cases of deficient kidney *yang*, deficiency and cold in the spleen and stomach, vomiting, poor appetite, frigidity, uterine bleeding, leukorrhagia, hemorrhage due to external injury, boils and ulcers. The recommended dosage is 10-15 g.

271. Morinda root (Bajitian)

Pharmaceutical Name: Radix Morindae officinalis
Botanical Name: Morinda officinalis How
Common Name: Morinda root
Source of Earliest Record: Shennong Bencao Jing
Part Used & Method for Pharmaceutical Preparations: The roots are dug in spring or winter. After the fibrous roots have been removed and the roots are dried in the sun, the dried roots are steamed or soaked. The core of the root is discarded, and the remaining root is cut into slices.
Properties & Taste: Pungent, sweet and slightly warm
Meridian: Kidney
Functions: 1. To tonify the kidneys and strengthen *yang*; 2. To dispel wind and transform dampness
Indications & Combinations:
1. Deficient kidney *yang* manifested as soreness and weakness in the lower back and knees, impotence, premature ejaculation, infertility, frigidity, irregular menstruation, and cold sensation and pain in the lower abdomen. a) Morinda root (Bajitian) is used with Ginseng (Ren-

shen), Cistanche (Roucongrong) and Dadder seed (Tusizi) for impotence, premature ejaculation and infertility; b) Morinda root (Bajitian) is used with Teasel root (Xuduan) and Eucommia bark (Duzhong) for soreness and weakness in lower back and knees; c) Morinda root (Bajitian) is used with Cinnamon bark (Rougui), Galangal rhizome (Gaoliangjiang) and Evodia fruit (Wuzhuyu) for irregular menstruation.

2. Morinda root (Bajitian) is used with Teasel root (Xuduan), Mulberry mistletoe (Sangjisheng) and Hypoglauca yam (Bixie) for cold sensation and pain in the lumbar region and knees or motor impairment.

Dosage: 10-15 g

Cautions & Contraindications: This herb is contraindicated in cases with deficient *yin* with excessive fire, or damp-heat.

272. Cistanche (Roucongrong)

Pharmaceutical Name: Herba cistanches
Botanical Name: Cistanche deserticola Y. C. Ma
Common Name: Cistanche
Source of Earliest Record: Shennong Bencao Jing.
Part Used & Method for Pharmaceutical Preparations: The fleshy stems are gathered in spring, dried in the sun and cut into slices.
Properties & Taste: Sweet, salty and warm
Meridians: Kidney and large intestine
Functions: 1. To tonify the kidneys and strengthen *yang*; 2. To moisten the intestines and move feces
Indications & Combinations:

1. Deficiency of the kidneys manifested as impotence. Cistanche (Roucongrong) is used with Prepared rehmannia root (Shudihuang), Dadder seed (Tusizi) and Schisandra fruit (Wuweizi) in the formula Roucongrong Wan.

2. Frigidity and infertility. Cistanche (Roucongrong) is used with Antler glue (Lujiaojiao), Human placenta (Ziheche) and Prepared rehmannia root (Shudihuang).

3. Pain in the lower back and knees and fragile bones and tendons due to kidney deficiency. Cistanche (Roucongrong) is used with Morinda root (Bajitian) and Eucommia bark (Duzhong) in the formula Jingang Wan.

4. Constipation due to dryness in the intestines. Cistanche (Rou-

congrong) is used with Hemp seed (Huomaren) in the formula Run-chang Wan.

Dosage: 10-20 g

Cautions & Contraindications: This herb is contraindicated in cases with deficiency of *yin* with excessive fire, diarrhea or constipation due to excessive heat in the stomach and intestine.

273. Curculigo rhizome (Xianmao)

Pharmaceutical Name: Rhizoma curculiginis
Botanical Name: Curculigo orchioides Gaertn.
Common Name: Curculigo rhizome, Golden-eye grass
Source of Earliest Record: Haiyao Bencao
Part Used & Method for Pharmaceutical Preparations: The rhizomes are dug in early spring. After the fibrous roots have been removed, the roots are dried in the sun and cut into slices.
Properties & Taste: Pungent, hot and toxic
Meridian: Kidney
Functions: 1. To warm the kidney and strengthen *yang*; 2. To dispel cold and dampness
Indications & Combinations:

1. Weakness of kidney *yang* manifested as impotence, frigidity and cold pain in the lower back and knees due to obstruction by invasion of wind-cold dampness. Curculigo rhizome (Xianmao) is used with Epimedium (Yinyanghuo).

Dosage: 10-15 g (It can be used as decoction, pill or ointment.)
Cautions & Contraindications: This herb is contraindicated in cases with deficient *yin* and excessive fire.

274. Epimedium (Yinyanghuo)

Pharmaceutical Name: Herba Epimedii
Botanical Name: 1. Epimedium koreanum Nakai; 2. Epimedium sagittatum (Sieb. et Zucc.) Maxim.; 3. Epimedium brevicornum Maxim.; 4. Epimedium pubescens Maxim.
Common Name: Epimedium
Source of Earliest Record: Haiyao Bencao
Part Used & Method for Pharmaceutical Preparations: The aerial part of the herb is gathered in spring and autumn, dried in the sun and cut into pieces.

Properties & Taste: Pungent, sweet and warm

Meridians: Liver and kidney

Functions: 1. To tonify the kidneys and strengthen *yang*; 2. To expel wind and dampness

Indications & Combinations:

1. Deficient kidney *yang* manifested as impotence, weakness of the lower back and knees and frequent urination. Epimedium (Yinyanghuo) is used with Curculigo rhizome (Xianmao) and Prepared rehmannia root (Shudihuang).

2. Cold pain in the lower back and knees and numbness of limbs due to obstruction by invasion of wind-cold-damp. Epimedium (Yinyanghuo) is used with Clematis root (Weilingxian), Eucommia bark (Duzhong) and Cinnamon twigs (Guizhi).

Dosage: 10-15 g

Cautions & Contraindications: This herb is contraindicated in cases with deficiency of *yin* with excessive fire.

275. Eucommia bark (Duzhong)

Pharmaceutical Name: Cortex Eucommiae

Botanical Name: Eucommia ulmoides oliv.

Common Name: Eucommia bark

Source of Earliest Record: Shennong Bencao Jing

Part Used & Method for Pharmaceutical Preparations: The bark is gathered in summer and autumn. The rough bark is removed and discarded, and then the smooth bark is dried in the sun.

Properties & Taste: Sweet and warm

Meridians: Liver and kidney

Functions: 1. To tonify liver and kidneys and strengthen bones and tendons; 2. To calm the fetus to prevent miscarriage

Indications & Combinations:

1. Deficiency of liver and kidneys manifested as soreness and pain in the lower back and knees. Eucommia bark (Duzhong) is used with Psoralea fruit (Buguzhi) and Walnut seed (Hutaoren).

2. Impotence due to deficient kidneys. Eucommia bark (Duzhong) is used with Dogwood fruit (Shanzhuyu), Dadder seed (Tusizi) and Schisandra fruit (Wuweizi).

3. Threatened abortion or restlessness of fetus manifested as lower abdominal pain and uterine bleeding. Eucommia bark (Duzhong) is

used with Teasel root (Xuduan) and Dioscorea (Shanyao).

Dosage: 10-15 g

Cautions & Contraindications: The fried herb is more effective than the raw herb. Eucommia bark (Duzhong) is contraindicated in cases with deficiency of *yin* with excessive fire.

276. Teasel root (Xuduan)

Pharmaceutical Name: Radix Dipsaci

Botanical Name: 1. Dipsacus asper Wall.

Common Name: Dipsacus root, Teasel root

Source of Earliest Record: Shennong Bencao Jing

Part Used & Method for Pharmaceutical Preparations: The roots are dug in the period from July to August. After the fibrous roots have been removed, the roots are cut into slices and dried in the sun.

Properties & Taste: Bitter, sweet, pungent and slightly warm

Meridians: Liver and kidney

Functions: 1. To tonify the liver and kidneys; 2. To promote the circulation of blood; 3. To strengthen the bones and tendons

Indications & Combinations:

1. Deficiency of the liver and kidneys manifested as soreness and pain in the lower back and knees or weakness of the legs. Teasel root (Xuduan) is used with Eucommia bark (Duzhong) and Cyathula root (Niuxi).

2. Derangement of Chong and Ren meridians due to deficient liver and kidneys manifested as profuse menstrual flow, uterine bleeding and threatened abortion (restless fetus). Teasel root (Xuduan) is used with Eucommia bark (Duzhong), Donkey hide gelatin (Ejiao), Mugwort leaf (Aiye), Astragalus root (Huangqi) and Chinese angelica root (Danggui).

3. External injury. Teasel root (Xuduan) is used with Drynaria (Gusuibu) and Dragon's blood (Xuejie) for reducing swelling and stopping pain.

Dosage: 10-20 g

Cautions & Contraindications: The fried herb is used for uterine bleeding and the powdered herb for external use.

277. Cibot rhizome (Gouji)

Pharmaceutical Name: Rhizoma Cibotii

Botanical Name: Cibotium barometz (L.) J. Sm.

Common Name: Cibot rhizome, Chain fern

Source of Earliest Record: Shennong Bencao Jing

Part Used & Method for Pharmaceutical Preparations: The rhizomes are dug in autumn. After the fibrous roots have been removed, the rhizomes are soaked in wine for one day, steamed, cut into slices and dried in the sun.

Properties & Taste: Bitter, sweet and warm

Meridians: Liver and kidney

Functions: 1. To tonify liver and kidneys; 2. To strengthen bones and tendons; 3. To expel wind and dampness

Indications & Combinations:

1. Deficiency of the liver and kidneys manifested as soreness and pain in the lower back and knees. Cibot rhizome (Gouji) is used with Eucommia bark (Duzhong), Teasel root (Xuduan) and Cyathula root (Niuxi).

2. Deficient liver and kidneys accompanied by invasion of wind and dampness manifested as soreness and pain in the lower back and knees and motor impairment. Cibot rhizome (Gouji) is used with Cinnamon twigs (Guizhi), Large-leaf gentian root (Qinjiao) and Futokadsura stem (Haifengteng).

Dosage: 10-15 g

Cautions & Contraindications: This herb is contraindicated in cases with dysuria, scanty, yellow or brown urine, bitter taste in the mouth or dryness of the tongue.

278. Drynaria (Gusuibu)

Pharmaceutical Name: Rhizoma Drynariae

Botanical Name: 1. Drynaria frotunei (Kunze) J. Sm.; 2. Drynaria baronii (Christ) Diels

Common Name: Drynaria, Davallia

Source of Earliest Record: Kaibao Bencao

Part Used & Method for Pharmaceutical Preparations: The rhizomes are dug in any season. After they have been cleaned, the rhizomes are cut into slices and dried.

Properties & Taste: Bitter and warm

Meridians: Liver and kidney

Functions: 1. To tonify the kidneys; 2. To invigorate blood and stop bleeding; 3. To heal wounds

Indications & Combinations:

1. Deficient kidneys manifested as lower back pain, weakness of the legs, tinnitus, deafness or toothache. Drynaria (Gusuibu) is used with Psoralea fruit (Buguzhi), Cyathula root (Niuxi) and Walnut seed (Hutaoren) for lower back pain and weakness of the legs. Drynaria (Gusuibu) can also be used with Prepared rehmannia root (Shudihuang) and Dogwood fruit (Shanzhuyu) for tinnitus, deafness and toothache.

2. Swelling and pain due to external trauma or injury. Drynaria (Gusuibu) is used with Tiger bone (Hugu), Tortoise plastron (Guiban) and Myrrh (Moyao).

Dosage: 10-20 g

Cautions & Contraindications: This herb is contraindicated in cases with deficiency of *yin* with internal heat and symptoms without blood stasis.

279. Psoralea fruit (Buguzhi)

Pharmaceutical Name: Fructus Psoraleae

Botanical Name: Psoralea corylifolia L.

Common Name: Psoralea fruit

Source of Earliest Record: Yaoxing Lun

Part Used & Method for Pharmaceutical Preparations: The ripe fruit is gathered in autumn, and then it is dried in the sun.

Properties & Taste: Bitter, pungent and very warm

Meridians: Kidney and spleen

Functions: 1. To tonify kidneys and strengthen *yang*; 2. To prevent emissions and nocturnal urination; 3. To warm the spleen and stop diarrhea

Indications & Combinations:

1. Deficient kidneys manifested as impotence and soreness and weakness of the lower back and knees. Psoralea fruit (Buguzhi) is used with Dadder seed (Tusizi), Cistanche (Roucongrong) and Eucommia bark (Duzhong).

2. Nocturnal urination and emissions due to kidney deficiency. Psoralea fruit (Buguzhi) is used with Bitter cardamom (Yizhiren) and Dioscorea (Shanyao).

3. Diarrhea due to deficiency of *yang* of the spleen and kidneys. Psoralea fruit (Buguzhi) is used with Evodia fruit (Wuzhuyu), Nutmeg

(Roudoukou) and Schisandra fruit (Wuweizi) in the formula Sishen Wan.

Dosage: 5-10 g

Cautions & Contraindications: This herb is contraindicated in cases with deficiency of *yin* with excessive fire as well as constipation.

280. Bitter cardamom (Yizhiren)

Pharmaceutical Name: Fructus Alpiniae oxyphyllae
Botanical Name: Alpinia oxyphylla Miq.
Common Name: Black cardamom, Bitter cardamom
Source of Earliest Record: Bencao Shiyi
Part Used & Method for Pharmaceutical Preparations: The fruit is gathered in summer. It is dried in the sun, fried with sand and peeled.
Properties & Taste: Pungent and warm
Meridians: Spleen and kidney
Functions: 1. To warm and tonify the spleen and kidneys; 2. To prevent emissions and stop diarrhea
Indications & Combinations:

1. Invasion of cold in the spleen and kidneys manifested as abdominal pain and vomiting. Bitter cardamom (Yizhiren) is used with Pilose asiabell root (Dangshen), White atractylodes (Baizhu) and Dried ginger (Ganjiang).

2. Kidney deficiency manifested as enuresis and seminal emissions. Bitter cardamom (Yizhiren) is used with Dioscorea (Shanyao) and Lindera root (Wuyao) in the formula Suoquan Wan.

3. Diarrhea and excessive salivation due to spleen deficiency. Bitter cardamom (Yizhiren) is used with Poria (Fuling), Dioscorea (Shanyao), Pilose asiabell root (Dangshen) and Pinellia tuber (Banxia).

Dosage: 3-6 g

Cautions & Contraindications: This herb is contraindicated in cases with deficiency of *yin* with excessive fire, seminal emissions, frequent urination and uterine bleeding caused by heat.

281. Cordyceps (Dongchongxiacao)

Pharmaceutical Name: Cordyceps
Botanical Name: Cordyceps sinensis (Berk.) Sacc
Common Name: Cordyceps, Chinese caterpillar fungus
Source of Earliest Record: Bencao Congxin

Part Used & Method for Pharmaceutical Preparations: The fungus and the carcass of the larvae of various insects are collected in the period of the Summer Solstice (tenth solar term). They are cleaned and dried in the sun or baked.

Properties & Taste: Sweet and warm

Meridians: Kidney and lung

Functions: 1. To tonify lungs and kidneys; 2. To stop bleeding; 3. To resolve phlegm

Indications & Combinations:

1. Deficient kidneys manifested as impotence, seminal emissions and soreness and pain in the lower back and knees. Cordyceps (Dongchongxiacao) is used with Dogwood fruit (Shanzhuyu), Dioscorea (Shanyao) and Dadder seed (Tusizi). The herb can also be used alone.

2. Chronic cough and asthma or cough with bloody sputum due to lung deficiency. Cordyceps (Dongchongxiacao) is used with Glehnia root (Shashen), Donkey hide gelatin (Ejiao) and Tendrilled fritillary bulb (Chuanbeimu).

3. Spontaneous sweating and aversion to cold due to weakness of the body or illness. Cordyceps (Dongchongxiacao) is cooked with chicken, duck or pork.

Dosage: 5-10 g

Cautions & Contraindications: This substance should be used cautiously in cases with exterior syndromes.

282. Gecko (Gejie)

Pharmaceutical Name: Gecko

Zoological Name: Gekko gecko L.

Common Name: Gecko, Toad-headed lizard

Source of Earliest Record: Leigong Paozhi Lun

Part Used & Method for Pharmaceutical Preparations: The gecko is caught in summer. The internal organs are removed, and the eyes are cut and drained. Pieces of bamboo are used to fix the body, and then the gecko is baked and put in a dry place.

Properties & Taste: Salty and neutral

Meridians: Lung and kidney

Functions: 1. To tonify lungs and kidneys; 2. To stop cough and asthma; 3. To replenish blood and essence

Indications & Combinations:

1. Cough and asthma due to deficiency of lungs and kidneys. Gecko (Gejie) is used with Ginseng (Renshen), Apricot seed (Xingren) and Tendrilled fritillary bulb (Chuanbeimu) in the formula Renshen Gejie San.

2. Impotence due to kidney deficiency. Gecko (Gejie) is used with Ginseng (Renshen), Pilose antler (Lurong) and Epimedium (Yinyanghuo). Also, Gecko (Gejie) can be used alone for this treatment.

Dosage: 3-7 g (for decoction), 1-2 g (for powder)

Cautions & Contraindications: This substance is contraindicated in patients with cough and asthma due to excessive internal heat or invasion by exogenous pathogenic wind and cold.

283. Walnut seed (Hutaoren)

Pharmaceutical Name: Semen Juglandis
Botanical Name: Juglans regia L.
Common Name: Walnut seed, Walnut kernel
Source of Earliest Record: Kaibao Bencao
Part Used & Method for Pharmaceutical Preparations: The ripe walnuts are gathered in the period from September to October, dried in the sun and shelled.
Properties & Taste: Sweet and warm
Meridians: Kidney, lung and large intestine
Functions: 1. To tonify the lungs and kidneys; 2. To moisten the intestines and move feces
Indications & Combinations:

1. Lower back pain and weakness of the legs due to deficient kidneys. Walnut seed (Hutaoren) is used with Eucommia bark (Duzhong) and Psoralea fruit (Buguzhi) in the formula Qing'e Wan.

2. Cough and asthma due to deficient lungs. Walnut seed (Hutaoren) is used with Ginseng (Renshen).

3. Constipation due to dryness in the intestines. Walnut seed (Hutaoren) is used with Hemp seed (Huomaren) and Cistanche (Roucongrong).

Dosage: 10-30 g

Cautions & Contraindications: This herb is contraindicated in cases with deficiency of *yin* with excessive fire, cough due to phlegm-heat or diarrhea.

284. Dadder seed (Tusizi)

Pharmaceutical Name: Semen Cuscutae
Botanical Name: 1. Cuscuta chinensis Lam.; 2. Cuscuta japonica Choisy
Common Name: Dadder seed, Cuscuta seed
Source of Earliest Record: Shennong Bencao Jing
Part Used & Method for Pharmaceutical Preparations: The ripe seeds are collected in autumn, and then they are dried in the sun or boiled.
Properties & Taste: Pungent, sweet and neutral
Meridians: Liver and kidney
Functions: 1. To tonify kidneys and control essence; 2. To nourish liver and brighten the eyes
Indications & Combinations:

1. Deficient kidneys manifested as impotence, nocturnal emissions, premature ejaculation, lower back pain or leukorrhagia. Dadder seed (Tusizi) is used with Eucommia bark (Duzhong), Dioscorea (Shanyao) and Cibot rhizome (Gouji) for lower back pain or leukorrhagia; Dadder seed (Tusizi) is used with Schisandra fruit (Wuweizi), Cnidium fruit (Shechuangzi), Flattened milkvetch seed (Shayuanzi) and Grossy privet fruit (Nüzhenzi) for impotence.

2. Diarrhea due to deficient spleen. Dadder seed (Tusizi) is used with Pilose asiabell root (Dangshen), White atractylodes (Baizhu) and Dioscorea (Shanyao).

Dosage: 10-15 g
Cautions & Contraindications: This herb is contraindicated in cases with deficiency of *yin* with excessive fire, constipation and red, scanty urine.

285. Flattened milkvetch seed (Shayuanzi)

Pharmaceutical Name: Semen Astragali complanati (Leguminosae)
Botanical Name: Astragalus complanatus R. Br.
Common Name: Flatstem milkvetch seed
Source of Earliest Record: Bencao Yanyi
Part Used & Method for Pharmaceutical Preparations: The ripe seeds are collected in late autumn or early winter. The seeds are then fried with salt water.
Properties & Taste: Sweet and warm
Meridians: Liver and kidney

Functions: 1. To tonify the kidneys and control essence; 2. To nourish the liver and brighten the eyes

Indications & Combinations:

1. Deficient kidneys manifested as impotence, seminal emissions, premature ejaculation or leukorrhea. Flattened milkvetch seed (Shayuanzi) is used with Dragon's bone (Longgu), Oyster shell (Muli) and Euryale seed (Qianshi).

2. Blurred vision due to deficiency of liver blood. Flattened milkvetch seed (Shayuanzi) is used with Dadder seed (Tusizi), Chrysanthemum flower (Juhua), Wolfberry fruit (Gouqizi) and Grossy privet fruit (Nüzhenzi).

Dosage: 10-20 g

Cautions & Contraindications: This herb is contraindicated in cases with deficiency of *yin* with excessive fire, as well as dysuria.

286. Dog testis (Huanggoushen)

Pharmaceutical Name: Testis et Penis Canis familiaris

Zoological Name: Canis familiaris L.

Common Name: Dog testis

Source of Earliest Record: Shennong Bencao Jing

Part Used & Method for Pharmaceutical Preparations: The penis or testis can be obtained at any time. After removing the fat, the testis is dried in the shade.

Properties & Taste: Salty and warm

Meridian: Kidney

Functions: To tonify the kidneys and strengthen *yang*

Indications & Combinations: Deficiency of kidney *yang* manifested as impotence, aversion to cold and cold extremities. Dog testis (Huanggoushen) is used with Wolfberry fruit (Gouqizi), Morinda root (Bajitian) and Dadder seed (Tusizi).

Dosage: 1.5-3 g (for pills)

Cautions & Contraindications: This substance is contraindicated in cases with internal heat with excessive fire.

287. Chinese chive seed (Jiuzi)

Pharmaceutical Name: Semen Allii tuberosi

Botanical Name: Allium tuberosum Rottl.

Common Name: Chinese leek, Chinese chive seed

Source of Earliest Record: Bencao Jingji Zhi

Part Used & Method for Pharmaceutical Preparations: The seeds are collected in autumn, and then dried in the sun or fried.

Properties & Taste: Pungent, sweet and warm

Meridians: Liver and kidney

Functions: 1. To tonify the liver and kidneys; 2. To strengthen *yang* and control the essence

Indications & Combinations:

1. Deficiency of kidney *yang* manifested as impotence and cold pain in the lower back and knees. Chinese chive seed (Jiuzi) is used with Cistanche (Roucongrong) and Morinda root (Bajitian).

2. Frequent urination or leukorrhea due to deficient kidneys. Chinese chive seed (Jiuzi) is used with Psoralea fruit (Buguzhi), Dioscorea (Shanyao) and Bitter cardamom (Yizhiren).

Dosage: 5-10 g (for decoction or pills)

Cautions & Contraindications: The herb is contraindicated in cases with deficiency of *yin* with excessive fire.

288. Cnidium fruit (Shechuangzi)

Pharmaceutical Name: Fructus Cnidii

Botanical Name: Cnidium monnieri (L.) Cuss.

Common Name: Cnidium fruit

Source of Earliest Record: Shennong Bencao Jing

Part Used & Method for Pharmaceutical Preparations: The ripe fruit is collected in autumn, and then dried in the sun.

Properties & Taste: Pungent, bitter and warm

Meridian: Kidney

Functions: 1. To warm the kidneys and strengthen the *yang*; 2. To dispel dampness and kill worms

Indications & Combinations:

1. Deficient *yang* of the kidneys manifested as impotence or infertility. Cnidium fruit (Shechuangzi) is used with Schisandra fruit (Wuweizi) and Dadder seed (Tusizi).

2. Vaginal trichomoniasis. The decoction of Cnidium fruit (Shechuangzi) is used as a douche.

Dosage: 3-10 g

Cautions & Contraindications: This herb is contraindicated in cases with deficiency of *yin* with excessive fire or damp-heat.

c) Herbs That Tonify the Blood

Herbs that tonify the blood are mainly used for deficiency of blood syndrome manifested as sallow complexion, pale lips and nails, dizziness, blurred vision, palpitations, anxiety, scanty and light-red menstrual flow, or amenorrhea. Because *"qi* can generate blood," herbs that tonify *qi* may enhance the therapeutic effect of tonifying the blood.

These herbs are characterized by viscosity, which may adversely affect digestion. For this reason, they are contraindicated in cases with poor appetite, abdominal distension and fullness due to turbid dampness in the spleen and stomach. For a person with such symptoms, herbs that strengthen the spleen and help digestion are often added to the combination.

289. Chinese angelica root (Danggui)

Pharmaceutical Name: Radix Angelicae sinensis
Botanical Name: Angelica sinensis (oliv.) Diels
Common Name: Chinese angelica root
Source of Earliest Record: Shennong Bencao Jing
Part Used & Method for Pharmaceutical Preparations: The roots are dug in late autumn. After the fibrous roots have been removed, the roots are laced, or smoked, with sulfur and cut into slices.
Properties & Taste: Sweet, pungent and warm
Meridians: Liver, heart and spleen
Functions: 1. To replenish blood; 2. To invigorate blood and stop pain; 3. To moisten the intestines
Indications & Combinations:

1. Syndromes due to deficiency of blood. Chinese angelica root (Danggui) is used with White peony root (Baishao), Prepared rehmannia root (Shudihuang) and Astragalus root (Huangqi) in the formula Siwu Tang or Danggui Buxue Tang.

2. Irregular menstruation. Chinese angelica root (Danggui) is used with Prepared rehmannia root (Shudihuang), White peony root (Baishao) and Chuanxiong rhizome (Chuanxiong) in the formula Siwu Tang.

3. Dysmenorrhea. Chinese angelica root (Danggui) is used with Cyperus tuber (Xiangfu), Corydalis tuber (Yanhusuo) and Motherwort (Yimucao).

4. Amenorrhea. Chinese angelica root (Danggui) is used with Peach seed (Taoren) and Safflower (Honghua).

5. Uterine bleeding. Chinese angelica root (Danggui) is used with Donkey hide gelatin (Ejiao), Mugwort leaf (Aiye) and Fresh rehmannia root (Shengdihuang).

6. Pains due to stagnation of blood: a) pain caused by external injuries—Chinese angelica root (Danggui) is used with Safflower (Honghua), Peach seed (Taoren), Frankincense (Ruxiang) and Myrrh (Moyao); b) pain caused by carbuncles and furuncles—Chinese angelica root (Danggui) is used with Moutan bark (Mudanpi), Red peony (Chishao), Honeysuckle flower (Jinyinhua) and Forsythia fruit (Lianqiao); c) postpartum abdominal pain—Chinese angelica root (Danggui) is used with Motherwort (Yimucao), Peach seed (Taoren) and Chuanxiong rhizome (Chuanxiong); d) wind-damp obstruction (rheumatic pain)—Chinese angelica root (Danggui) is used with Cinnamon twigs (Guizhi), Spatholobus stem (Jixueteng) and White peony root (Baishao).

7. Constipation due to dryness in the intestines. Chinese angelica root (Danggui) is used with Cistanche (Roucongrong) and Hemp seed (Huomaren).

Dosage: 5-15 g

Cautions & Contraindications: The head of the herb is more effective for nourishing blood; the tail is good for moving blood; and the body is used to invigorate and nourish blood. Chinese angelica root (Danggui), when mixed with wine, can enhance the function of invigorating blood. It is contraindicated in cases of excessive dampness in the stomach and spleen, and of diarrhea or loose stool.

290. Prepared rehmannia root (Shudihuang)

Pharmaceutical Name: Radix Rehmanniae praeparata
Botanical Name: Rehmannia gultinosa Libosch.
Common Name: Prepared rehmannia root
Source of Earliest Record: Bencao Tujing

Part Used & Method for Pharmaceutical Preparations: The rehmannia roots are prepared with wine, Amomum fruit (Sharen) and Tangerine peel (Chenpi). The roots are steamed and dried in the sun several times until they become black, soft and sticky; then they are cut into slices.

Properties & Taste: Sweet and slightly warm
Meridians: Liver and kidney
Functions: To nourish blood and replenish *yin*
Indications & Combinations:

1. Deficient blood syndrome manifested as sallow complexion, dizziness, vertigo, palpitations, insomnia, irregular menstruation and uterine bleeding. Prepared rehmannia root (Shudihuang) is used with Chinese angelica root (Danggui) and White peony root (Baishao) in the formula Siwu Tang.

2. Deficient kidney syndrome manifested as afternoon fever, night sweating, noctural emissions, diabetes, dizziness and blurred vision. Prepared rehmannia root (Shudihuang) is used with Dogwood fruit (Shanzhuyu) and Dioscorea (Shanyao) in the formula Liuwei Dihuang Wan.

3. Deficient *yin* and excessive fire syndrome manifested as afternoon fever, feverish sensation on the palms, soles and in the chest, night sweating, noctural emissions, red tongue proper with scanty coating and thready, rolling and rapid pulse. Prepared rehmannia root (Shudihuang) is used with Tortoise plastron (Guiban), Anemarrhena rhizome (Zhimu) and Phellodendron bark (Huangbai) in the formula Zhi Bai Dihuang Wan.

Dosage: 10-30 g

Cautions & Contraindications: This herb is contraindicated in cases with *qi* stagnation and profuse phlegm, with epigastric and abdominal distension and pain, and with poor appetite and diarrhea.

291. Fleeceflower root (Heshouwu)

Pharmaceutical Name: Radix Polygoni multiflori
Botanical Name: Polygonum multiflorum Thunb.
Common Name: Fleeceflower root
Source of Earliest Record: Kaibao Bencao
Part Used & Method for Pharmaceutical Preparations: The tuberous roots are dug in autumn or spring. They are cleaned, cut into slices and dried in the sun.

Properties & Taste: Bitter, sweet, astringent and slightly warm
Meridians: Liver and kidney
Functions: 1. To nourish blood and replenish essence; 2. To moisten the intestines and move stool; 3. To release toxins

Indications & Combinations:

1. Deficient blood syndrome manifested as sallow complexion, dizziness, vertigo, insomnia, early graying of hair and soreness and weakness in the lumbar region and knees. Fleeceflower root (Heshouwu) is used with Prepared rehmannia root (Shudihuang), Grossy privet fruit (Nüzhenzi), Wolfberry fruit (Gouqizi), Dadder seed (Tusizi) and Mulberry mistletoe (Sangjisheng).

2. Constipation due to dryness in the intestines. Fleeceflower root (Heshouwu) is used with Chinese angelica root (Danggui) and Hemp seed (Huomaren).

3. Chronic malaria due to weakness of the body. Fleeceflower root (Heshouwu) is used with Ginseng (Renshen) and Chinese angelica root (Danggui) in the formula He Ren Yin.

4. Scrofula. Fleeceflower root (Heshouwu) is used with Prunella spike (Xiakucao) and Tendrilled fritillary bulb (Chuanbeimu).

Dosage: 10-30 g

Cautions & Contraindications: This herb is contraindicated in cases with severe phlegm-damp or diarrhea.

292. White peony root (Baishao)

Pharmaceutical Name: Radix Paeoniae alba
Botanical Name: Paeonia lactiflora pall.
Common Name: White peony root
Source of Earliest Record: Shennong Bencao Jing
Part Used & Method for Pharmaceutical Preparations: The white peony roots are dug in summer. The fibrous roots are cleaned and their bark is removed. The roots are then soaked in hot boiled water and dried in the sun. They are soaked again before being cut into slices.
Properties & Taste: Bitter, sour and slightly cold
Meridians: Liver and spleen
Functions: 1. To nourish blood and consolidate the *yin*; 2. To pacify the liver and stop pain; 3. To soothe liver *yang*
Indications & Combinations:

1. Deficiency of blood manifested as irregular menstruation, dysmenorrhea and uterine bleeding. White peony root (Baishao) is used with Chinese angelica root (Danggui), Prepared rehmannia root (Shudihuang) and Chuanxiong rhizome (Chuanxiong) in the formula Siwu Tang.

2. Deficient blood and *yin* leading to the *yang* floating to the surface manifested as night sweating and spontaneous sweating. White peony root (Baishao) is used with Dragon's bone (Longgu), Oyster shell (Muli) and Light wheat (Fuxiaomai).

3. Weakness of the body due to invasion by exogenous pathogenic wind and cold manifested as spontaneous sweating and aversion to wind. White peony root (Baishao) is used with Cinnamon twigs (Guizhi) in the formula Guizhi Tang.

4. Liver *qi* stagnation manifested as hypochondriac pain, breast distension and irregular menstruation. White peony root (Baishao) is used with Bupleurum root (Chaihu) and Chinese angelica root (Danggui) in the formula Xiaoyao San.

5. Muscle spasms and pain of hands and feet or abdominal pain. White peony root (Baishao) is used with Licorice root (Gancao).

6. Abdominal pain and tenesmus in dysentery. White peony root (Baishao) is used with Coptis root (Huanglian), Costus root (Muxiang) and Bitter orange (Zhiqiao).

7. Headache and dizziness caused by hyperactivity of liver *yang*. White peony root (Baishao) is used with Cyathula root (Niuxi), Uncaria stem (Gouteng) and Chrysanthemum flower (Juhua).

Dosage: 5-10 g

Cautions & Contraindications: This herb is contraindicated in cases with cold or deficiency of *yang* syndromes. It counteracts the herb Black false bellebore (Lilu).

293. Donkey hide gelatin (Ejiao)

Pharmaceutical Name: Colla Corii Asini
Zoological Name: Equus asinnus L.
Common Name: Gelatin, Donkey hide gelatin, Ass hide glue
Source of Earliest Record: Shennong Bencao Jing
Part Used & Method for Pharmaceutical Preparations: The glue is fried from the skin of a donkey.
Properties & Taste: Sweet and neutral
Meridians: Lung, liver and kidney
Functions: 1. To nourish blood; 2. To stop bleeding; 3. To replenish *yin* and moisten the lungs
Indications & Combinations:
1. Blood deficiency manifested as dizziness, blurred vision and

palpitations. Donkey hide gelatin (Ejiao) is used with Ginseng (Ren-shen), Chinese angelica root (Danggui) and Prepared rehmannia root (Shudihuang).

2. Hemorrhage manifested as vomiting with blood, epistaxis, bloody stool, excessive menstrual flow, bleeding during pregnancy and uterine bleeding. Donkey hide gelatin (Ejiao) is used with Mugwort leaf (Aiye), Fresh rehmannia root (Shengdihuang), Cattail pollen (Puhuang) and Lotus node (Oujie).

3. *Yin* consumed by febrile disease manifested as irritability and insomnia or spasms and trembling of hands and feet. Donkey hide gelatin (Ejiao) is used with Coptis root (Huanglian), White peony root (Baishao), Uncaria stem (Gouteng) and Oyster shell (Muli).

4. Cough due to deficient *yin* manifested as cough with scanty sputum or cough with bloody sputum, dry mouth, irritability and a thready and rapid pulse. Donkey hide gelatin (Ejiao) is used with Glehnia root (Shashen), Ophiopogon root (Maidong), Apricot seed (Xingren) and Tendrilled fritillary bulb (Chuanbeimu).

Dosage: 5-10 g

Cautions & Contraindications: This herb is contraindicated in cases with weakness of the spleen and stomach manifested as poor appetite and indigestion, or vomiting and diarrhea.

294. Longan aril (Longyanrou)

Pharmaceutical Name: Arillus longan
Botanical Name: Euphoria longan (Lour.) steud.
Common Name: Longan aril, Arillus fruit
Source of Earliest Record: Shennong Bencao Jing
Part Used & Method for Pharmaceutical Preparations: The aril can be collected from the ripe longan in early autumn. Then it is baked or dried in the sunshine.
Properties & Taste: Sweet and warm
Meridians: Heart and spleen
Functions: 1. To nourish blood and tranquilize the mind; 2. To strengthen the spleen and replenish *qi*

Indications & Combinations: Deficiency of *qi* and blood manifested as palpitations, insomnia and forgetfulness. Longan aril (Longyanrou) is used with Ginseng (Renshen), Astragalus root (Huangqi), Chinese angelica root (Danggui) and Wild jujube seed (Suanzaoren) in the formula

Guipi Tang.

Dosage: 10-30 g

Cautions & Contraindications: This herb is contraindicated in cases of phlegm-fire or dampness in the middle *jiao* (spleen and stomach).

d) Herbs That Tonify *Yin*

Herbs that tonify *yin* are used mainly for deficient *yin* syndromes which occur at the later stage of febrile diseases or in chronic diseases. Deficient *yin* syndromes can often be seen as deficient lung *yin*, deficient stomach *yin*, deficient liver *yin* and deficient kidney *yin*. In deficient lung *yin*, manifestations commonly are dry cough, cough with scanty sputum or cough with blood, fever due to *yin* deficiency, and dry mouth and tongue. In deficient stomach *yin*, manifestations are dark red tongue with peeled coating, dry throat, thirst, absence of hunger and constipation. In deficient liver *yin*, the resulting manifestations are dry eyes, blurred vision, dizziness and vertigo. In deficient kidney *yin*, manifestations include soreness and pain in the lower back and knees, feverish sensation on the palms, soles and chest, irritability, insomnia, seminal emissions, and afternoon fever.

In treating these syndromes, herbs that tonify *yin* can be used with herbs that clear heat where manifestations of deficient heat are present. When there is deficient *yin* with excessive heat in the interior, herbs that clear heat due to *yin* deficiency should be added to the combination of herbs. When there is deficient *yin* with hyperactivity of *yang*, herbs that subdue *yang* should be added. In the conditions where deficiency of *yin* is complicated by deficiency of *qi*, herbs that tonify *qi* and herbs that tonify *yin* should be combined.

In general, herbs which are cold or sweet in nature are contraindicated for a person with weakness of the spleen and stomach, internal blockage of phlegm and dampness, abdominal distension or diarrhea.

295. Glehnia root (Shashen)

Pharmaceutical Name: Radix Glehniae

Botanical Name: 1. Glehnia littoralis Fr. Sehmidt ex Miq; 2. Adenophora tetraphylla (Thunb.) Fisch

Common Name: Glehnia root

Source of Earliest Record: Shennong Bencao Jing

Part Used & Method for Pharmaceutical Preparations: The roots are dug in summer or autumn. After the fibrous roots have been removed, the roots are washed in boiled water and the bark peeled off. Then the roots are soaked again before being cut into pieces or slices.

Properties & Taste: Sweet and slightly cold

Meridians: Lung and stomach

Functions: 1. To clear the lungs and tonify *yin*; 2. To strengthen the stomach and promote the production of body fluids

Indications & Combinations:

1. Deficient *yin* of the lungs with heat manifested as dry cough or cough with scanty sputum, hoarse voice from a chronic cough, dry throat and thirst. Glehnia root (Shashen) is used with Ophiopogon root (Maidong) and Tendrilled fritillary bulb (Chuanbeimu).

2. Body fluids consumed by febrile diseases manifested as dry tongue and poor appetite. Glehnia root (Shashen) is used with Ophiopogon root (Maidong), Fresh rehmannia root (Shengdihuang) and Fragrant solomonseal rhizome (Yuzhu) in the formula Yiwei Tang.

Dosage: 10-15 g (15-30 g for the fresh herb)

Cautions & Contraindications: This herb is contraindicated in cases with deficient cold syndrome. Also, it counteracts the herb Black false bellebore (Lilu).

296. Ophiopogon root (Maidong)

Pharmaceutical Name: Radix Ophiopogonis

Botanical Name: 1. Ophiopogon japonicus (Thunb.) Ker-Gawl.; 2. Liriope spicata

Common Name: Ophiopogon root, Lilyturf root

Source of Earliest Record: Shennong Bencao Jing

Part Used & Method for Pharmaceutical Preparations: The tuberous roots are dug in summer. After the fibrous roots have been removed, the roots are dried in the sun.

Properties & Taste: Sweet, slightly bitter and slightly cold

Meridians: Lung, heart and stomach

Functions: 1. To nourish the *yin* and moisten the lungs; 2. To strengthen the stomach and promote the production of body fluids; 3. To clear heat in the heart and relieve irritability

Indications & Combinations:

1. Dryness and heat in the lungs due to deficiency of *yin* manifested as cough with scanty and sticky sputum or cough with bloody sputum.

Ophiopogon root (Maidong) is used with Glehnia root (Shashen), Asparagus root (Tianmendong), Tendrilled fritillary bulb (Chuanbeimu) and Fresh rehmannia root (Shengdihuang).

2. Deficient *yin* of the stomach manifested as dry tongue and thirst. Ophiopogon root (Maidong) is used with Fragrant solomonseal rhizome (Yuzhu), Glehnia root (Shashen) and Fresh rehmannia root (Shengdihuang).

3. Irritability and insomnia: a) nutritive (*ying*) system invaded by pathogenic heat—Ophiopogon root (Maidong) is used with Fresh rehmannia root (Shengdihuang), Bamboo leaf (Zhuye) and Coptis root (Huanglian) in the formula Qingying Tang; b) heart *yin* deficiency with internal heat causing insomnia—Ophiopogon root (Maidong) is used with Fresh rehmannia root (Shengdihuang) and Wild jujube seed (Suanzaoren) in the formula Tianwang Buxin Dan.

4. Constipation caused by dryness in the intestines. Ophiopogon root (Maidong) is used with Fresh rehmannia root (Shengdihuang) and Scrophularia (Xuanshen) in the formula Zengye Tang.

Dosage: 6-15 g

Cautions & Contraindications: This herb is contraindicated in cases with cough due to wind-cold type of common cold, with presence of phlegm fluid and turbid dampness, with diarrhea due to deficiency, and cold in the spleen and stomach.

297. Asparagus root (Tianmendong)

Pharmaceutical Name: Radix Asparagi
Botanical Name: Asparagus cochinchinensis (Lour.) Merr.
Common Name: Asparagus root
Source of Earliest Record: Shennong Bencao Jing
Part Used & Method for Pharmaceutical Preparations: The tuberous roots are dug in autumn. After the fibrous roots have been removed, the roots are boiled in hot water or steamed, and soaked again in clear water. The roots are then dried in the sun or baked. Finally, they are cut into slices.
Properties & Taste: Sweet, bitter and very cold
Meridians: Lung and kidney
Functions: 1. To clear the lungs and descend fire; 2. To nourish the *yin* and moisten dryness
Indications & Combinations:

1. Flaring up of fire caused by deficient *yin* of the lungs and kidneys manifested as scanty and sticky sputum or cough with bloody sputum. Asparagus root (Tianmendong) is used with Ophiopogon root (Maidong) in the formula Erdong Gao.

2. Consumption of *yin* and *qi* by febrile disease manifested as thirst, shortness of breath or diabetes. Asparagus root (Tianmendong) is used with Fresh rehmannia root (Shengdihuang) and Ginseng (Renshen) in the formula Sancai Tang.

3. Constipation due to dryness in the intestines. Asparagus root (Tianmendong) is used with Chinese angelica root (Danggui) and Cistanche (Roucongrong).

Dosage: 6-15 g

Cautions & Contraindications: The herb is contraindicated in cases with deficiency and cold in the spleen and stomach, poor appetite or diarrhea.

298. Dendrobium (Shihu)

Pharmaceutical Name: Herba Dendrobii

Botanical Name: 1. Dendrobium nobile Lindl.; 2. Dendrobium loddigesii Rolfe.; 3. Dendrobium candidum Wall. ex Lindl.; 4. Dendrobium chrysanthum Wall.; 5. Dendrobium fimbriatum Hook. var. oculatum Hook.

Common Name: Dendrobium

Source of Earliest Record: Shennong Bencao Jing

Part Used & Method for Pharmaceutical Preparations: The stems are gathered in the period between summer and autumn, dried in the sun and cut into pieces.

Properties & Taste: Sweet and slightly cold

Meridians: Lung and kidney

Functions: 1. To tonify the *yin* and clear heat; 2. To promote the production of body fluids and nourish the stomach

Indications & Combinations:

1. *Yin* consumed by febrile diseases or deficient *yin* in the stomach manifested as dry tongue, thirst and red tongue proper with scanty coating. Dendrobium (Shihu) is used with Ophiopogon root (Maidong), Glehnia root (Shashen) and Fresh rehmannia root (Shengdihuang).

2. Afternoon fever caused by deficient *yin* and internal heat. Dendrobium (Shihu) is used with Fresh rehmannia root (Shengdihuang),

Swallowwort root (Baiwei) and Asparagus root (Tianmendong).

Dosage: 6-15 g

Cautions & Contraindications: This herb should be cooked first before the other herbs are added to the decoction. It is contraindicated for a person in the early stage of febrile disease.

299. Fragrant solomonseal rhizome (Yuzhu)

Pharmaceutical Name: Rhizoma Polygonati odorati

Botanical Name: Polygonatum odoratum (Mill.) Druce

Common Name: Polygonatum rhizome, Fragrant solomonseal rhizome

Source of Earliest Record: Shennong Bencao Jing

Part Used & Method for Pharmaceutical Preparations: The rhizomes are dug in summer and autumn. After the fibrous roots have been removed, the rhizomes are dried in the sun or steamed, and cut into pieces.

Properties & Taste: Sweet and neutral

Meridians: Lung and stomach

Functions: 1. To nourish the *yin* and moisten the lungs; 2. To promote the production of body fluids and strengthen the stomach

Indications & Combinations: Dry cough with scanty sputum due to lung *yin* deficiency or thirst and intense hunger due to stomach *yin* deficiency. Fragrant solomonseal rhizome (Yuzhu) is used with Glehnia root (Shashen), Ophiopogon root (Maidong) and Asparagus root (Tianmendong).

Dosage: 10-15 g

Cautions & Contraindications: This herb is contraindicated in cases with deficient spleen or phlegm-damp.

300. Siberian solomonseal (Huangjing)

Pharmaceutical Name: Rhizome Polygonati

Botanical Name: 1. Polygonatum sibiricum Red.; 2. Polygonatum cyrtonema Hua; 3. Polygonatum kingianum Coll., et Hemsl.

Common Name: Siberian solomonseal rhizome

Source of Earliest Record: Mingyi Bielu

Part Used & Method for Pharmaceutical Preparations: The rhizomes are dug in autumn. After the fibrous root have been removed, the rhizomes are dried in the sun and cut into slices.

244

Properties & Taste: Sweet and neutral

Meridians: Spleen, lung and kidney

Functions: 1. To nourish the *yin* and moisten the lungs; 2. To tonify the spleen and promote *qi*

Indications & Combinations:

1. Cough due to lung *yin* deficiency. Siberian solomonseal (Huangjing) is used with Glehnia root (Shashen), Tendrilled fritillary bulb (Chuanbeimu) and Anemarrhena rhizome (Zhimu).

2. Kidney essence deficiency manifested as soreness in the lower back, dizziness and heat in the feet. Siberian solomonseal (Huangjing) is used with Wolfberry fruit (Gouqizi) and Grossy privet fruit (Nüzhenzi).

3. Deficient *qi* of the spleen and stomach manifested as lassitude, poor appetite and weak and forceless pulse. Siberian solomonseal (Huangjing) is used with Pilose asiabell root (Dangshen) and White atractylodes (Baizhu).

4. Deficient *yin* of the spleen and stomach manifested as poor appetite, dry mouth, constipation and red tongue proper with no coating. Siberian solomonseal (Huangjing) is used with Glehnia root (Shashen), Ophiopogon root (Maidong) and Germinated millet (Guya).

5. Diabetes. Siberian solomonseal (Huangjing) is used with Astragalus root (Huangqi), Trichosanthes root (Tianhuafen), Ophiopogon root (Maidong) and Fresh rehmannia root (Shengdihuang).

Dosage: 10-20 g (30-60 g for the fresh herb)

Cautions & Contraindications: This herb is contraindicated in cases of deficient spleen with dampness or cough with profuse sputum or diarrhea due to cold in the spleen and stomach.

301. Lily bulb (Baihe)

Pharmaceutical Name: Bulbus Lilii

Botanical Name: 1. Lilium brownii var. viridulum Baker; 2. Lilium pumilum DC.; 3. Lilium lancifolium Thunb.

Common Name: Lily bulb

Source of Earliest Record: Shennong Bencao Jing

Part Used & Method for Pharmaceutical Preparations: The bulbs are gathered in autumn. After they are cleaned, the bulbs are washed in boiled water or steamed, then dried in the sun or baked.

Properties & Taste: Sweet and slightly cold

Meridians: Lung and heart

Functions: 1. To moisten the lungs and stop cough; 2. To clear heat in the heart and calm the mind

Indications & Combinations:

1. Deficient *yin* of the lung with excessive fire manifested as cough and hemoptysis. Lily bulb (Baihe) is used with Scrophularia (Xuanshen), Tendrilled fritillary bulb (Chuanbeimu) and Fresh rehmannia root (Shengdihuang) in the formula Baihe Gujin Tang.

2. The later stage of febrile diseases with residual heat manifested as irritability, palpitations, insomnia and dreamful sleep. Lily bulb (Baihe) is used with Anemarrhena rhizome (Zhimu) and Fresh rehmannia root (Shengdihuang) in the formula Baihe Dihuang Tang.

Dosage: 10–30 g

Cautions & Contraindications: This herb is contraindicated in cases of cough due to invasion by wind-cold or diarrhea due to cold in the spleen and stomach.

302. Wolfberry fruit (Gouqizi)

Pharmaceutical Name: Fructus Lycii

Botanical Name: Lycium barbarum L.

Common Name: Wolfberry fruit, Lycium fruit

Source of Earliest Record: Shennong Bencao Jing

Part Used & Method for Pharmaceutical Preparations: The ripe fruit is gathered in the period around the Summer Solstice (tenth solar term), and then it is dried in the shade.

Properties & Taste: Sweet and neutral

Meridians: Liver, kidney and lung

Functions: 1. To tonify kidneys and promote the production of essence; 2. To nourish the liver and brighten the eyes; 3. To moisten the lungs

Indications & Combinations:

1. Deficient *yin* of the liver and kidneys manifested as dizziness, blurred vision and decreased eyesight. Wolfberry fruit (Gouqizi) is used with Chrysanthemum flower (Juhua) and Prepared rehmannia root (Shudihuang) in the formula Qiju Dihuang Wan.

2. Deficient *yin* of the liver and kidneys manifested as soreness of the lower back and knees and nocturnal emissions. Wolfberry fruit (Gouqizi) is used with Prepared rehmannia root (Shudihuang) and

Asparagus root (Tianmendong).

3. Deficient *yin* of the lungs manifested as cough. Wolfberry fruit (Gouqizi) is used with Ophiopogon root (Maidong), Anemarrhena rhizome (Zhimu) and Tendrilled fritillary bulb (Chuanbeimu).

Dosage: 5-10 g

Cautions & Contraindications: This herb is contraindicated in cases of diarrhea due to deficient spleen.

303. Mulberry (Sangshen)

Pharmaceutical Name: Fructus Mori

Botanical Name: Morus alba L.

Common Name: Mulberry, Morus fruit

Source of Earliest Record: Xinxiu Bencao

Part Used & Method for Pharmaceutical Preparations: The ripe fruit is gathered from April to June. It is cleaned and dried in the sun.

Properties & Taste: Sweet and cold

Meridians: Heart, liver and kidney

Functions: 1. To nourish the *yin* and replenish the blood; 2. To promote the production of body fluids and stop thirst; 3. To moisten the intestines and move feces

Indications & Combinations:

1. Deficient *yin* and blood manifested as dizziness, vertigo, blurred vision, tinnitus, deafness, insomnia and early graying of hair. Mulberry (Sangshen) is used with Fleeceflower root (Heshouwu), Grossy privet fruit (Nüzhenzi) and Eclipta (Mohanlian) in the formula Shouwu Yanshou Dan.

2. Thirst and dry mouth due to deficient body fluids or diabetes manifested as thirst with desire to drink, profuse urine and lassitude. Mulberry (Sangshen) is used with Ophiopogon root (Maidong), Grossy privet fruit (Nüzhenzi) and Trichosanthes root (Tianhuafen).

3. Constipation due to dryness in the intestines. Mulberry (Sangshen) is used with Black sesame seed (Heizhima), raw Fleeceflower root (Heshouwu) and Hemp seed (Huomaren).

Dosage: 10-15 g

Cautions & Contraindications: This herb is contraindicated in cases with diarrhea due to cold and deficiency of the spleen and stomach.

304. Eclipta (Mohanlian)

Pharmaceutical Name: Herba Ecliptae
Botanical Name: Eclipta prostrata L.
Common Name: Eclipta
Source of Earliest Record: Xinxiu Bencao
Part Used & Method for Pharmaceutical Preparations: The aerial parts of the plant are gathered in early autumn, dried in the sun and cut into pieces.

Properties & Taste: Sweet, sour and cold
Meridians: Liver and kidney
Functions: 1. To nourish *yin* and tonify the kidneys; 2. To cool the blood and stop bleeding
Indications & Combinations:

1. Deficient *yin* of the liver and kidneys manifested as early graying of hair, dizziness, vertigo and blurred vision. Eclipta (Mohanlian) is used with Grossy privet fruit (Nüzhenzi) in the formula Erzhi Wan.

2. Deficient *yin* with internal heat causing extravasation of blood manifested as vomiting with blood, epistaxis, hematuria, bloody stool and uterine bleeding. Eclipta (Mohanlian) is used with Fresh rehmannia root (Shengdihuang), Donkey hide gelatin (Ejiao), Imperata rhizome (Baimaogen) and Cattail pollen (Puhuang).

3. Hemorrhage due to external injuries. Eclipta (Mohanlian) is used alone for external use to stop bleeding.

Dosage: 10-15 g (double dosage for the fresh herb)
Cautions & Contraindications: This herb is contraindicated in cases with diarrhea due to cold and deficiency of the spleen and stomach.

305. Grossy privet fruit (Nüzhenzi)

Pharmaceutical Name: Fructus Ligustri lucidi
Botanical Name: Ligustrum lucidum Ait.
Common Name: Ligustrum seed, Grossy privet fruit
Source of Earliest Record: Shennong Bencao Jing
Part Used & Method for Pharmaceutical Preparations: The ripe fruit is gathered in autumn, then steamed and dried in the sun.

Properties & Taste: Sweet, bitter and cool
Meridians: Liver and kidney
Functions: 1. To tonify the liver and kidneys; 2. To clear heat and brighten the eyes

Indications & Combinations:

1. Deficient *yin* of the liver and kidneys manifested as early graying of hair, decreased eyesight, dryness of eyes, tinnitus and soreness and weakness of the lower back and knees. Grossy privet fruit (Nüzhenzi) is used with Mulberry (Sangshen), Eclipta (Mohanlian) and Wolfberry fruit (Gouqizi).

2. Deficient *yin* and heat. Grossy privet fruit (Nüzhenzi) is used with Wolfberry bark (Digupi), Moutan bark (Mudanpi) and Fresh rehmannia root (Shengdihuang).

Dosage: 10-15 g

Cautions & Contraindications: This herb is contraindicated in cases with diarrhea due to cold and deficiency of the spleen and stomach, or *yang* deficiency.

306. Tortoise plastron (Guiban)

Pharmaceutical Name: Plastrum Testudinis
Zoological Name: Clinemys reevesii (Gray)
Common Name: Tortoise plastron
Source of Earliest Record: Shennong Bencao Jing
Part Used & Method for Pharmaceutical Preparations: The plastron of a freshwater tortoise can be obtained all year round. It is cleaned and dried in the sun.

Properties: Sweet, salty and cold
Meridians: Liver, kidney and heart
Functions: 1. To nourish *yin* and subdue *yang*; 2. To tonify the kidneys and strengthen the bones

Indications & Combinations:

1. Hyperactivity of liver *yang* due to deficient *yin* of the liver and kidneys manifested as dizziness, distension and pain in the head and blurred vision. Tortoise plastron (Guiban) is used with White peony root (Baishao), Cyathula root (Niuxi), Sea-ear shell (Shijueming) and Uncaria stem (Gouteng).

2. Malnutrition of tendons and muscles due to *yin* consumed by febrile diseases manifested as spasms and convulsions of hands and feet. Tortoise plastron (Guiban) is used with Donkey hide gelatin (Ejiao), Fresh rehmannia root (Shengdihuang) and Oyster shell (Muli).

3. Deficient *yin* of the liver and kidney manifested as soreness and weakness of the lower back and knees and fragile bones and tendons.

Tortoise plastron (Guiban) is used with Cyathula root (Niuxi), Dragon's bone (Longgu) and Prepared rehmannia root (Shudihuang).

4. Deficient *yin* and excessive fire manifested as afternoon fever, cough with blood, night sweating and seminal emissions. Tortoise plastron (Guiban) is used with Prepared rehmannia root (Shudihuang) in the formula Da Buyin Wan.

5. Derangement of mind by deficiency of *yin* and blood manifested as insomnia, forgetfulness, palpitations and fright. Tortoise plastron (Guiban) is used with Dragon's bone (Longgu), Grass-leaved sweetflag (Shichangpu) and Polygala root (Yuanzhi) in the formula Kongsheng Zhenzhong Dan.

6. Deficient *yin* and heat in the blood manifested as excessive menstruation and uterine bleeding. Tortoise plastron (Guiban) is used with Fresh rehmannia root (Shengdihuang) and Eclipta (Mohanlian).

Dosage: 10-30 g (The herb is cooked first, then additional herbs are added for decoction.)

Cautions & Contraindications: This herb should be used with caution during pregnancy.

307. Turtle shell (Biejia)

Pharmaceutical Name: Carapax Trionycis
Zoological Name: Trionyx sinensis Wiegmann
Common Name: Fresh-water turtle shell
Source of Earliest Record: Shennong Bencao Jing
Part Used & Method for Pharmaceutical Preparations: The shell can be removed after the turtle has been boiled for one or two hours.
Properties & Taste: Salty and cold
Meridian: Liver
Functions: 1. To nourish *yin* and subdue *yang*; 2. To soften hardness and disperse nodules
Indications & Combinations:

1. Internal stirring of endogenous wind following the later stage of febrile disease in which *yin* and body fluids are consumed or tendons and muscles are not nourished manifested as tremulous fingers, spasms and convulsions, thready and rapid pulse and dry tongue proper with scanty coating. Turtle shell (Biejia) is used with Oyster shell (Muli), Fresh rehmannia root (Shengdihuang), Donkey hide gelatin (Ejiao) and White peony root (Baishao) in the formula Erjia Fumai Tang.

2. Deficient *yin* with fever: a) deficient *yin* and body fluids at the later stage of febrile disease manifested as night fever and subsiding in the morning without sweating and red tongue with scanty coating. Turtle shell (Biejia) is used with Sweet wormwood (Qinghao) and Moutan bark (Mudanpi) in the formula Qinghao Biejia Tang; b) deficient *yin* with internal heat manifested as afternoon fever and night sweating. Turtle shell (Biejia) is used with Stellaria root (Yinchaihu) and Wolfberry bark (Digupi) in the formula Qinggu San.

3. Chronic malaria with amenorrhea manifested as hypochondriac pain and hard, palpable masses in the epigastric and abdominal regions. Turtle shell (Biejia) is used with Burreed tuber (Sanleng), Zedoary (Ezhu), Moutan bark (Mudanpi) and Rhubarb (Dahuang).

Dosage: 10-30 g

Cautions & Contraindications: This herb is contraindicated in cases with deficiency and cold in the spleen and stomach with poor appetite and diarrhea, and during pregnancy.

308. Black sesame seed (Heizhima)

Pharmaceutical Name: Semen Sesami
Botanical Name: Sesamum indicum nigrum L.
Common Name: Black sesame seed
Source of Earliest Record: Shennong Bencao Jing
Part Used & Method for Pharmaceutical Preparations: The ripe sesame seeds are gathered in autumn, then they are dried in the sun.
Properties & Taste: Sweet and neutral
Meridians: Liver and kidney
Functions: 1. To tonify the essence and blood; 2. To moisten the intestines and move feces
Indications & Combinations:

1. Deficient essence and blood manifested as dizziness, blurred vision and early graying of the hair. Black sesame seed (Heizhima) is used with Mulberry leaf (Sangye) in the formula Sang Ma Wan.

2. Constipation due to dryness in the intestines. Black sesame seed (Heizhima) is used with Chinese angelica root (Danggui), Cistanche (Roucongrong) and Arborvitae seed (Baiziren).

Dosage: 10-30 g (The herb is most effective when fried.)

Cautions & Contraindications: This herb should not be used in cases with diarrhea.

XVIII. Astringent Herbs

Astringent herbs, being sour and astringent in nature, stop sweating, check diarrhea, control essence, hold in urine and stop leukorrhea, bleeding and coughing. They are indicated in cases with weakness from chronic disease or unconsolidated anti-pathogenic factors which lead to spontaneous sweating, night sweating, chronic diarrhea, chronic dysentery, seminal emissions, nocturnal emissions, enuresis, frequent urination, chronic cough and asthma, or uterine bleeding, leukorrhea and prolapse of the uterus or rectum.

Astringent herbs relieve symptoms so as to prevent the anti-pathogenic factor from weakening. In order to treat the symptoms and the root cause simultaneously, corresponding tonifying herbs should be added to the combination.

Astringent herbs should not be used while pathogenic factors are in the exterior, there is interior accumulation of dampness or accumulated heat exists.

309. Schisandra fruit (Wuweizi)

Pharmaceutical Name: Fructus Schisandrae

Botanical Name: 1. Schisandra chinensis (Turcz.) Baill.; 2. Schizandra sphenanthera Rehd. et Wils.

Common Name: Schisandra fruit

Source of Earliest Record: Shennong Bencao Jing

Part Used & Method for Pharmaceutical Preparations: The ripe fruit is gathered in autumn and dried in the sun.

Properties & Taste: Sour and warm

Meridians: Lung, kidney and heart

Functions: 1. To astringe the lungs and nourish the kidneys; 2. To promote the production of body fluids and astringe sweat; 3. To restrain the essence and stop diarrhea; 4. To calm the heart and soothe the mind

Indications & Combinations:

1. Chronic cough and asthma due to rebellion of lung *qi* caused by deficiency of the lungs and kidneys manifested as cough with scanty sputum and asthma aggravated by slight exertion. Schisandra fruit (Wuweizi) is used with Dogwood fruit (Shanzhuyu), Prepared rehmannia root (Shudihuang) and Ophiopogon root (Maidong) in the formula Baxian Changshou Wan.

2. Deficiency of *qi* and body fluids manifested as spontaneous sweating, night sweating, thirst, palpitations, shortness of breath and deficient and forceless pulse. Schisandra fruit (Wuweizi) is used with Ginseng (Renshen) and Ophiopogon root (Maidong) in the formula Shengmai San.

3. Diabetes manifested as thirst, preference for excessive fluid intake, shortness of breath, lassitude and deficient and forceless pulse. Schisandra fruit (Wuweizi) is used with Astragalus root (Huangqi), Fresh rehmannia root (Shengdihuang), Ophiopogon root (Maidong) and Trichosanthes root (Tianhuafen) in the formula Huangqi Tang.

4. Seminal emissions and nocturnal emissions caused by deficiency of the kidneys. Schisandra fruit (Wuweizi) is used with Dragon's bone (Longgu) and Mantis egg case (Sangpiaoxiao).

5. Chronic diarrhea caused by deficiency of the spleen and kidneys. Schisandra fruit (Wuweizi) is used with Nutmeg (Roudoukou) and Evodia fruit (Wuzhuyu) in the formula Sishen Wan.

6. Deficient *yin* and blood of the heart and kidneys manifested as palpitations, irritability, insomnia, dreamful sleep and forgetfulness. Schisandra fruit (Wuweizi) is used with Fresh rehmannia root (Shengdihuang), Ophiopogon root (Maidong) and Wild jujube seed (Suanzaoren) in the formula Tianwang Buxin Dan.

Dosage: 2-6 g

Cautions & Contraindications: This herb is contraindicated in the early stage of cough or rubella and in excessive internal heat with unrelieved exterior syndrome.

310. Black plum (Wumei)

Pharmaceutical Name: Fructus Mume
Botanical Name: Prunus mume (Sieb.) Sieb. et Zucc.
Common Name: Black plum, Mume
Source of Earliest Record: Shennong Bencao Jing
Part Used & Method for Pharmaceutical Preparations: The unripe fruit is gathered in the period at the Beginning of Summer (seventh solar term). It is baked at a low temperature until the skins turn black. The plum stone is removed.
Properties & Taste: Sour and neutral
Meridians: Spleen, lung and large intestine
Functions: 1. To astringe the lungs and stop cough; 2. To restrain

the intestines and stop diarrhea; 3. To promote the production of body fluids; 4. To expel roundworms

Indications & Combinations:

1. Chronic cough due to deficiency of the lungs. Black plum (Wumei) is used with Poppy capsule (Yingsuqiao), Donkey hide gelatin (Ejiao) and Apricot seed (Xingren).

2. Chronic diarrhea or dysentery. Black plum (Wumei) is used with Nutmeg (Roudoukou), Chebula fruit (Hezi) and Poppy capsule (Yingsuqiao).

3. Acute dysentery. Black plum (Wumei) is used with Coptis root (Huanglian).

4. Diabetes. Black plum (Wumei) is used with Trichosanthes root (Tianhuafen), Ophiopogon root (Maidong), Ginseng (Renshen) and Pueraria root (Gegen).

5. Roundworms in the biliary tract manifested as abdominal pain, nausea and vomiting. Black plum (Wumei) is used with Asarum herb (Xixin) and Coptis root (Huanglian) in the formula Wumei Wan.

Dosage: 3-30 g

Cautions & Contraindications: This herb is contraindicated in cases with exterior syndrome or accumulation of excessive heat in the interior.

311. Light wheat (Fuxiaomai)

Pharmaceutical Name: Fructus Tritici levis

Botanical Name: Triticum aestivum

Common Name: Light wheat

Source of Earliest Record: Bencao Mengquan

Part Used & Method for Pharmaceutical Preparations: The light grain is first soaked in water and then dried.

Properties & Taste: Sweet and cool

Meridian: Heart

Functions: 1. To tonify *qi* and clear heat; 2. To stop sweating

Indications & Combinations: Weakness of the body manifested as spontaneous sweating or night sweating. Light wheat (Fuxiaomai) is used with Oyster shell (Muli), Astragalus root (Huangqi) and Ephedra root (Mahuanggen) in the formula Muli San.

Dosage: 15-30 g

312. Ephedra root (Mahuanggen)

Pharmaceutical Name: Radix Ephedrae
Botanical Name: 1. Ephedra sinica stapf; 2. Ephedra equisetina Bge.; 3. Ephedra intermedia schrenk et C. A. Mey.
Common Name: Ephedra root
Source of Earliest Record: Mingyi Bielu
Part Used & Method for Pharmaceutical Preparations: The roots are dug in the period of the Beginning of Autumn (thirteenth solar term). After the fibrous roots have been removed, the roots are cleaned and cut into pieces.
Properties & Taste: Sweet and neutral
Meridian: Lung
Functions: To stop sweating
Indications & Combinations:

1. Spontaneous sweating. Ephedra root (Mahuanggen) is used with Astragalus root (Huangqi) and Chinese angelica root (Danggui).

2. Night sweating. Ephedra root (Mahuanggen) is used with Fresh rehmannia root (Shengdihuang) and Oyster shell (Muli).

Dosage: 3-10 g
Cautions & Contraindications: This herb is contraindicated in cases with exterior syndromes.

313. Ailanthus bark (Chunpi)

Pharmaceutical Name: Cortex ailanthi
Botanical Name: Ailanthus altissima (Mill.) Swingle
Common Name: Ailanthus bark, Tree of heaven bark
Source of Earliest Record: Xinxiu Bencao
Part Used & Method for Pharmaceutical Preparations: The bark of roots or stems of the tree are obtained year round. After the superficial rough bark has been removed, the remaining bark is dried in the sun and then cut into pieces.
Properties & Taste: Bitter, astringent and cold
Meridians: Large intestine, stomach and liver
Functions: 1. To clear heat, dry dampness and stop leukorrhea; 2. To astringe the intestines; 3. To stop bleeding; 4. To kill worms
Indications & Combinations:

1. Damp-heat type of diarrhea or dysentery. Ailanthus bark (Chunpi) is used with Coptis root (Huanglian), Scutellaria root (Huangqin)

and Costus root (Muxiang).

2. Yellow leukorrhea due to damp-heat. Ailanthus bark (Chunpi) is used with Phellodendron bark (Huangbai).

3. Menorrhagia or uterine bleeding caused by heat in the blood. Ailanthus bark (Chunpi) is used with Tortoise plastron (Guiban), White peony root (Baishao) and Scutellaria root (Huangqin).

Dosage: 3-5 g

314. Chebula fruit (Hezi)

Pharmaceutical Name: Fructus Chebulae
Botanical Name: 1. Terminalia chebula Retz.; 2. Terminalia chebula Retz. var. tomentella Kurt.
Common Name: Terminalia fruit, Chebula fruit
Source of Earliest Record: Yaoxing Lun
Part Used & Method for Pharmaceutical Preparations: The ripe fruit is gathered from July to August and dried in the sun.
Properties & Taste: Bitter, sour, astringent and neutral
Meridians: Lung and large intestine
Functions: 1. To astringe the intestines; 2. To astringe the lungs
Indications & Combinations:

1. Chronic diarrhea, chronic dysentery and prolapsed anus: a) heat syndrome—Chebula fruit (Hezi) is used with Coptis root (Huanglian) and Costus root (Muxiang) in the formula Hezi San; b) deficiency and cold syndrome—Chebula fruit (Hezi) is used with Dried ginger (Ganjiang) and Poppy capsule (Yingsuqiao).

2. Cough and asthma due to deficiency in lungs or chronic cough with hoarse voice. Chebula fruit (Hezi) is used with Platycodon root (Jiegeng), Licorice root (Gancao) and Apricot seed (Xingren).

Dosage: 3-10 g (The raw herb is used for hoarse voice, the baked herb for diarrhea.)

Cautions & Contraindications: This herb is contraindicated in cases with exterior syndrome and during accumulation of damp-heat in the interior.

315. Nutmeg (Roudoukou)

Pharmaceutical Name: Semen Myristicae
Botanical Name: Myristica fragrans Houtt.
Common Name: Nutmeg

Source of Earliest Record: Yaoxing Lun

Part Used & Method for Pharmaceutical Preparations: The seeds are removed from the ripe fruit and dried in the sun.

Properties & Taste: Pungent and warm

Meridians: Spleen, stomach and large intestine

Functions: 1. To warm the spleen and stomach and promote circulation of *qi*; 2. To astringe the intestines and stop diarrhea

Indications & Combinations:

1. Chronic diarrhea. Nutmeg (Roudoukou) is used with Chebula fruit (Hezi), White atractylodes (Baizhu) and Pilose asiabell root (Dangshen).

2. *Qi* stagnation due to deficiency and cold in the spleen and stomach manifested as epigastric and abdominal pain, vomiting and nausea. Nutmeg (Roudoukou) is used with Costus root (Muxiang), Fresh ginger (Shengjiang) and Pinellia tuber (Banxia).

Dosage: 3-10 g (1.5-3 g for pills or powder form)

Cautions & Contraindications: This herb is contraindicated in cases with damp-heat diarrhea or dysentery.

316. Poppy capsule (Yingsuqiao)

Pharmaceutical Name: Pericarpium Papaveris

Botanical Name: Papaver somniferum L.

Common Name: Opium poppy capsule, Poppy capsule

Source of Earliest Record: Kaibao Bencao

Part Used & Method for Pharmaceutical Preparations: The capsules are gathered in summer. After the seeds are removed, the capsules are dried in the sun, and then they are fried with honey.

Properties & Taste: Sour, astringent, neutral and toxic

Meridians: Lung, large intestine and kidney

Functions: 1. To astringe the lungs; 2. To astringe the intestines; 3. To stop pain

Indications & Combinations:

1. Chronic cough due to deficiency of the lungs. Poppy capsule (Yingsuqiao) is used with Black plum (Wumei).

2. Chronic diarrhea or chronic dysentery. Poppy capsule (Yingsuqiao) is used with Coptis root (Huanglian), Costus root (Muxiang) and Dried ginger (Ganjiang).

3. Pain. Poppy capsule (Yingsuqiao) is used alone for the treatment

of pain.

Dosage: 3-10 g (Fried with honey, the herb is used for cough; prepared with vinegar, for diarrhea with pain.)

Cautions & Contraindications: This herb is contraindicated in the early stage of cough and dysentery. Care should be taken to avoid overdosing.

317. Lotus seed (Lianzi)

Pharmaceutical Name: Semen Nelumbinis
Botanical Name: Nelumbo nucifera Gaertn.
Common Name: Lotus seed
Source of Earliest Record: Shennong Bencao Jing
Part Used & Method for Pharmaceutical Preparations: The lotus seeds are collected from August to September. After the skins of the seeds have been removed, the seeds are dried in the sun.
Properties & Taste: Sweet, astringent and neutral
Meridians: Spleen, kidney and heart
Functions: 1. To tonify the spleen and stop diarrhea; 2. To reinforce the kidneys and control the essence; 3. To nourish the blood and tranquilize the mind
Indications & Combinations:

1. Palpitations, insomnia and irritability. Lotus seed (Lianzi) is used with Wild jujube seed (Suanzaoren), Arborvitae seed (Baiziren) and Poria with hostwood (Fushen).

2. Kidney deficiency manifested as seminal emissions or leukorrhagia. Lotus seed (Lianzi) is used with Dadder seed (Tusizi), Dioscorea (Shanyao) and Euryale seed (Qianshi).

3. Chronic diarrhea due to deficiency of the spleen. Lotus seed (Lianzi) is used with White atractylodes (Baizhu), Dioscorea (Shanyao) and Poria (Fuling).

Dosage: 6-15 g

Cautions & Contraindications: This herb is contraindicated in cases with constipation.

318. Euryale seed (Qianshi)

Pharmaceutical Name: Semen Euryales
Botanical Name: Euryale ferox Salisb.
Common Name: Euryale seed

Source of Earliest Record: Shennong Bencao Jing

Part Used & Method for Pharmaceutical Preparations: The ripe seeds are collected from August to September. The seeds are shelled, dried in the sun and pounded into pieces.

Properties & Taste: Sweet, astringent and neutral

Meridians: Spleen and kidney

Functions: 1. To tonify the spleen and stop diarrhea; 2. To strengthen the kidneys and control essence; 3. To dispel dampness and relieve leukorrhea

Indications & Combinations:

1. Chronic diarrhea due to deficiency of the spleen. Euryale seed (Qianshi) is used with White atractylodes (Baizhu) and Dioscorea (Shanyao).

2. Seminal emissions or leukorrhea. Euryale seed (Qianshi) is used with Flattened milkvetch seed (Shayuanzi) and Cherokee rose hips (Jinyingzi).

Dosage: 10-15 g

319. Dogwood fruit (Shanzhuyu)

Pharmaceutical Name: Fructus Corni

Botanical Name: Cornus officinalis Sieb. et Zucc.

Common Name: Cornus fruit, Dogwood fruit

Source of Earliest Record: Shennong Bencao Jing

Part Used & Method for Pharmaceutical Name: The ripe fruit is gathered from October to November. The fruit is baked or boiled, after which the fruit pit is removed. The fruit is then dried in the sun or baked again.

Properties & Taste: Sour and slightly warm

Meridians: Liver and kidney

Functions: 1. To tonify the liver and kidneys; 2. To astringe the essence; 3. To stop sweating

Indications & Combinations:

1. Deficiency of the liver and kidneys manifested as dizziness, blurred vision, soreness in the lower back, weakness of the legs, seminal emissions and impotence. Dogwood fruit (Shanzhuyu) is used with Prepared rehmannia root (Shudihuang), Dadder seed (Tusizi), Wolfberry fruit (Gouqizi) and Eucommia bark (Duzhong).

2. Spontaneous sweating due to weakness of the body. Dogwood

fruit (Shanzhuyu) is used with Ginseng (Renshen), Prepared aconite root (Fuzi) and Oyster shell (Muli).

Dosage: 5-10 g

Cautions & Contraindications: This herb is contraindicated in cases with damp-heat or dysuria.

320. Cherokee rose hips (Jinyingzi)

Pharmaceutical Name: Fructus Rosae laevigatae
Botanical Name: Rosa laevigata Michx.
Common Name: Rosa fruit, Cherokee rose hips
Source of Earliest Record: Shu Bencao
Part Used & Method for Pharmaceutical Preparations: The ripe fruit is gathered from September to October. After the fruit pits have been removed, the fruit is cleaned and dried in the sun.
Properties & Taste: Sour, astringent and neutral
Meridians: Kidney, urinary bladder and large intestine
Functions: 1. To control the essence; 2. To astringe the intestines and stop diarrhea; 3. To decrease urination
Indications & Combinations:

1. Deficiency of the kidneys manifested as seminal emissions, nocturnal enuresis or leukorrhagia. Cherokee rose hips (Jinyingzi) is used with Euryale seed (Qianshi) and Dadder seed (Tusizi).

2. Chronic diarrhea due to deficiency of the spleen. Cherokee rose hips (Jinyingzi) is used with Pilose asiabell root (Dangshen), White atractylodes (Baizhu) and Dioscorea (Shanyao).

Dosage: 6-18 g

Cautions & Contraindications: This herb is contraindicated in cases with excessive fire or excessive pathogenic factors.

321. Mantis egg case (Sangpiaoxiao)

Pharmaceutical Name: Oötheca Mantidis
Zoological Name: 1. Tenodera sinensis Saussure; 2. Statilia maculata (Thunb.); 3. Hierodula patellifera (Serville)
Common Name: Mantis egg case
Source of Earliest Record: Shennong Bencao Jing
Part Use & Method for Pharmaceutical Preparations: The egg case is collected in late autumn or spring, and then boiled or steamed and dried in the sun.

260

Properties & Taste: Sweet, salty and neutral

Meridians: Liver and kidney

Functions: 1. To tonify the kidneys and strengthen *yang*; 2. To control essence and decrease urination

Indications & Combinations: Deficient *yang* of the kidneys manifested as seminal emissions, nocturnal enuresis or leukorrhea. Mantis egg case (Sangpiaoxiao) is used with Dragon's bone (Longgu), Oyster shell (Muli), Dadder seed (Tusizi) and Psoralea fruit (Buguzhi).

Dosage: 3-10 g

Cautions & Contraindications: This substance is contraindicated in cases with deficient *yin* with excessive fire, or heat in the urinary bladder with frequent urine.

322. Cuttlefish bone (Wuzeigu)

Pharmaceutical Name: Os Sepiae seu Sepiellae

Zoological Name: 1. Sepiella maindroni de Rochebrune; 2. Sepia esculenta Hoyle

Common Name: Cuttlefish bone, Cuttlebone

Source of Earliest Record: Shennong Bencao Jing

Part Used & Method for Pharmaceutical Preparations: The cuttlefish is caught from April to August. The bone is removed from the fish and dried for twenty-four hours.

Properties & Taste: Salty, astringent and slightly warm

Meridians: Liver and kidney

Functions: 1. To astringe and stop bleeding; 2. To control the essence and relieve leukorrhea; 3. To restrain hyperacidity and stop pain; 4. To promote healing of ulcers

Indications & Combinations:

1. Hemorrhage. Cuttlefish bone (Wuzeigu) is used with Rubia root (Qiancao), Carbonized petiole of windmill palm (Zonglütan) and Donkey hide gelatin (Ejiao). Cuttlefish bone (Wuzeigu) can be used alone for bleeding due to external injuries.

2. Deficiency of the kidneys manifested as seminal emissions or leukorrhea. Cuttlefish bone (Wuzeigu) is used with Dogwood fruit (Shanzhuyu), Dioscorea (Shanyao), Dadder seed (Tusizi) and Oyster shell (Muli).

3. Stomach pain and acid regurgitation. Cuttlefish bone (Wuzeigu) is used with Tendrilled fritillary bulb (Chuanbeimu) in the formula Wu

Bei San.

4. Eczema or chronic ulcers. Cuttlefish bone (Wuzeigu) is used with Phellodendron bark (Huangbai) and Natural indigo (Qingdai) for external use in powder form.

Dosage: 6-12 g

Cautions & Contraindications: This substance is contraindicated in cases with deficient *yin* and excessive heat.

APPENDIX

I. Index of the Serial
Medicinal Herbs

263

Cinnabar (Zhusha 朱砂)

Cinnamon bark (Rougui 肉桂), 126

Cinnamon twigs (Guizhi 桂枝), 2

Cistanche (Roucongrong 肉苁蓉), 272

Citron (Xiangyuan 香橼), 137

Clematis root (Weilingxian 威灵仙), 78

Clematis stem (Mutong 木通), 110

Cloves (Dingxiang 丁香), 130

Cnidium fruit (Shechuangzi 蛇床子), 288

Cockroach (Chechong 䗪虫), 194

Coix seed (Yiyiren 薏苡仁), 107

Coltsfoot flower (Kuandonghua 款冬花), 227

Common knotgrass (Bianxu 萹蓄), 121

Coptis root (Huanglian 黄连), 40

Cordyceps (Dongchongxiacao 冬虫夏草), 281

Coriander (Husui 胡荽), 14

Corydalis tuber (Yanhusuo 延胡索), 182

Costazia bone (Haifushi 海浮石), 217

Costus root (Muxiang 木香), 138

Cyperus tuber (Xiangfu 香附), 139

Croton seed (Badou 巴豆), 76

Curculigo rhizome (Xianmao 仙茅), 273

Curcuma root (Yujin 郁金), 183

Cuttlefish bone (Wuzeigu 乌贼骨), 322

Cyathula root (Niuxi 牛膝), 192

Daburian angelica root (Baizhi 白芷), 9

Dadder seed (Tusizi 菟丝子), 284

Dalbergia wood (Jiangxiang 降香), 197

Dandelion herb (Pugongying 蒲公英), 52

Datura Flower (Yangjinhua 洋金花), 231

Deglued antler powder (Lujiaoshuang 鹿角霜), 270b

Dendrobium (Shihu 石斛), 298

Dichroa root (Changshan 常山), 222

Dioscorea (Shanyao 山药), 266

Dittany bark (Baixianpi 白藓皮), 57

Dog testis (Huanggoushen 黄狗肾), 286

Dogbane (Luobuma 罗布麻), 255

Dogwood fruit (Shanzhuyu 山茱萸), 319

Donkey hide gelatin (Ejiao 阿胶), 293

Dragon's blood (Xuejie 血竭), 204

Dragon's bone (Longgu 龙骨), 235

Dried ginger (Ganjiang 干姜), 125

Drynaria (Gusuibu 骨碎补), 276

Eagle wood (Chenxiang 沉香), 141

Earthworm (Dilong 地龙), 254

Eclipta (Mohanlian 墨旱莲), 304

Elsholtzia (Xiangru 香薷), 5

Ephedra (Mahuang 麻黄), 1

Ephedra root (Mahuanggen 麻黄根), 312

Epimedium (Yinyanghuo 淫羊藿), 274

Erythrina bark (Haitongpi 海桐皮), 90

Eucommia bark (Duzhong 杜仲), 275

Eupatorium (Peilan 佩兰), 99

Euryale seed (Qianshi 芡实), 318

Evodia fruit (Wuzhuyu 吴茱萸), 127

Fennel fruit (Xiaohuixiang 小茴香), 132

Finger citron (Foshou 佛手), 136

II. A List of Applicable Formulas

Angong Niuhuang Wan (安宫牛黄丸)
— Ox-gallstone Pills for Resurrection
Anshen Dingzhi Wan (安神定志丸)
— Pills to Soothe the Mind
Baihe Dihuang Tang (百合地黄汤)
— Decoction of Lily Bulb and Rehmannia Root
Baihe Gujin Tang (百合固金汤)
— Lily Bulb Decoction to Strengthen the Lungs
Baihu Jia Renshen Tang (白虎加人参汤)
— White Tiger Decoction with Ginseng
Baihu Tang (白虎汤)
— White Tiger Decoction
Baijiangcan San (白僵蚕散)
— Powder of White-stiff Silkworm
Baiqian Tang (白前汤)
— Decoction of Swallowwort Rhizome
Baitouweng Tang (白头翁汤)
— Decoction of Pulsatilla Root Combination
Bali San (八厘散)
— Eight *Li* Powder
Banxia Baizhu Tianma Tang (半夏白术天麻汤)
— Decoction of Pinellia Tuber, White Atractylodes and Gastrodia Tuber
Banxia Houpo Tang (半夏厚朴汤)
— Decoction of Pinellia Tuber and Magnolia Bark Combination
Baochi San (保赤散)

271

— Powder to Keep Red Face

Baohe Wan (保和丸)

— Pills to Keep the Function of the Stomach in Good Condition

Baxian Changshou Wan (八仙长寿丸)

— Pills of Eight Noble Ingredients for Longevity

Bazheng San (八正散)

— Powder of Eight Ingredients to Clear Heat and Dampness

Biejia Jian Wan (鳖甲煎丸)

— Decocted Turtle Shell Pills

Bing Peng San (冰硼散)

— Powder of Borneol and Sodium Borate

Bixie Fenqing Yin (萆薢分清饮)

— Hypoglauca Yam Decoction to Clear the Turbid Urine

Buhuanjin Zhenqi San (不换金正气散)

— Powder for Strengthening Body Resistance Which Is Worth More Than Gold

Buwang San (不忘散)

— The Never Forgetful Powder

Buyang Huanwu Tang (补阳还五汤)

— Decoction to Tonify *Yang* and Restore Normal Function of the Five Viscera

Buzhong Yiqi Tang (补中益气汤)

— Decoction to Reinforce the Middle *Jiao* and Tonify *Qi*

Cang'er San (苍耳散)

— Powder of Xanthium Fruit

Canshi Tang (蚕矢汤)

— Decoction of Silkworm Excrement

Chai Ge Jieji Tang (柴葛解肌汤)

— Decoction of Bupleurum Root and Pueraria Root

Chaihu Qinggan Tang (柴胡清肝汤)

— Decoction of Bupleurum Root for Asthenia-heat Due to Malnutrition in Children

Chaihu Sugan San (柴胡疏肝散)

— Powder of Bupleurum Root to Disperse *Qi* in the Liver

Chan Hua San (蝉花散)

— Powder of Cicada Slough and Chrysanthemum Flower

Changpu Yujin Tang (菖蒲郁金汤)

— Decoction of Grass-leaved Sweetflag and Curcuma Root

Chuanxiong Cha Tiao San (川芎茶调散)

— Powder of Chuanxiong Rhizome Combination with Tea

Chuanxiong San (川芎散)

— Powder of Chuanxiong Rhizome

Cong Chi Tang (葱豉汤)

— Decoction of Chinese Green Onion and Prepared Soybean

Da Buyin Wan (大补阴丸)

— Pills for Replenishing the *Yin*

Da Chengqi Tang (大承气汤)

— Drastic Purgative Decoction

Da Jianzhong Tang (大建中汤)

— Major Decoction for Restoring the Normal of Middle *Jiao*

Da Xianxiong Tang (大陷胸汤)

— Major Decoction for Removing Phlegm-heat from the Chest

Dahuang Zhechong Wan (大黄䗪虫丸)

— Pills of Rhubarb and Cockroach

Dahuang Mudangpi Tang (大黄牡丹皮汤)

— Decoction of Rhuberb and Moutan Bark Combination

Danggui Buxue Tang (当归补血汤)

— Decoction with Chinese Angelica Root Combination to Tonify Blood

Danggui Liuhuang Tang (当归六黄汤)

— Decoction of Chinese Angelica Root and Six Yellow Ingredients

Danggui Luhui Wan (当归芦荟丸)

— Pills of Chinese Angelica Root and Aloes

Danshen Yin (丹参饮)

— Decoction of Red Sage Root

Daochi San (导赤散)

— Powder of Fresh Rehmannia Root and Clematis Stem to Conduct the Fire Downward

Daoqi Tang (导气汤)

— Decoction to Promote *Qi*

Daotan Tang (导痰汤)

— Decoction to Resolve Phlegm

Dingchuan Tang (定喘汤)

    — Decoction to Relieve Asthma

Donggua Wan (冬瓜丸)

    — Pills of Benincasa

Duhuo Jisheng Tang (独活寄生汤)

    — Decoction of Pubescent Angelica Root and Mulberry Mistletoe Combination

Duoming Dan (夺命丹)

    — Pills to Save Life

Erchen Tang (二陈汤)

    — Decoction of Two Old Ingredients, Tangerine Peel and Pinellia Tuber Combination

Erdong Gao (二冬膏)

    — Asparagus Root and Ophiopogon Root Plaster

Erjia Fumai Tang (二甲复脉汤)

    — Promoting Pulse Decoction with Two Shells

Ermu San (二母散)

    — Powder of Anemarrhena Rhizome and Tendrilled Fritillary Bulb

Erqi Tang (二气汤)

    — Decoction of Pharbitis Seed and Kansui Root

Erzhi Wan (二至丸)

    — Pills of Grossy Privet Fluit and Eclipta

Ezhu Wan (莪术丸)

    — Pills of Zedoary

Fangji Huangqi Tang (防己黄芪汤)

    — Decoction of Tetrandra Root and Astragalus Root Combination

Feier Wan (肥儿丸)

    — Baby-fattening Pills

Fuzi Lizhong Wan (附子理中丸)

    — Pills of Prepared Aconite Root to Regulate the Middle *Jiao* (Spleen and Stomach)

Gancao Fuzi Tang (甘草附子汤)

    — Decoction of Licorice Root and Prepared Aconite Root

Gan Mai Dazao Tang (甘麦大枣汤)

APPENDIX

— Decoction of Licorice Root, Light Wheat and Jujube

Gegen Huangqin Huanglian (葛根黄芩黄连汤)

   — Decoction of Pueraria Root, Scutellaria Root and Coptis Root Combination

Gegen Tang (葛根汤)

   — Decoction of Pueraria Root

Gualou Xiebai Baijiu Tang (瓜蒌薤白白酒汤)

   — Decoction of Trichosanthes Fruit, Macrostem Onion and White Wine Combination

Gualou Xiebai Banxia Tang (瓜蒌薤白半夏汤)

   — Decoction of Trichosanthes Fruit, Macrostem Onion and Pinellia Tuber

Guanxin Suhexiang Wan (冠心苏合香丸)

   — Storax Pills to Treat Coronary Heart Disease

Gui Fu Bawei Wan (桂附八味丸)

   — Pills of Cinnamon Twigs, Aconite Root and Six Other Ingredients

Gui Fu Lizhong Wan (桂附理中丸)

   — Pills of Cinnamon Bark and Prepared Aconite Root to Regulate the Middle *Jiao* (Spleen and Stomach)

Guipi Tang (归脾汤)

   — Decoction to Strengthen the Spleen and Heart

Guizhi Fuling Wan (桂枝茯苓丸)

   — Pills of Cinnamon Twigs and Poria

Guizhi Jia Houpo Xingzi Tang (桂枝加厚朴杏子汤)

   — Cinnamon Twigs Decoction with Magnolia Bark and Apricot Seed

Guizhi Tang (桂枝汤)

   — Decoction of Cinnamon Twigs Combination

Haifu San (海浮散)

   — Powder of Frankincense and Myrrh

Haizao Yuhu Tang (海藻玉壶汤)

   — The Seaweed Decoction

Hanhua Wan (含化丸)

   — Pills for Goiter

Hanjiang Tang (寒降汤)

   — Decoction for Cooling and Descending

Hao Qin Qingdan Tang (蒿芩清胆汤)

275

— Febrifugal Decoction of Sweet Wormwood and Scutellaria Root Combination

He Ren Yin（何人饮）

— Decoction of Fleeceflower Root and Ginseng

Hezi San（诃子散）

— Powder of Chebula Fruit Combination to Treat Chronic Dysentery

Hu Qian Wan（虎潜丸）

— The Tiger Pills to Nourish *Yin* and Strengthen the Bones

Huangqin Huashi Tang（黄芩滑石汤）

— Decoction of Scutellaria Root and Talc

Huangqi Tang（黄芪汤）

— Decoction of Astragalus Root

Huaxue Dan（化血丹）

— Pellets to Remove Blood Stasis and Check Bleeding

Hugu Mugua Jiu（虎骨木瓜酒）

— Wine of Tiger's Bone and Chaenomeles Fruit

Huoxiang Zhengqi San（霍香正气散）

— Decoction of Agastache Combination to Regulate *Qi*

Hupo San（琥珀散）

— Powder of Amber

Ji Jiao Li Huang Wan（己椒苈黄丸）

— Pills of Tetrandra Root, Prickly Ash Seed, Lepidium Seed and Rhubarb

Jiao Ai Tang（胶艾汤）

— Decoction of Donkey-hide Gelatin and Mugwort Leaf Combination

Jiming San（鸡鸣散）

— Cock Crowing Powder

Jingang Wan（金刚丸）

— Diamond Pills

Jinlingzi San（金铃子散）

— Powder of Sichuan Chinaberry

Jinsuo Gujing Wan（金锁固精丸）

— Pills to Control Seminal Emission

Jiuwei Qianghuo Tang（九味羌活汤）

— Decoction of Nine Ingredients with Notopterygium Root

Juanbi Tang（**蠲痹汤**）

— Decoction for Treating Rheumatism

Kongsheng Zhenzhong Dan (孔圣枕中丹)

    — Pellets in Confucius Pillow

Kuanxiong Wan (宽胸丸)

    — Pills to Ease the Chest

Kunbu Wan (昆布丸)

    — Pills of Laminaria

Liang Fu Wan (良附丸)

    — Pills of Galangal Rhizome and Cyperus Tuber

Liang Jing Wan (凉惊丸)

    — Pills to Relieve Spasm by Clearing Heat

Ling Gui Zhu Gan Tang (苓桂术甘汤)

    — Decoction of Poria, Cinnamon Twigs, White Atractylodes and Licorice Root

Lingjiao Gouteng Tang (羚角钩藤汤)

    — Decoction of Antelope's Horn and Uncaria Stem

Lingyangjiao San (羚羊角散)

    — Powder of Antelope's Horn

Liuwei Dihuang Wan (六味地黄丸)

    — Pills of Six Ingredients with Prepared Rehmannia Root Combination

Liu Yi San (六一散)

    — Powder of Ingredients Six to One in Ratio

Lizhong Wan (理中丸)

    — Pills to Regulate the Middle *Jiao* (Spleen and Stomach)

Ma Xing Shi Gan Tang (麻杏石甘汤)

    — Decoction of Ephedra, Apricot Seed, Gypsum and Licorice Root Combination

Mahuang Fuzi Xixin Tang (麻黄附子细辛汤)

    — Decoction of Ephedra, Prepared Aconite Root and Asarum Herb

Mahuang Tang (麻黄汤)

    — Decoction of Ephedra

Maziren Wan (麻子仁丸)

    — Pills of Hemp Seed Combination

Mugua Jian (木瓜煎)

    — Decoction of Chaenomeles Fruit

Muli San (牡蛎散)
— Powder of Oyster Shell Combination

Muxiang Binglang Wan (木香槟榔丸)
— Pills of Costus Root and Areca Seed Combination

Neixiao Lei Li Wan (内消瘰疬丸)
— Pills to Relieve Scrofula

Neixiao San (内消散)
— Powder to Relieve Poisoning Swelling

Niubang Tang (牛蒡汤)
— Decoction of Arctium Fruit

Niuxi Tang (牛膝汤)
— Decoction of Cyathula Root

Nuangan Jian (暖肝煎)
— Decoction for Warming the Liver

Pingwei San (平胃散)
— Powder to Neutralize the Stomach

Qi Ju Dihuang Wan (杞菊地黄丸)
— Prepared Rehmannia Root Pills with Wolfberry Fruit and Chrysanthemum Flower

Qianghuo Shengshi Tang (羌活胜湿汤)
— Decoction of Notopterygium Root Combination to Eliminate Dampness

Qianhu San (前胡散)
— Powder of Peucedanum Root

Qianjin San (千金散)
— Powder Worth a Thousand Gold

Qianzhen San (牵正散)
— Powder to Restore to Normal Position

Qili San (七厘散)
— Seven *Li* Powder

Qingdai Haishi Wan (青黛海石丸)
— Pills of Natural Indigo and Costazia Bone

Qingdai Shigao Tang (青黛石膏汤)
— Decoction of Natural Indigo and Gypsum

Qing'e Wan (青娥丸)
— Pills for Lumbago in Kidney Deficiency

Qinggu San (清骨散)
— Powder to Clear Heat in the Bone

Qinghao Biejia Tang (青蒿鳖甲汤)
— Decoction of Sweet Wormwood and Turtle Shell

Qingpi Wan (青皮丸)
— Pills of Green Tangerine Peel

Qingqi Huatan Wan (清气化痰丸)
— Pills to Clear *Qi* and Resolve Phlegm

Qingwei San (清胃散)
— Powder to Clear Heat in the Stomach

Qingying Tang (清营汤)
— Decoction to Dispel Pathogenic Heat from Ying System

Qinjiao Biejia Tang (秦艽鳖甲汤)
— Decoction of Large-leaf Gentian Root and Turtle Shell

Qiwei Baizhu San (七味白术散)
— Powder of Seven Medicinal Herbs

Renshen Gejie San (人参蛤蚧散)
— Powder of Ginseng and Gecko

Roucongrong Wan (肉苁蓉丸)
— Cistanche Pills

Runchang Wan (润肠丸)
— Pills to Moisten the Intestines

Sancai Tang (三才汤)
— Decoction of Three Herbs

Sang Ju Yin (桑菊饮)
— Decoction of Mulberry Leaf and Chrysanthemum Flower Combination

Sang Ma Wan (桑麻丸)
— Pills of Mulberry Leaf and Sesame Seed

Sang Xing Tang (桑杏汤)
— Decoction of Mulberry Leaf and Apricot Seed

Sanjia Fumai Tang (三甲复脉汤)
— Decoction of Three Shells to Promote the Pulse

Sanjin Tang (三金汤)
— Decoction of Three Gold

Sanmiao Wan (三妙丸)

— Pills of Three Wonder Ingredients

Sanniu Tang (三拗汤)

— Decoction of Three Crude Ingredients

Sanren Tang (三仁汤)

— Decoction of Three Kinds of Seeds

Sanwu Beiji Wan (三物备急丸)

— Pills of Three Ingredients for Emergency

Sanzi Yangqing Tang (三子养亲汤)

— Three Seeds Decoction for the Aged Asthma by Damp-phlegm

Shen Fu Tang (参附汤)

— Decoction of Ginseng and Prepared Aconite Root

Shen Ling Baizhu San (参苓白术散)

— Powder of Ginseng, Poria and White Atractylodes

Shengji Yuhong Gao (生肌玉红膏)

— Adhesive Plaster to Promote Tissue Regeneration

Shengma Gegen Tang (升麻葛根汤)

— Decoction of Cimicifuga Rhizome and Pueraria Root

Shengmai San (生脉散)

— Powder to Activate Vitality

Shexiang Tang (麝香汤)

— Decoction of Musk

Shihui San (十灰散)

— Ten Carbonized Ingredients for Bleeding

Shijueming Wan (石决明丸)

— Pills of Sea-ear Shell

Shixiao San (失笑散)

— Powder to Stop Pain by Dissipating Blood Stasis

Shizao Tang (十枣汤)

— Decoction of Ten Jujubes Combination

Shouwu Yanshou Dan (首乌延寿丹)

— Fleeceflower Root Pills to Prolong the Life

Shujing Tang (舒筋汤)

— Decoction to Relax Muscles

Sijunzi Tang (四君子汤)

— The Four Noble Ingredients Decoction

Siling San (四苓散)
— Powder of Four Ingredients Containing Poria

Sini Tang (四逆汤)
— Decoction to Treat Cold Limbs

Sishen Wan (四神丸)
— Pills of Four Miraculous Ingredients

Sisheng Wan (四生丸)
— Pills of Four Fresh Ingredients

Siwu Tang (四物汤)
— The Four Ingredients Decoction

Su Bing Diwan (苏冰滴丸)
— Pills of Storax and Borneol

Suhexiang Wan (苏合香丸)
— Storax Pills

Suoquan Wan (缩泉丸)
— Pills for Enuresis

Tao Hong Siwu Tang (桃红四物汤)
— The Four Ingredients Decoction with Peach Seed and Safflower

Tianma Gouteng Yin (天麻钩藤饮)
— Decoction of Gastrodia Tuber and Uncaria Stem

Tianma Wan (天麻丸)
— Pills of Gastrodia Tuber

Tiantai Wuyao San (天台乌药散)
— Powder of Lindera Root from Tiantai

Tianwang Buxin Dan (天王补心丹)
— The Heavenly King's Tonic Pills

Tingli Dazao Xiefei Tang (葶苈大枣泻肺汤)
— Decoction to Purge the Lungs with Lepidium Seed and Jujube

Tuoli Huangqi Tang (托里黄芪汤)
— Astragalus Root Decoction to Relieve Boils

Weijing Tang (苇茎汤)
— Decoction of Reed Stem Combination

Wendan Tang (温胆汤)
— Decoction to Warm the Gallbladder

Wenpi Tang (温脾汤)

— Decoction to Warm the Spleen

Wu Bei San（乌贝散）
— Powder of Cuttlefish Bone and Tendrilled Fritillary Bulb

Wu Ji San（乌芨散）
— Powder of Cuttlefish Bone and Bletilla Tuber

Wuhu Zhuifeng San（五虎追风散）
— Five Tigers Powder for Expelling Wind

Wuling San（五苓散）
— Powder of Five Ingredients with Poria

Wumei Wan（乌梅丸）
— Pills of Black Plum Combination

Wupi Yin（五皮饮）
— Decoction of Five Peels of Drugs

Wuren Wan（五仁丸）
— Pills of Five Kernels of Drugs

Wuzhuyu Tang（吴茱萸汤）
— Decoction of Evodia Fruit Combination

Xi Tong Wan（豨桐丸）
— Pills of Siegesbeckia and Glorybower Leaf

Xia Yuxue Tang（下瘀血汤）
— Decoction of Removing Blood Stagnation

Xianfang Huoming Yin（仙方活命饮）
— Decoction of Fairy Formula for Life

Xiang Gui San（香桂散）
— Powder of Musk and Cinnamon Bark

Xiang Lian Wan（香连丸）
— Pills of Costus Root and Coptis Root

Xiang Sha Liujunzi Wan（香砂六君子丸）
— Six Noble Ingredients Decoction with Costus Root and Amomum Fruit

Xiang Sha Zhi Zhu Wan（香砂枳术丸）
— Pills of Immature Bitter Orange and White Atractylodes with Costus Root
and Amomum Fruit

Xiangru San（香薷散）
— Decoction of Elsholtzia Combination

Xiao Banxia Tang（小半夏汤）

— Decoction of Smaller Amount of Pinellia Tuber

Xiao Qinglong Tang (小青龙汤)

— Decoction of Minor Blue Dragon Combination

Xiao Xianxiong Tang (小陷胸汤)

— Minor Decoction for Phlegm-heat Sinking into the Chest

Xiaofeng San (消风散)

— Powder to Dispel Wind

Xiao Huoluo Dan (小活络丹)

— Small Pills for Invigorating Circulation

Xiaoji Yinzi (小蓟饮子)

— Decoction of Small Thistle Combination

Xiaolei Wan (消瘰丸)

— Pills for Scrofula

Xiaoru Tang (消乳汤)

— Decoction for Mastitis

Xiaoyao San (逍遥散)

— The Ease Powder

Xiebai San (泻白散)

— Powder to Purge the White (Lungs)

Xiexin Tang (泻心汤)

— Decoction to Reduce Heat from the Heart

Xing Su San (杏苏散)

— Powder of Apricot Seed and Perilla Leaf Combination

Xingxiao Wan (醒消丸)

— Pills for Reducing Boils and Swellings

Xuanfu Daizhe Tang (旋复代赭汤)

— Decoction of Inula Flower and Red Ochre Combination

Xuanbi Tang (宣痹汤)

— Decoction to Relieve Pain from the Meridian Obstruction

Yanghe Tang (阳和汤)

— Decoction of Prepared Rehmannia Root, Cinnamon Bark and Ephedra Combination

Yihuang Tang (易黄汤)

— Decoction to Treat Yellow Leukorrhea

Yin Qiao San (银翘散)

— Powder of Honeysuckle Flower and Forsythia Fruit Combination

Yinchen Sini Tang (茵陈四逆汤)

— Oriental Wormwood Decoction to Treat Cold Limbs

Yinchenhao Tang (茵陈蒿汤)

— Decoction of Oriental Wormwood Combination

Yiwei Tang (益胃汤)

— Decoction to Strengthen the Stomach

Yixue Runchang Wan (益血润肠丸)

— Pills to Promote the Blood and Moisten the Intestines

Yiyi Fuzi Baijiang San (薏苡附子败酱散)

— Powder of Coix Seed, Prepared Aconite Root and Patrinia Herb

Yuebi Tang (越婢汤)

— Decoction for Edema

Yuliren Tang (郁李仁汤)

— Decoction of Bush-cherry Seed

Yunü Jian (玉女煎)

— The Fair Maiden Decoction of Fresh Rehmannia Root and Gypsum Combination

Yupingfeng San (玉屏风散)

— The Jade Screen Powder

Yuye Tang (玉液汤)

— Jade Fluid Decoction

Yuzhen San (玉真散)

— Real Healing Powder

Zengye Chengqi Tang (增液承气汤)

— Purgative Decoction by Increasing Body Fluids

Zengye Tang (增液汤)

— Decoction to Increase Body Fluids

Zhengan Xifeng Tang (镇肝熄风汤)

— Decoction to Subdue the Endogenous Wind in the Liver

Zhenling Dan (震灵丹)

— Pills for Wakening the Mind

Zhenwu Tang (真武汤)

— Decoction of Prepared Aconite Root, White Atractylodes and Poria Combination

Zhi Bai Dihuang Wan (知柏地黄丸)

— Prepared Rehmannia Root Pills with Anemarrhena Rhizome and Phellodendron Bark

Zhi Zhu Wan (枳术丸)

— Pills of Immature Bitter Orange and White Atractylodes

Zhibao Dan (至宝丹)

— The Most Precious Pellets

Zhishi Daozhi Wan (枳实导滞丸)

— Immature Bitter Orange Pills to Relieve Stagnation

Zhishi Xiebai Guizhi Tang (枳实薤白桂枝汤)

— Decoction of Immature Bitter Orange, Macrostem Onion and Cinnamon Twigs

Zhisou San (止嗽散)

— Powder to Stop Cough

Zhizi Chi Tang (栀子豉汤)

— Decoction of Capejasmine and Prepared Soybean

Zhuye Liu Bang Tang (竹叶柳蒡汤)

— Decoction of Bamboo Leaf, Tamarisk Tops and Arctium Fruit

Zhuye Shigao Tang (竹叶石膏汤)

— Decoction of Bamboo Leaf and Gypsum Combination

Zijin Ding (紫金锭)

— Purplish Gold Lozenge

Zijing San (止痉散)

— Powder to Relieve Spasm

Zitong Linbao San (止痛灵宝散)

— Treasured Powder to Alleviate Pain

Ziwan Tang (紫菀汤)

— Decoction of Aster Root

Zixue Dan (紫雪丹)

— Purple Snowy Powder

Zuojin Wan (左金丸)

— Pills of Coptis Root and Evodia Fruit

III. Bibliography

Bencao Congxin (《本草从新》)
— New Compendium of Materia Medica
Bencao Gangmu (《本草纲目》)
— Compendium of Materia Medica
Bencao Gangmu Shiyi (《本草纲目拾遗》)
— A Supplement to the Compendium of Materia Medica
Bencao Jingji Zhi (《本草经籍志》)
— Collection of Classics on Materia Medica
Bencao Mengquan (《本草蒙荃》)
— Primary Study of Materia Medica
Bencao Shiyi (《本草拾遗》)
— A Supplementary Study of Materia Medica
Bencao Tujing (《本草图经》)
— A Collection of Materia Medica with Illustrations
Bencao Yanyi (《本草衍义》)
— Amplified Materia Medica
Bencao Zaixin (《本草再新》)
— New Compilation of Materia Medica
Benjing Jizhu (《本经集注》)
— Collected Notes on Shennong's Canon of Materia Medica
Diannan Bencao (《滇南本草》)
— Medicinal Herbs from Southern Yunnan
Haiyao Bencao (《海药本草》)
— Materia Medica from Abroad
Jiayou Bencao (《嘉佑本草》)

— Jiayou Materia Medica

Kaibao Bencao (《开宝本草》)

— Kaibao Materia Medica

Leigong Paozhi Lun (《雷公炮炙论》)

— Lei's Theory on Preparing Drugs

Lingnan Caoyao Lu (《岭南草药录》)

— Recording of Medicinal Herbs Produced in Guangdong and Guangxi

Mingyi Bielu (《名医别录》)

— Transactions of Famous Physicians

Rihuazi Bencao (《日华子本草》)

— Rihuazi Materia Medica

Shennong Bencao Jing (《神农本草经》)

— Shennong's Cannon of Materia Medica

Shiwu Bencao (《食物本草》)

— Dietary Materia Medica

Shu Bencao (《蜀本草》)

— Sichuan Materia Medica

Xiandai Shiyong Zhongyao (《现代实用中药》)

— Modern Practical Chinese Medicinal Herbs

Xinxiu Bencao (《新修本草》)

— Newly Revised Materia Medica

Yaoxing Lun (《药性论》)

— On Nature of Drugs

Yaoxue Dacidian (《药学大辞典》)

— A Dictionary of Pharmacology

Yinshan Zhenyao (《饮膳正要》)

— True Essence of Dietary

Zhiwu Mingshi Tukao (《植物名实图考》)

— An Illustrated Book on Plants

Zhongguo Yaoyong Zhiwu Zhi (《中国药用植物志》)

— Recording of Chinese Materia Medica

Zhonghua Yixue Zazhi (《中华医学杂志》)

— Chinese Medical Journal

Zhongyao Zhi (《中药志》)

— Recording of Chinese Medicinal Herbs

图书在版编目（CIP）数据

实用中草药：英文/耿俊英等著
－北京：新世界出版社，1997.6 重印
ISBN 7－80005－119－6

Ⅰ．实… Ⅱ．耿… Ⅲ．中草药－基本知识－英文
Ⅳ．R28

实 用 中 草 药

耿俊英 等著

*

新世界出版社出版

（北京百万庄路 24 号）

北京大学印刷厂印刷

中国国际图书贸易总公司发行

（中国北京车公庄西路 35 号）

北京邮政信箱第 399 号　邮政编码 100044

1991 年（英文）第一版　1997 年第二次印刷

ISBN 7－80005－119－6

04200

14－E－2522P